Collaborative Case Conceptualization

Collaborative Case Conceptualization

Working Effectively with Clients
in Cognitive-Behavioral Therapy

Willem Kuyken
Christine A. Padesky
Robert Dudley

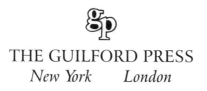

THE GUILFORD PRESS
New York   London

Published by The Guilford Press
A Division of Guilford Publications, Inc.
72 Spring Street, New York, NY 10012
www.guilford.com

Printed in the United States of America

This book is printed on acid-free paper.

Last digit is print number: 9   8   7   6   5   4   3   2   1

Library of Congress Cataloging-in-Publication Data

Kuyken, W. (Willem), 1968–
    Collaborative case conceptualization : working effectively with clients in
cognitive-behavioral therapy / Willem Kuyken, Christine A. Padesky, Robert
Dudley.
        p. ; cm.
    Includes bibliographical references and index.
    ISBN 978-1-60623-072-5 (hardcover : alk. paper)
    1. Cognitive therapy. 2. Psychiatry—Case formulation.   I. Padesky,
Christine A.   II. Dudley, Robert (Robert E. J.)   III. Title.
    [DNLM: 1. Cognitive Therapy.   2. Cooperative Behavior.
 3. Psychological Theory.   WM 425.5.C6 K965c 2009]
    RC489.C63K89 2009
    616.89′1425—dc22
                                                              2008042357

—

About the Authors

Willem Kuyken, PhD, is Professor of Clinical Psychology at the University of Exeter, United Kingdom; Cofounder of the Mood Disorders Centre; and a Fellow of the Academy of Cognitive Therapy. His primary research and clinical interests are case conceptualization and cognitive-behavioral approaches to depression, and he has published more than 50 articles and book chapters. Dr. Kuyken is a recipient of the May Davidson Award from the British Psychological Society.

Christine A. Padesky, PhD, is a Distinguished Founding Fellow of the Academy of Cognitive Therapy and recipient of its Aaron T. Beck Award. She is an internationally renowned speaker, consultant, and coauthor of six books, including the bestselling *Mind Over Mood*. Dr. Padesky's numerous awards include the Distinguished Contribution to Psychology Award from the California Psychological Association. Through her website, *www.padesky.com,* she produces audiovisual programs on case conceptualization and other topics that provide CBT training for therapists in more than 45 countries.

Robert Dudley, PhD, is a Consultant Clinical Psychologist for the Early Intervention in Psychosis Service at the Northumberland, Tyne, and Wear Mental Health NHS Trust, United Kingdom. He is currently serving as a Beck Institute Scholar at the Beck Institute for Cognitive Therapy and Research. Dr. Dudley's primary clinical and research focus is the understanding and treatment of psychotic symptoms. As a clinician, trainer, and supervisor, he developed an interest in case conceptualization and has undertaken several research projects in this area.

Preface

Cognitive-behavioral therapy (CBT) is both art and science. Nowhere is this truer than during case conceptualization, when therapists stay attuned to clients' unique experiences while also attending to the scientific theories and research that underpin CBT. Like many cognitive therapists, we deeply appreciate CBT precisely because it bridges art and science, practice and theory, idiosyncratic experiences and the commonalities encapsulated by cognitive and behavioral theories of emotion. We stand on this bridge with our clients working together to relieve distress and build resilience.

The three of us first met in 2002 in Warwick, England, at a CBT conference symposium entitled "Case Conceptualization: Is the Emperor Clothed?" The conference organizers had scheduled the symposium in a relatively small seminar room. The topic generated so much interest that the room was full, with many people standing at the back or sitting in the aisles. Rather like Hans Christian Andersen's allegorical tale alluded to in the symposium's title, the symposium highlighted several important "facts." First, case conceptualization is considered a fundamental therapy skill. Even so, many therapists lack confidence in how to conceptualize. Second, therapist interest in case conceptualization outstrips the sparse evidence base. Third, the little research that exists challenges assumptions about the positive value of CBT case conceptualization. The symposium concluded that the case conceptualization emperor appeared to be unclothed!

At the end of the symposium the three of us lingered in conversation and began talking about case conceptualization. As we talked, we realized we shared a keen interest in case conceptualization and each of us brought different, valuable, and complementary perspectives to the topic. While the three of us teach, supervise, consult, and conduct CBT research, each of us has acquired special expertise in at least one of these areas. Robert offers keen clinical insights gleaned from his years of experience as a therapist and supervisor working with complex clinical cases. Christine is an internationally recognized CBT instructor and innovator. Willem is a leading case conceptualization researcher and teacher. We thought this combination of experience and knowledge could advance understanding of how to make case conceptualization more effective in CBT.

This book is the result of an ongoing collaboration that began at that conference. Our ideas evolved in stages over the past 6 years. First we *made explicit* the unresolved implicit research and clinical challenges to case conceptualization. These are summarized for the reader in Chapter 1. As we jointly struggled with how to respond to these challenges, we realized many of our solutions were insufficient. We generated fresh ideas and tested these out with each other; in discussions with peers; in our clinical work; in our work as supervisors, consultants, and instructors; and in relation to the emerging research. We distilled useful ideas down to their simplest form using collaborative empiricism as a check and balance to guard against heuristic biases. After a few years, we reached consensus on a model for case conceptualization that we felt adequately addressed the existing challenges.

Our model is described in Chapter 2 along with three principles to guide its practice: collaborative empiricism, incorporation of client strengths, and evolving levels of conceptualization. This model has its roots in the conceptual and empirical traditions of Aaron T. Beck, the founder of CBT as well as a mentor and friend to each of us. We draw on the rich empiricism of behavioral therapy, especially functional analysis. In addition, our ideas are informed by contemporary research on resilience and strengths. Throughout, our aim is to provide a conceptualization approach that therapists can use collaboratively with clients to more effectively relieve distress and build resilience.

This book teaches our approach to case conceptualization and brings it to life with case examples, practical clinical tips, and sample dialogues. Step by step, we show how to develop a conceptualization that first describes client presenting issues and then deepens in explanatory power as treatment progresses. Client strengths are identified and harnessed throughout the process of conceptualization to help create effective and lasting improvement. We describe how therapist and client can truly collaborate to explicitly co-create and test conceptualizations throughout the course of therapy.

Chapter 3 delineates our first conceptualization principle, *collaborative empiricism*, and shows readers how a collaborative and empirical approach to therapy leads to effective resolution of a number of conceptualization challenges. In Chapter 4 we show how our second principle, *incorporation of client strengths*, expands the emphasis of case conceptualization to encompass goals of restoring and building client resilience. Chapters 5 through 7 illustrate our third principle, *levels of conceptualization*, by following a client, Mark, over the course of therapy as he tackles depression, obsessive–compulsive disorder, health worries, work difficulties, and family struggles.

Although Mark is a composite of many clients, his case portrays a common clinical presentation that requires individualized conceptualization: he experiences high levels of distress in the context of many overlapping diagnostic issues. Readers learn how Mark and his therapist progress from simpler, descriptive case conceptualizations (Chapter 5), to explanatory conceptualizations of what triggers and maintains his presenting issues (Chapter 6), to a longitudinal account of what predisposed him to this particular set of presenting issues and what strengths protected him from worse difficulties (Chapter 7). Mark's in-depth case illustration demonstrates how our approach can simultaneously help decrease psychological distress and promote resilience.

As CBT instructors, supervisors, and consultants we observe that learning to use case conceptualization effectively is one of the biggest challenges faced by therapists. In Chapter 8 we demystify the learning process and suggest a systematic approach for therapists and instructors to learn and teach case conceptualization skills. In our closing chapter we consider some of the issues therapists might face in using our model in a variety of therapeutic settings. Consistent with our commitment to empiricism, we also propose a program of research to test the assumptions and principles central to our model.

One of the measures of a worthwhile collaboration is how engaged the parties remain throughout the process. By this standard, our collaboration as authors has held great value. Each of us is even more enthusiastic and interested in case conceptualization now than we were at the outset of this project. We have done our best to capture for readers the essence of the spirited discussions and debates that infused our interactions over the last several years. Now this book is in readers' hands. We hope it enhances your understanding of case conceptualization, shows you how to actively collaborate with your clients during these processes, and stimulates research to evaluate our ideas. In the years ahead we look forward to a broader conversation that includes many of you as we continue to explore the boundaries and depths of collaborative case conceptualization.

Acknowledgments

A number of people have shaped and contributed to this book and we gratefully acknowledge their input. At various stages we have tested the ideas in this book on colleagues whose opinions we greatly value. The book has benefited from the ideas and comments of Peter Bieling, Gillian Butler, Paul Chadwick, Tracy Eells, Melanie Fennell, Mark Freeston, Kevin Meares, Kathleen Mooney, Ed Watkins, and Kim Wright. We are grateful for the artistic talents of Bruce Lim, who created original illustrations throughout the book, including the case conceptualization crucible, an image central to our model. We thank Bibiana Rojas for her excellent graphic design work on the figures. We appreciate Seymour Weingarten at The Guilford Press for his constructive support of this work at every stage of its development. Finally, we are indebted to our Guilford editor, Barbara Watkins, whose professional and insightful commentary on a series of drafts significantly enhanced the clarity and cohesion of the book.
—WILLEM KUYKEN, CHRISTINE A. PADESKY, ROBERT DUDLEY

I am grateful to my mentors, collaborators, and clients, who have helped me cross the divide between science and practice so many times that I no longer regard it as a divide but rather as a creative dialectic! I thank Professors Aaron T. Beck, Chris Brewin, Tony Lavender, and Paul Webley, who, in different and important ways, provided inspiration, challenge, and support during my professional development. I have been very lucky to be able to work with superb collaborators, including Peter Bieling, Sarah Byford, Paul Chadwick, Tim Dalgleish, Emily Holden, Rachael Howell, Michelle Moulds, Eugene Mullan, Rod Taylor, Ed Watkins, Kat White, and the World Health Organization Quality of Life (WHOQOL) Group. Collaboration is at the heart of my professional work. In my opinion, the challenges faced by clinical researchers are often best met by multidisciplinary teams. I am fortunate to have had productive collaborations with colleagues and students whose creativity and hard work helped me envision, articulate, and realize new ideas. The faculty and staff of the Exeter Mood Disorders Centre are an exemplar of this process.

I am grateful to the research staff and postgraduate students who have worked with me on case conceptualization: Rachel Day, Claire Fothergill, and Meyrem Musa. As is true for many cognitive-behavioral therapists, working with my clients is a two-way learning process. I have learned a great deal from the many clients whom I have had the privilege of working alongside in a range of therapeutic settings. I have been supported and learned much from my parents, Jan and Miets Kuyken; my wife, Halley; and friends Andy, Edoardo, Emmanuelle, and Tim. Finally, I want to thank my two coauthors, Christine Padesky and Robert Dudley. At every phase of this book my respect for their unique strengths has grown and deepened. Writing a book together has been an enormously rewarding experience, and I cherish it as a highlight of my professional career.

—WILLEM KUYKEN

Early in my career, I presented a case to Aaron T. (Tim) Beck. After asking a few clarifying questions, Tim effortlessly summarized my client's central issues. Then he articulated a succinct explanatory case conceptualization that struck me as more accurate than my own understanding of a person I had been treating for several months. Tim's conceptualization skills were so superior to my own that I thought, "He seems to understand my client so well. Why didn't I see that? I'll never be good at case conceptualization. I must not have the case conceptualization gene." I thought skillful case conceptualization was an innate talent rather than a skill that would develop over time. Fortunately, I was wrong. I did acquire skills and learned principles that helped me conceptualize cases more effectively. Even so, I was right to recognize that Tim Beck conceptualizes cases better than anyone else I've ever met. Nearly every good idea and principle I've "discovered" in my career as a psychologist owes a debt to him. His wisdom, compassion, and scientific rigor infuse this book.

My development as a psychologist, instructor, and writer owes an equal debt to Kathleen Mooney, whose perceptive comments, contributions, and questions continue to energize my thinking after 27 years of collaboration and partnership. Other CBT therapists who inform my understanding of case conceptualization include Judith S. Beck, Gillian Butler, David M. Clark, Melanie Fennell, Kate Gillespie, Emily Holmes, Helen Kennerley, and Jacqueline Persons. Therapists who sought consultation for case conceptualization assistance over the past several years directly and indirectly contributed ideas that improved this book, including Monica Hill, Susan Reynolds, Jennifer Shannon, Ann Twomey, and Mary Beth Whittaker. Therapists from around the world who attend my workshops ask many provocative questions; the answers often take years to develop and appear in books like this one. Your curiosity often inspires new developments in my thinking and I am grateful for your interest in CBT. A special thanks to all the therapists who attended our many Winter Workshops and Camps Cognitive Therapy.

I hold a radical commitment to collaboration during therapy. This stance is encouraged by clients, who show me over and over again that the more I ask them to participate in every aspect of therapy, the more fruitful their participation becomes. Client enthusiasm for case conceptualization led me to believe it was important to write this book. I thank my clients for teaching me that every therapy activity can be improved through client collaboration.

Finally, my appreciation of Willem and Robert deepens each year. Collaboration with you is a rich and enjoyable experience. I hope you don't mind if I continue to telephone you on Tuesdays at 8 P.M. to carry on the conversation it seems we began only yesterday.

—CHRISTINE A. PADESKY

I trace the onset of my interest in the purpose and process of conceptualization to a very specific and key moment. I was fortunate enough to be supervised by Professor Ivy Blackburn and I asked her about a case study she had published 12 years earlier. When I began to describe the case details she interrupted me, "Do not tell me the details, tell me the formulation. I never forget a formulation." I outlined the key elements from her published formulation and immediately she was able to remember the case in rich clinical detail. I knew at that moment what a powerful organizing framework a coherent conceptualization could be.

The value of case conceptualization for clinicians was obvious. Over the years I strove to learn how to use this powerful tool effectively with my clients. I have been aided in this process by many excellent colleagues who supported my clinical work, including Peter Armstrong, Paul Cromarty, Kevin Gibson, Carolyn John, Brian Scott, Vivien Twaddle, Douglas Turkington, and members of the Newcastle Cognitive and Behavioural Therapies Centre and the South of Tyne Early Intervention in Psychosis Service. My research regarding conceptualization has been undertaken with the valuable contribution of colleagues including Stephen Barton, Mark Freeston, Ian James, Kevin Meares, Guy Dodgson, Isabelle Park, Pauline Summerfield, Jaime Dixon, Clare Maddison, Jonna Siitarinen, Barry Ingham, and Katy Sowerby. Many of my clients provided feedback and ideas that shaped how I approach the process of conceptualization. I am indebted to many people but especially my wife, Joy, who supported my efforts to complete this book. I also express deep appreciation to my coauthors who made this process a pleasure.

—ROBERT DUDLEY

Contents

Chapter 1   The Procrustean Dilemma   *1*

Chapter 2   The Case Conceptualization Crucible: *25*
              A New Model

Chapter 3   Two Heads Are Better Than One: *59*
              Collaborative Empiricism

Chapter 4   Incorporating Client Strengths   *93*
              and Building Resilience

Chapter 5   "Can You Help Me?":   *121*
              Descriptive Case Conceptualization

Chapter 6   "Why Does This Keep Happening to Me?":   *171*
              Cross-Sectional Explanatory Conceptualizations

Chapter 7   "Does My Future Look Like My Past?":   *217*
              Longitudinal Explanatory Conceptualizations

Chapter 8   Learning and Teaching Case Conceptualization   *248*

Chapter 9   Appraising the Model   *306*

Appendix   Aid to History Taking Form   *327*

References   *341*

Index   *355*

Chapter 1

The Procrustean Dilemma

The mythological character Procrustes was a host who invited guests to his house, claiming that all visitors, whatever their size, would fit the bed in his guest room. Such a grand and magical claim attracted a lot of attention. What Procrustes did not tell his guests was that he was willing to either cut off his guest's legs or stretch them on a rack to make them fit the bed. The story of Procrustes could be a cautionary tale for psychotherapy clients. Although there are many empirically tested models for understanding psychological distress, few clients want to see a therapist who cuts off or distorts client experience in order to fit preexisting theories.

Clients present with complex and comorbid presentations for which no single approach is a 100% fit. This book teaches therapists how to become skilled in methods of case conceptualization that offer custom-made hospitality for clients seeking help. Readers learn how to shape case conceptualizations that synthesize individual aspects of a given case with relevant theory and research without the need to resort to Procrustean measures.

As a case illustration, Steve is a single 28-year-old man referred to an outpatient clinic for cognitive-behavioral therapy (CBT). The referral notes that Steve experiences difficulties adjusting to his enjoyment of cross-dressing. At the assessment Steve confirms that cross-dressing is something he wants to discuss in therapy but it is a greater priority to talk about having been "terrorized in the city where I lived until recently ... and ... I'm having a lot of trouble getting over it even though I have relocated." Steve suffered repeated violent physical attacks in the city where he used to live and he moved because there was no sign that these attacks

1

would stop. Steve is slight in build, soft-spoken, and unassertive. In the diagnostic work-up Steve meets criteria for posttraumatic stress disorder (PTSD), major depressive disorder, and agoraphobia with panic. In terms of Axis II there is some evidence of avoidant personality traits. His therapist hypothesized that Steve's slight build and soft-spoken, unassertive style led the bullies in his neighborhood to victimize him. His PTSD was a reaction to repeated physical assaults that he felt powerless to prevent. Withdrawal to his apartment exacerbated the PTSD symptoms and contributed to Steve's becoming depressed and agoraphobic.

Steve and the therapist agreed to begin therapy by focusing on Steve's PTSD symptoms. In the sixth session Steve disclosed that neighbors had seen him the previous year in his home dressed in women's clothing. Word quickly spread through the neighborhood that Steve was a cross-dresser. With this revelation, a group of youths began a campaign of violence against him. Repeated physical assaults led to Steve's decision to relocate.

The issues Steve's therapist faced are similar to the issues therapists face with each client at the beginning of therapy:

- "Given the various presenting issues and Axis I and/or II diagnoses, what should be the primary focus for the work?"
- "Do I address Axis I or Axis II problems, or both? If both, in what order?"
- "How do Steve's presenting issues relate to one another, if at all?"
- "What CBT protocol do I use here? What do I do when no particular protocol seems appropriate?"
- "How should I work with his cross-dressing?' How do I do this without exacerbating his fear?"
- "How do I work collaboratively with Steve to weave his priorities and my clinical judgment into our decision making about therapy?"
- "How do I work with my own beliefs, values, and reactions if these are sometimes different than my client's?"

In short, Steve's therapist is faced with the question that faces all therapists at the beginning of therapy: "How do I best use my training and experience along with evidence-based therapy approaches to help these particular issues presented by this person?" This book answers this question by showing how skillful case conceptualization provides ways to work collaboratively with clients to (1) describe presenting issues, (2) understand them in cognitive-behavioral terms, and then (3) find constructive ways to relieve distress and build client resilience.

WHAT IS CASE CONCEPTUALIZATION?

We define CBT case conceptualization as follows:

Case conceptualization is a process whereby therapist and client work collaboratively first to describe and then to explain the issues a client presents in therapy. Its primary function is to guide therapy in order to relieve client distress and build client resilience.

We use the metaphor of a crucible to emphasize several aspects of our definition (Figure 1.1). A crucible is a strong container for synthesizing different substances so that they are changed into something new. Typically, heating the crucible facilitates the process of change. The case conceptualization process is like that insofar as it synthesizes a client's presenting issues and experiences with CBT theory and research to form a new understanding that is original and unique to the client. CBT theory and research are essential ingredients in the crucible; it is the integration of empirical knowledge that differentiates case conceptu-

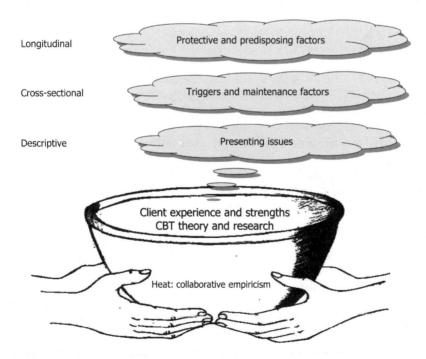

Figure 1.1. The case conceptualization crucible.

alization from the natural processes of deriving meaning from experience in which people engage all the time.

The crucible metaphor further illustrates three key defining principles of case conceptualization developed in detail throughout this book and shown in Figure 1.1. First, heat drives chemical reactions in a crucible. In our model, collaborative empiricism drives the conceptualization process. The hands in Figure 1.1 represent collaborative empiricism between therapist and client; they generate the heat that encourages transformation within the crucible. Collaboration helps ensure that the right ingredients are mixed in a useful way. The perspectives of therapist and client combine to develop a shared understanding that fits, is useful to the client, and informs therapy. Empiricism is a fundamental principle in CBT (J. S. Beck, 1995). It refers to the empirical research and relevant theory that grounds therapy as well as to the use of empirical methods within day-to-day practice. An empirical approach is one in which hypotheses are continually developed based on client experience, theory, and research. These hypotheses are tested and then revised based on observations and client feedback.

Second, like the chemical reaction in a crucible, a conceptualization develops over time. Typically, it begins at more descriptive levels (e.g., describing Steve's problems in cognitive and behavioral terms), moves to include explanatory models (e.g., a theory-based understanding of how his posttraumatic stress symptoms are maintained), and, if necessary, develops further to include a historical explanation of how predisposing and protective factors played a role in the development of Steve's issues (e.g., incorporating Steve's developmental history into the conceptualization).

Third, new substances formed in a crucible depend on the characteristics of the materials put into it. A client's experiences along with CBT theory and research are key ingredients in a conceptualization. Traditionally, the emphasis has been on client problems. Rather than simply look at these, our model incorporates client strengths at every stage of the conceptualization process. Regardless of their presentation and history, all clients have strengths that they have used to cope effectively in their lives. Incorporation of client strengths into conceptualizations increases the odds that the outcome will both relieve distress and build client resilience. As illustrated in Figure 1.1, client strengths are part of the crucible's mix.

This book responds to the Procrustean dilemma by proposing a new approach to case conceptualization that joins theory and research with the particularities of an individual's life experience. Three principles guide this approach: (1) collaborative empiricism, (2) levels of conceptualization that evolve over time from the descriptive to the explanatory, and (3) incorporation of client strengths. Each chapter in this book offers specific "how-to" guidelines for the development of case conceptualizations that can improve therapy's effectiveness.

In this opening chapter we suggest that case conceptualization has become central to CBT practice because it serves the 10 key functions outlined below. However, we also go on to consider some important empirical challenges to the centrality of case conceptualization in CBT practice. These challenges have been important in shaping the case conceptualization approach proposed in this book.

FUNCTIONS OF CBT CASE CONCEPTUALIZATION

We propose that therapy has two overarching goals: (1) to alleviate clients' distress and (2) to build resilience. There is an emerging consensus that CBT case conceptualization helps achieve these two goals when it fulfills the following 10 functions (see Box 1.1; Butler, 1998; Denman, 1995; Eells, 2007; Flitcroft, James, Freeston, & Wood-Mitchell, 2007; Needleman, 1999; Persons, 2005; Tarrier, 2006).

1. *Case conceptualization synthesizes client experience, relevant CBT theory, and research.* As articulated in our definition, a primary function of case conceptualization is to meaningfully integrate client experiences with relevant CBT theory and research. In Steve's case CBT theories of PTSD (Ehlers & Clark, 2000), depression (Clark, Beck, & Alford, 1999), anxiety (Beck, Emery, & Greenberg, 1985), and personality (Beck et al., 2004) can all usefully inform the case conceptualization. These theoretical ideas are integrated with related research and key aspects of Steve's personal history, current life situation, beliefs, and ways of coping to create a unique case conceptualization. Evidence-based theory and research ensure that the best available knowledge informs our emerging understanding of the presenting issues.

2. *Case conceptualization normalizes clients' presenting issues and is validating.* Many clients worry that their presenting issues are stigmatizing, set them apart from others, and make them somehow "abnormal." Clients sometimes say, "I thought I was crazy," or "I am so ashamed to have these problems." Case conceptualization describes problems in constructive language and helps clients understand how problems are maintained. While there still is real social stigma regarding many mental health problems, the process of collaborative case conceptualization can helpfully validate and normalize client experience. As Steve said later in therapy, "There are other people like me and I am not a freak. I know I am not the only person who cross-dresses, and I don't need

---

Box 1.1. Functions of Case Conceptualization in CBT

1. Synthesizes client experience, CBT theory, and research.
2. Normalizes presenting issues and is validating.
3. Promotes client engagement.
4. Makes numerous complex problems more manageable.
5. Guides the selection, focus, and sequence of interventions.
6. Identifies client strengths and suggests ways to build client resilience.
7. Suggests the simplest and most cost-efficient interventions.
8. Anticipates and addresses problems in therapy.
9. Helps understand nonresponse in therapy and suggests alternative routes for change.
10. Enables high-quality supervision.

---

to blame myself or expect to be attacked." Normalization of the issues clients present in therapy can instill hope, help clients see the personal relevance of the cognitive model, and provide a platform for change.

    3. Case conceptualization promotes client engagement. Engagement with CBT is a prerequisite for change. Case conceptualization often generates curiosity and interest, which lead to client engagement. Most clients enjoy case conceptualization because it offers a sense of mastery over difficulties and suggests pathways for reaching goals. Even when struggles persist, clients experience mastery when situations unfold in expected ways: "Just as we discussed last week, when my daughter began to whine I found my chest tightening and I felt ashamed. Even though I couldn't stop myself from this reaction, for once it made sense to me. I didn't feel so crazy. And that felt really good!"

    Occasionally, clients begin therapy with beliefs that affect therapy engagement negatively. This was the case with Steve, who avoided revealing relevant information about his cross-dressing to the therapist. Once Steve chose to disclose more of his history, the therapist used this as an opportunity to uncover beliefs that might interfere with engagement:

THERAPIST: Thank you, Steve, for being honest with me—this will help us work together better. (*Steve looks uncomfortable and afraid. The therapist uses this nonverbal information as a prompt to ask*): What do you think will happen now that you have told me how the victimization started in your last neighborhood?

STEVE: (*hesitantly and avoiding eye contact*) You will despise me and not want to work with me any more. I feel so ashamed. (*Looks afraid and begins to sob.*)

This example illustrates how an unanticipated problem in therapy is used to sharpen the case conceptualization, clearing the way for greater therapy progress and client engagement. When handled well, moments like this can be a real breakthrough because important client beliefs, emotions, and behaviors are uncovered and integrated into a conceptualization. His therapist helped Steve understand that feelings of shame and fear surrounding cross-dressing were understandable in the context of his previous experiences and associated beliefs. As a child, his mother supported Steve when he expressed a desire to cross-dress, yet his father reacted violently, threatening to throw him out of the house unless Steve stopped. Later neighborhood harassment and violent attacks affirmed his father's perspective. These experiences were linked with his fear that the therapist would despise him if his behavior was revealed. Collaboratively constructing this case conceptualization with the therapist dissolved many of Steve's fears regarding engagement in therapy.

4. *Case conceptualization can make complex and numerous problems seem more manageable for clients and therapists.* Clients, particularly those with complex and long-standing difficulties, can feel overwhelmed by the sheer number of issues they face. Steve's list of presenting issues and comorbid diagnoses exemplifies this phenomenon. Therapists also can feel overwhelmed when faced with clients' complex and long-standing problems. When done skillfully, case conceptualization can help problems become more manageable for clients *and for therapists.* One therapist described it as the process of "making the soupy mess into something more palatable." A client described it as, "All these bits of the puzzle fit together now."

5. *Case conceptualization guides the selection, focus, and sequence of interventions.* Arguably the most important function of case conceptualization is to inform the therapy. The number of CBT interventions that are potentially appropriate with any given client is large and expanding (J. S. Beck, 1995, 2005). Moreover, it is not always obvious which protocol to select for those clients with comorbid presentations or for those presentations that do not fit a particular model. How does a cognitive therapist choose from this vast array of choices? Case conceptualization helps the therapist select, focus, and sequence interventions. It helps clients understand why they are doing what they are doing, emphasizes the need for change, and provides a clearer therapy focus.

Once the therapist and client have a working understanding of the presenting issues, they can begin to consider which concern(s) to address first. CBT involves numerous choice points for therapists and clients. Case conceptualizations provide explicit rationales for making particular choices. When therapist and client agree on a conceptualization, a clear rationale can be made for following particular therapeutic approaches. Furthermore, a shared case conceptualization allows clients to fully participate in making decisions about the prioritization of presenting issues and therapy choice points.

For example, the most pressing issues for Steve at the beginning of therapy were his fear of revictimization and terrifying daily flashbacks to the violence he had experienced. In the early stages of conceptualization it became clear that Steve's cognitive and behavioral avoidance were maintaining his fear. This led Steve and his therapist to focus initially on the PTSD symptoms. However, as this work progressed Steve disclosed that he had not taken enough care to ensure the privacy of his cross-dressing in the neighborhood where he lived, thereby risking negative reactions from others. At this juncture the therapist decided to develop a fuller description and understanding of Steve's cross-dressing behavior. The emerging conceptualization led to a better description and understanding of his cross-dressing so that Steve could be supported in safe expressions of this behavior.

This process of sequencing interventions continues throughout therapy. Evolving case conceptualizations provide the road map to help the therapist and client decide together on the best routes toward therapy goals.

6. *Case conceptualization can identify client strengths and suggest ways to help build client resilience.* Conceptualization that attends to client strengths and uses a resilience lens to understand how clients respond adaptively to challenge has a number of advantages. It provides a description and understanding of the whole person, not just problematic issues. A strengths focus broadens potential therapy outcomes from alleviation of distress and resumption of normal functioning to improvement of the client's quality of life and bolstering client resilience. Discussion of client strengths often enhances a positive therapeutic alliance and can lead to the incorporation of positive client values into therapy goals.

7. *Case conceptualization often suggests the most cost-efficient interventions.* There are many drivers toward cost-effectiveness in health care delivery. Clients and other parties paying for CBT want a cost-effective approach. A case conceptualization approach can provide this by helping therapists and clients select the most efficient way of working toward therapy goals. It may be that a particular cognitive or behavioral mechanism is a linchpin that connects the client's main issues. Drawing out, loosening, and remediating this mechanism could, rather like a stone dropping into

a pond, ripple out to other areas of a client's life. For example, someone who is depressed, has stopped working, and no longer answers the phone or door has greatly diminished opportunities for mastery or pleasure. For such a person, behavioral activation reintroduces reinforcing contingencies that can lead to other positive changes (e.g., sense of self-efficacy) that in turn might lead to further changes (e.g., the confidence to engage in more reinforcing activities).

8. *Case conceptualization anticipates and addresses problems in therapy.* Therapeutic impasses and difficulties provide opportunities to test or develop the conceptualization. A good conceptualization offers an understanding of therapeutic difficulties as well as ways to address them. Ideally, every conceptualization enables a therapist to hypothesize issues that are likely to arise in therapy. For example, a client assessed for group CBT who suffers from depression and comorbid social phobia can be expected to have beliefs and fears that may interfere with participation in group therapy. Possible beliefs include "Group therapy won't help me because I am less capable than others," "People in the group will see how inadequate I am," or "I will get so anxious I will want to escape." Assessment of these beliefs as part of an initial conceptualization allows the therapist to address these client concerns, making group therapy accessible for someone who might otherwise avoid a group or drop out after a few sessions.

9. *Case conceptualization helps us to understand nonresponse to therapy and suggests alternative routes to change.* CBT outcome research studies report that a significant proportion of cases respond either partially or not at all (Butler, Chapman, Forman, & Beck, 2006). At best, a case conceptualization suggests ways to address partial or nonresponse by targeting the cognitive and behavioral mechanisms that maintain clients' problems. For example, residual depressive symptoms are excellent predictors of depressive relapse (Judd et al., 1999), and CBT innovations are beginning to inform our practice of working to prevent relapse (Hollon et al., 2005). However, there will always be cases that are not successful. For these, a case conceptualization should provide some understanding of nonresponse. Nonresponse could, for example, be a result of stable hopelessness or entrenched avoidance (Kuyken, Kurzer, DeRubeis, Beck, & Brown, 2001; Kuyken, 2004). The case conceptualization crucible provides a framework for therapists and clients to explore the various factors that might explain nonresponse in terms of the client's presentation and history, relevant theory, or research (Hamilton & Dobson, 2002).

10. *Case conceptualization enables high-quality supervision and consultation.* During case conceptualization we begin to understand what triggers, maintains, and predisposes the client's presenting issues. We also

begin to understand the factors that protect clients and foster resilience. Just as these realizations unfold in therapy, there is a parallel process in supervision and consultation. Case conceptualization structures supervisor and supervisee thinking and discussion. The collaborative conceptualization process between supervisor and supervisee can be a tremendous learning experience because it provides a model for curiosity and guided discovery that the supervisee can emulate in therapy with the client. Treatment plans, therapy progress, outcomes of particular interventions, therapeutic impasses, and therapist reactions are discussed in supervision. Each of these supervisory discussions can be viewed through a case conceptualization lens to test its "fit," better understand what has occurred, and then plan a way forward.

Like many therapists, we are drawn to CBT because of the creative dialogue that exists between clinical experience, theory, and research. Our clinical experience resonates with the mainstream position (cf. Eells, 2007) that case conceptualization can indeed function in the 10 ways just described. But the existing research tells a less certain story. The following sections review the evidence base for CBT case conceptualization and the challenges it raises. In Chapter 2, we describe why we believe our model resolves the key challenges posed by both research and clinical practice.

WHAT THE EVIDENCE FOR CASE CONCEPTUALIZATION TELLS US

The case conceptualization research literature has been reviewed comprehensively elsewhere (see Bieling & Kuyken, 2003; Kuyken, 2006). This synopsis highlights important challenges to the claim that CBT case conceptualization is "evidence based."

Can Case Conceptualization Be Subjected to Research?

Some therapists maintain that case conceptualization cannot be subjected to research. In psychodynamic psychotherapy there is a compelling repost to this critique that comes in the form of a research program that examines a particular case conceptualization framework, the Core Conflictual Relationship Theme (CCRT; Luborsky & Crits-Christoph, 1998). To illustrate that case conceptualization can be evidence based we present a synopsis of this research program.

Patients' descriptions of their relationships are used in the CCRT method to infer core themes in relationship conflicts (i.e., wishes toward the self, wishes toward others, responses from others, and responses from the self). The authors (Luborsky & Crits-Christoph, 1998) make explicit links to underlying psychodynamic theory and have developed a systematic and transparent scoring methodology.

The CCRT has proven reliable. A review of eight studies examining judges' agreement about patients' core relationship themes found agreement in the moderate to good range (kappa = .6 –.8; Luborsky & Diguer, 1998). Reliability was better for some aspects of the CCRT than for others, and more skilled and systematic judges tended to show higher rates of agreement with one another. Evidence of test–retest reliability has been established from the assessment to early treatment phase (Barber, Luborsky, Crits-Christoph, & Diguer, 1998). In studies of validity, pervasiveness of core conflictual relationship themes have been associated in predicted ways with defensive functioning (Luborsky, Crits-Christoph, & Alexander, 1990). Furthermore, changes in CCRT pervasiveness have been associated with symptom changes during therapy (Crits-Christoph, 1998), although the size of changes in CCRT pervasiveness was small (especially for wishes toward self or others) and the size of the association modest. The CCRT has been linked to therapy outcome. Accurate interpretations based on CCRT-derived case conceptualizations have been associated with patient improvements in a study of 43 patients in brief psychodynamic psychotherapy (Crits-Christoph, Cooper, & Luborsky, 1988).

Thus the CCRT appears to be a case conceptualization method that is reliable, valid, and related to improved outcomes. In summary, the CCRT method suggests that a systematic and coherent case conceptualization approach used by well-trained and skilled therapists can be evidence based.

Is There an Evidence Base for CBT Case Conceptualization?

Is CBT case conceptualization evidence based in the same way as the psychodynamic CCRT? Peter Bieling and Willem Kuyken set out criteria to evaluate whether case conceptualization deserves its emerging mantle as "the heart of evidence-based practice" (Bieling & Kuyken, 2003, p. 53), "the lynch pin that holds theory and practice together" (Butler, 1998, p. 1), and a key principle underpinning cognitive therapy (J. S. Beck, 1995). As set out below, the criteria for evidence-based case conceptualization can be broadly classed as top-down and bottom-up:

Top-down criterion

- Is the theory on which the conceptualization is founded evidence based?

Bottom-up criteria

- Is conceptualization reliable? That is,
  —Is the process of conceptualization reliable?
  —Can clinicians agree on the conceptualization?
- Is the conceptualization valid? Does it triangulate with the client's experience, any standardized measures, therapist and clinical supervisor's impressions?
- Does the conceptualization improve the intervention and the therapy outcomes?
- Is the conceptualization acceptable and useful to clients and therapists?

Top-Down Criterion for Evidence-Based Conceptualization

The top-down criterion is satisfied by affirmative responses to two questions: "Is the theory from which case conceptualization is derived based on sound clinical observation?" and "Are the descriptive and explanatory elements of cognitive theory upheld by research?" To consider these two questions we briefly describe the elements of cognitive theory and the evidence base for CBT theories of emotional disorders.

Since its inception CBT theory has been appreciated for its systematic descriptions and explanations of emotional difficulties. While CBT was developing between the late 1950s and the late 1970s, the dominant accounts of emotional disorders were biological and psychoanalytic. Pioneers such as Aaron T. Beck and Albert Ellis were trained in psychoanalytic therapy but discovered that when they tried to apply these theories to their clients it proved to be Procrustean. To make psychoanalytic theory fit they had to disregard the ways people described their depression and anxiety. This mismatch led Aaron T. Beck to articulate a model of emotional disorders that was grounded in how people described their distress (Beck, 1967) and which continues to evolve (Beck, 2005). The current model recognizes modes of information processing (Barnard & Teasdale, 1991; Power & Dalgleish, 1997) as well as two levels of belief: core beliefs and conditional underlying assumptions (Beck, 1996, 2005; J. S. Beck, 1995, 2005). The strategies that people use in various situations are assumed to be linked to the operating mode and activated beliefs and assumptions. Modes, core beliefs, underlying assumptions, and favored behavioral strategies are linked to one another and to a person's developmental history. Finally, automatic thoughts describe the thoughts and images that spontaneously arise in the mind moment to moment.

Modes

Modes are the broadest of these concepts. Modes describe whole patterns of information processing that help people adapt to changing demands. They become activated when orienting schema identify these demands. A classic example of a mode in action is when a person *instantaneously* orients and selectively attends to threat, bringing on line finely attuned cognitive processes (e.g., where, who, what, how bad), emotional reactions (e.g., fear), physiological states (e.g., autonomic arousal), and behavioral reactions (e.g., freeze, fight, or flight).

The content of modes is organized around core themes and mirrors the themes associated with particular emotional disorders. Loss, defeat, and deenergizing are associated with depressive disorders. Threat, fear, and energizing are associated with anxiety disorders. A person in the depressive mode conserves resources; in anxiety, immediate safety seeking is emphasized. In this sense some modes are "primal" and are experienced as reflex reactions to stimuli (e.g., threat triggers escape behavior). Other modes are more differentiated (e.g., hostility and prejudice) and associated with more complex behavioral reactions.

Core Beliefs

Core beliefs are central beliefs a person holds about the self, others, and the world. Unlike modes, which represent whole patterns of information processing and response, core beliefs refer to specific cognitive constructs or content such as "I am lovable" or "People can't be trusted." Core beliefs are often formed at an early age. Most people will form paired core beliefs such as "I am strong" and "I am weak" (Padesky, 1994a). Only one of these paired core beliefs is activated at a time. When anxious, the core belief "I am weak" is likely to be activated. In less threatening circumstances, the core belief "I am strong" may be activated. When activated, core beliefs are experienced as absolute truths; as such, they are typically affectively charged.

Sometimes people do not develop paired core beliefs in all domains. Whether due to adverse developmental circumstances, traumatic events, or biological factors, some people hold strongly developed core beliefs that are not balanced by an alternative core belief (Beck et al., 2004). For example, people diagnosed with personality disorders or those with chronic depression and anxiety often hold highly emotionally charged core beliefs that generalize unconditionally across situations and moods. A person with histrionic personality disorder is likely to view others as "needing to be entertained" and the self as "dull and unlovable," even under conditions of safety. Thus one way to detect the presence of a core belief is to notice thoughts that are accompanied by intense emotion and that do not shift in the face of contradictory evidence.

Underlying Assumptions

Underlying assumptions are intermediate-level beliefs that (1) maintain core beliefs by explaining life experiences that otherwise might contradict the activated core belief, (2) offer cross-situational rules for living that are consistent with core beliefs, and (3) protect the person from the negative affect associated with activation of core beliefs. They are called intermediate because they lie between core beliefs, which are absolute, and automatic thoughts, which are situation specific. Box 1.2

Box 1.2. Case Examples Linking Modes, Core Beliefs, Underlying Assumptions, and Strategies

	Suzette: "I'm always acting."	Bob: "You have to take care of number 1!"
Modes	Hyperarousal	Fight mode
Core beliefs	"I am dull and unlovable."	"I am powerful and superior."
	"Others need to be entertained."	"Others exploit me and deserve to be exploited."
Underlying assumptions	"If I entertain people, then they will find me interesting/love me."	"As long as I stay on top of other people, they won't be able to take advantage of me."
	"If I am not special and different, then no one will find me interesting or lovable."	"If I don't exploit people first, they will exploit me."
Strategies	Act, entertain, charm, and seduce.	Manipulate and lie.
	When this isn't met with appreciation, self-injury, and suicide attempts.	Vigilant to others' behavior.
Automatic thoughts	Thought: "I'm not special."	Thought: "My boss is just using me."
	Image of herself disappearing into a crowd.	Image of himself telling a story to colleagues and seeing them being "won over" by him.

illustrates the links among modes, core beliefs, underlying assumptions, and strategies for two people, Suzette and Bob.

Cognitive therapists offer a variety of terminology to describe underlying assumptions. Judith S. Beck (1995) calls them associated beliefs and distinguishes between assumptions (e.g., "If I am not special and different, then no one will find me interesting or lovable"), rules for living (e.g., "The 'show' must go on"), and attitudes (e.g., "Only people who are entertaining are likeable"). Padesky uses the term *underlying assumption* to highlight that these beliefs operate beneath the surface of automatic thoughts and behaviors (Padesky & Greenberger, 1995). She makes the case that it is helpful whenever possible to state underlying assumptions as "if ... then ..." conditional beliefs. Her reasoning is that beliefs stated in an "if ... then ..." form are predictive and thus can be more easily tested in therapy via behavioral experiments. Also there can be many different reasons for a particular rule for living. The " 'show' must go on" rule could just as likely result from the underlying assumptions "If I am not special and different then no one will find me interesting or lovable," or "If people fail to entertain me, they are not worth my attention." Stating underlying assumptions in an "if ... then ..." form fleshes out beliefs more clearly.

Whether they are called underlying assumptions, associated beliefs, or conditional assumptions, these beliefs form a network of generally consistent beliefs that support related core beliefs. Core beliefs are a primary way of construing the self, others, and the world; underlying assumptions support this primary construal. Even so, core beliefs do not predict which specific underlying assumptions a person will hold because there are a variety of assumptions that can sustain a core belief.

Strategies

Strategies describe what the person does when modes, core beliefs, and underlying assumptions are activated. They are closely linked to modes and the content of core beliefs and underlying assumptions. For example, in a primal threat mode, the strategy may be fight or flight. In a more differentiated paranoid mode, the behavioral reaction may be withdrawal and hypervigilance. Strategies can be both cognitive and behavioral, and their range is enormous; what is important is that they are understandable when we understand a person's modes and beliefs.

Even highly unusual strategies become understandable reactions once mode, core beliefs, and underlying assumptions are identified. For example, Suzette, one of the people conceptualized in Box 1.2, cut her wrist when a coworker warmly reassured her, "You are just like everyone else in this company." For Suzette, this inclusion in normality was devastating because she held an underlying assumption, "If I am not special and different, then no one will find me interesting or lovable." Her colleague's comment that Suzette was normal activated a high level of distress that she managed by cutting.

Strategies are activated by an affective thermostat; a person reacts cognitively or behaviorally when his/her internal state becomes deregulated. These reaction patterns often strengthen over time through processes of operant or classical conditioning. Strategies that become reflexive over time often seem dysfunctional until their origins are examined. It can be normalizing for clients to see how the unhelpful strategies they use now were highly adaptive at an earlier point in their lives.

Automatic Thoughts

Automatic thoughts describe thoughts and images that arise for everyone in the course of the day. They are called "automatic" because they arise routinely for people as they make sense of their experience. People are typically more aware of their emotional reactions than of the thoughts and images that precede or accompany them. Automatic thoughts are the focus of conceptualization when they explain the link between a situation and an emotional reaction. In the example above, Suzette's automatic thought when her colleague said, "You are just like everyone else in this company" was "I'm not special," with an associated image of herself disappearing into a crowd.

Since the publication of the seminal book *Cognitive Therapy and the Emotional Disorders* (Beck, 1976), Beck and his colleagues have developed formulations of a broad range of problem areas grounded in carefully listening to clients' accounts of their beliefs, emotions, and behaviors. Each CBT theory posits particular belief sets along with information-processing styles that describe and explain the disorder. The cognitive model of depression emphasizes negativity, specifically in relation to the self (Clark et al., 1999), and cognitive models of anxiety emphasize an overdeveloped sensitivity to threat (Beck et al., 1985). Cognitive models of personality disorder emphasize the beliefs and strategies associated with different personality disorders (Beck et al., 2004), with Suzette and Bob illustrating people with histrionic and antisocial traits, respectively (Box 1.2). Perhaps because cognitive-behavioral theories have their origins in careful observations from clinical practice, these theories tend to provide good descriptive accounts of emotional disorders that have high face validity with clients and are well supported in research. As shown in Box 1.3, there is a substantial empirical basis for cognitive theories of many Axis I and II disorders as well as growing empirical support for cognitive models of psychosis and more recently models of resiliency.

However, supporting research for the explanatory hypotheses con-

Box 1.3. Primary CBT Protocols and Evidence Summaries

Problem area	Protocol	Summary of evidence
Depression (unipolar)	Beck et al. (1979)	Clark et al. (1999)
Depression (bipolar)	Newman, Leahy, Beck, Reilly-Harrington, & Gyulai (2002)	Beynon, Soares-Weiser, Woolacott, Duffy, & Geddes (2008)
Anxiety disorders	Beck et al. (1985)	Butler et al. (2006); Chambless & Gillis (1993)
PTSD	Ehlers, Clark, Hackmann, McManus, & Fennell (2005)	Harvey, Bryant, & Tarrier (2003)
Personality disorders	Beck & Rector (2003)	Beck & Rector (2003), but see Roth & Fonagy (2005)
Substance abuse and dependence	Beck, Wright, Newman, & Liese (1993)	No summary to date, but see Roth & Fonagy (2005)
Eating disorders	Fairburn, Cooper, & Shafran (2003)	No summary to date, but see Roth & Fonagy (2005)
Relationship problems	Beck (1989); Epstein & Baucom (1989)	Baucom, Shoham, Mueser, Daiuto, & Stickle (1998)
Resilience and health	Seligman & Csikszentmihalyi (2000); Wells-Federman, Stuart-Shor, & Webster (2001); Williams (1997)	No summary to date
Psychosis	Beck & Rector (2003); Fowler, Garety, & Kuipers (1995); Morrison (2002)	Tarrier & Wykes (2004)
Hostility and violence	Beck (2002)	R. Beck & Fernandez (1998)

Note. Several seminal reviews examine the empirical status of CBT across problems areas (Beck, 2005; Butler et al., 2006; Roth & Fonagy, 2005).

tained within CBT theories is more mixed. For example, the cognitive theory of panic disorder has solid research support for both the general model and many of its explanatory hypotheses (Clark, 1986). On the other hand, although there is substantial supporting research for the broad cognitive model of generalized anxiety disorder (GAD), there are fewer studies supporting its explanatory hypotheses; in fact, there are competing explanatory hypotheses. More specifically, the broad model is that persons with GAD overestimate dangers and underestimate their ability to cope with these threats (Beck et al., 1985). Of the models competing to explain the development and maintenance of GAD, Riskind postulates a "looming cognitive style," a specific danger schema that gives rise to worry and avoidance (Riskind, Williams, Gessner, Chrosniak, & Cortina, 2000). Wells offers a cognitive model of GAD that proposes maladaptive metacognitions, such as negative beliefs about worry (Wells, 2004). Borkovec (2002) suggests that an inflexible focus on the future might be a central cognitive problem in GAD. Each of these differing models has some empirical support. Therefore, clinicians looking for an evidence-based model to conceptualize a client's GAD-based worry have several different CBT models to consider as well as empirically supported behavioral models (e.g., Ost & Breitholtz, 2000).

In short, according to the top-down criterion for evidence-based case conceptualization, general cognitive theory provides a solid basis for working with clients to develop conceptualizations. Additional research is needed to examine the explanatory elements of cognitive theories of depression (Beck, 1967; Beck, Rush, Shaw, & Emery, 1979; Clark et al., 1999), anxiety (Beck et al., 1985; Clark, 1986; Craske & Barlow, 2001), and personality disorders (Beck et al., 2004; Linehan, 1993; Young, 1999). However, these theories already offer rich frameworks for therapists' use. Cognitive theories provide an evidence-based foundation for describing clients' presenting issues and generate testable hypotheses about triggers, maintenance, predisposing, and protective factors. We consider CBT theory a vital ingredient in the case conceptualization crucible because it is derived from grounded clinical observation and has extensive research support. When therapists have a robust theory with which they are familiar, they are much better equipped to integrate theory seamlessly into their conceptualization practice.

Bottom-Up Criteria for Evidence-Based Conceptualization

The remaining criteria for evaluating case conceptualization's evidence base are described by Bieling and Kuyken (2003) as "bottom up," referring to the process, utility, and impact of case conceptualization in clinical practice. A case conceptualization meets bottom-up criteria if it is reliable, valid (i.e., relates meaningfully to clients' experiences and can be cross-validated with other measures of clients' experiences and functioning), meaningfully and usefully affects the process and outcome of therapy, and if it is viewed as acceptable and useful to clients, therapists, and supervisors. Is there evidence that CBT conceptualizations meet these bottom-up criteria? In this section we provide a summary of evidence to date.

Is CBT Case Conceptualization Reliable?

Reliability studies answer one or both of these questions:

1. Is the process of case conceptualization reliable?
2. Can therapists agree with one another on the conceptualization for a given case?

To answer these questions, researchers presented CBT therapists with case material and a framework for conceptualization and asked them to formulate a case to see whether therapists agreed on key aspects of the conceptualization (Kuyken, Fothergill, Musa, & Chadwick, 2005; Mumma & Smith, 2001; Persons et al., 1995; Persons & Bertagnolli, 1999). These studies converge in suggesting that therapists generally agree on the descriptive aspects of the conceptualization (e.g., clients' problem list) but reliability breaks down as more inference is required to hypothesize underlying explanatory cognitive and behavioral mechanisms (e.g., key beliefs and associated strategies).

Higher rates of agreement on underlying cognitive mechanisms are achieved with more systematic case conceptualization frameworks although, even then, reliability is not high. In a study by Kuyken and his colleagues (Kuyken, Fothergill, et al., 2005), 115 therapists attending a 1-day workshop on case conceptualization formulated a case using J. S. Beck's (1995) Case Conceptualization Diagram. Judith Beck formulated the same case also using her diagram. Rates of agreement between her prototypical conceptualization and workshop participants' conceptualizations were high for descriptive information (e.g., relevant background information), moderate for easy-to-infer information (e.g., compensatory strategies), and poor for difficult-to-infer information (e.g., dysfunctional assumptions). Agreement was higher for more experienced therapists.

We propose that a systematic approach, focused training, and therapist experience will improve conceptualization as it moves from more descriptive levels to explanatory levels, which require much greater theory-based inference. More recent studies offer some support for this view (Eells, Lombart, Kendjelic, Turner, & Lucas, 2005; Kendjelic & Eells, 2007; Kuyken, Fothergill, et al., 2005).

Is CBT Case Conceptualization Valid?

The next bottom-up criterion asks "Is the conceptualization valid?" While reliability is normally a prerequisite for validity, there is value in considering validity in its own right, at least for more descriptive levels of conceptualization, where reliability has been established. Unlike with the dynamic CCRT approach reviewed earlier, evidence bearing on this criterion is only recently emerging. In a study varying the information available to therapists over time and asking them to account for changes in clients' distress, the clinicians with expertise in case conceptualization explained, on average, twice the proportion of variance in the distress variables (Mumma & Mooney, 2007). In a similar finding, when the quality of therapist-generated CBT conceptualizations are judged by outside raters, more experienced or accredited CBT therapists are judged to produce higher-quality conceptualizations (Kuyken, Fothergill, et al., 2005). Across therapy approaches, therapist expertise is consistently related to higher-quality conceptualizations in terms of their being more comprehensive, elaborated, complex, and systematic (Eells et al., 2005). A recent study (Kendjelic & Eells, 2007) demonstrates that training aimed at improving therapists' use of a systematic approach to conceptualization led to improvements in overall quality of conceptualization as well as improvements along dimensions of elaboration, comprehensiveness, and precision.

In summary, the paucity of data bearing on the validity of case conceptualization within the context of CBT is striking, although the emerging data suggest that high-quality conceptualizations require a high level of therapist expertise.

Does CBT Case Conceptualization Improve Therapy and Outcomes?

The next criterion is whether case conceptualization improves therapy interventions and outcomes. If case conceptualization does not satisfy this criterion, its utility for clinical practice is questionable. Clinical lore maintains that individualized case conceptualizations enhance the process and outcome of CBT because they guide interventions and help predict issues that need to be addressed in therapy (Flitcroft et al., 2007). There is a growing body of research that examines whether case conceptualization enhances the process and outcome of CBT. Most of this research posits that an individualized approach should outperform a manualized approach because the therapy is being tailored to the particular needs of a client.

A series of studies of behavior therapy, CBT, and cognitive-analytic therapy have consistently failed to provide support for this basic idea (Chadwick, Williams, & Mackenzie, 2003; Emmelkamp, Visser, & Hoekstra, 1994; Evans & Parry, 1996; Ghaderi, 2006; Jacobson et al., 1989; Nelson-Gray, Herbert, Herbert, Sigmon, & Brannon, 1989; Schulte, Kunzel, Pepping, & Shulte-Bahrenberg, 1992). A seminal early study by Dietmar Schulte and his colleagues (Schulte et al., 1992) randomly assigned 120 people diagnosed with phobias to either manualized behavioral therapy, individualized therapy (based on a functional analysis of the problem behaviors), or a yoked control in which they were offered a treatment package that had been tailored for someone else. Although the three groups differed significantly, the authors do not report pairwise comparisons even though the means suggest that the manualized approach outperformed the other two conditions. The individualized and yoked controls did not differ from each other.

We ran post hoc *t* tests comparing the standardized and individualized arms. The results suggest that the manualized arm was superior to the individualized arm on the anxiety reaction questionnaire ($t = 2.14$, $p < .05$) and the clients' own global ratings ($t = 2.39$, $p < .05$), and there was a trend for the fear thermometer ($t = 1.63$, $p = .1$). Taken at face value, these results suggest that conceptually individualized therapy (based on a functional analysis) conferred no advantages in terms of therapy outcome, was not significantly different from the wrong individualization, and on two dimensions was inferior to the manualized treatment! On the other hand, the authors' own post hoc analyses of the integrity of the individualized and manualized therapy arms suggest significant evidence of individualization in the manualized arm; that is, therapists adapted the manual for their clients and thus the manualized treatment was not identical across clients (Schulte et al., 1992).

In a more recent study involving a series of single-case designs applying CBT for psychosis, case conceptualization had no discernible impact on outcomes or client-rated process measures such as the therapeutic relationship (Chadwick et al., 2003). The only discernible effect of case conceptualization was for the therapist, who felt that the alliance had improved following the session in which the case conceptualization had been shared with the client. However, clients did not rate the alliance as being improved.

There are some exceptions to this general trend of findings (Ghaderi, 2006; Schneider & Byrne, 1987; Strauman et al., 2006). For example, in a small randomized controlled trial for clients reporting depressive symptoms, a tailored intervention (self-system therapy) specifically addressing clients' self-discrepancies and goals proved particularly effective with clients for whom these concerns were central to the presenting issues (Strauman et al., 2006). In another study, Ghaderi (2006) compared individualized and manualized approaches for clients with bulimia nervosa. Although there were few differences between conditions, some outcome measures favored the individualized condition and the majority of nonresponders were in the manualized condition.

These few studies offer promising preliminary evidence that theory-driven individualized treatment models can enhance outcomes. However, this promise is accompanied by two cautionary observations. First, differences between manualized and individualized conditions tend to emerge only in a small subset of the outcome measures, and the effect sizes for significant differences tend to be small. Second, the assessors doing the follow-up assessments have typically not been blind to treatment condition. In summary, studies that examine the relationship between case conceptualization and therapy outcomes offer little definitive support for the benefits often claimed for case conceptualization. We concur with other commentators (e.g., Eifert, Schulte, Zvolensky, Lejuez, & Lau, 1997) that individualized and manualized treatment are not mutually exclusive. In addition, we propose that manuals be used in a flexible, theory-driven fashion, guided as far as possible by an empirical approach to clinical decision making. Moreover, our model proposes that conceptualizations co-created with clients are more likely to provide compelling rationales for therapy interventions.

Is CBT Conceptualization Considered Acceptable and Useful?

The final bottom-up criterion for judging the evidence base of case conceptualization in CBT asks whether case conceptualization is helpful for CBT clients and is regarded as useful by therapists, supervisors, and clinical researchers. A few small-scale studies are beginning to address this question with fascinating results (Chadwick et al., 2003; Evans & Parry, 1996). Client reactions to case conceptualizations are both positive (led to better understanding, felt more hopeful) and negative (made me think I was "crazy," overwhelmed). This work is salutary because mainstream CBT typically describes case conceptualization as beneficial (as we do, above) and rarely mentions its potential negative impact. Negative reactions to a case conceptualization might impede therapy or, as Evans and Parry (1996) speculate in a post hoc way from the perspective of cognitive analytic therapy, motivate clients and facilitate change.

From the perspective of therapists, case conceptualization is increasingly viewed as a core aspect of CBT (Flitcroft et al., 2007). Basic and advanced CBT training programs typically include case conceptualization as a core skill. While a decade ago only a very small handful of empirical papers on case conceptualization existed, research in this area is growing steadily. The growth of commitment to case conceptualization suggests that therapists find case conceptualization helpful as a method for individualizing CBT manuals for particular clients. On the other hand, there is little evidence that clients experience case conceptualization as a core part of CBT.

Should We Eliminate Case Conceptualization from CBT?

Even though CBT therapists and training programs are very committed to case conceptualization, the evidence challenges the claimed roles of case conceptualization in CBT. We cannot strongly advocate existing case conceptualization approaches as an alternative to protocol-based approaches just because protocol-based approaches are sometimes not effective with comorbid or complex presentations. We argue, however, that the research to date is not cause for abandoning case conceptualization; rather, we believe it challenges us to develop models that are more likely to meet evidence-based standards.

From a top-down perspective, cognitive theories are based in careful clinical observation, have a strong evidence base, and offer many testable hypotheses. A good CBT therapist uses cognitive theories to plan and navigate therapy. However, unlike the evidence base for the psychodynamic CCRT case conceptualization approach, CBT therapists currently do not appear to use case conceptualization in a principle-driven and empirical way.

This text teaches an approach to CBT case conceptualization that bridges theory and practice, informs therapy, and potentially will stand up to empirical scrutiny. We believe it takes a step toward resolving some of the challenges presented by the research studies examining CBT case conceptualization. In the following chapters we present our model of CBT case conceptualization, provide a rationale for why therapists should follow it, and explain in detail how to apply it. We next examine the model's three foundation principles: evolving levels of conceptualization (Chapter 2), collaborative empiricism (Chapter 3), and incorporation of client strengths (Chapter 4). We then bring these three principles to life by showing how one particular client's case conceptualization evolves over the course of treatment and guides it (Chapters 5–7). Case conceptualization requires higher-order skills that can be developed through training and supervision; Chapter 8 offers ideas for both learning and teaching case conceptualization skills. In Chapter 9 we draw these themes together and suggest future directions for research on case conceptualization. By explicitly describing the processes and principles of case conceptualization we hope this book encourages CBT therapists to approach case conceptualization as a journey that is exciting, creative, dynamic, rewarding, and best enjoyed with the clients' full participation.

Chapter 1 Summary

- Case conceptualization is a process like that in a crucible; it synthesizes individual client experience with relevant theory and research.
- Collaborative empiricism is the "heat" that drives the conceptualization process.

- Conceptualization evolves over the course of CBT, progressing from descriptive to increasingly explanatory levels.
- Conceptualizations incorporate not only client problems but also client strengths and resilience.
- CBT case conceptualization serves 10 key functions that describe client-presenting issues in CBT terms, improve understanding of these presenting issues, and inform therapy.
- Case conceptualization helps achieve the two overarching goals of CBT: to relieve client distress and build resilience.
- The evidence base for CBT case conceptualization presents important challenges. This book responds to these challenges by providing a framework for how to conceptualize.

Chapter 2

The Case Conceptualization Crucible
A New Model

I know I should conceptualize with my clients, but I'm afraid I tend to fly by the seat of my pants.

—THERAPIST

While most therapists believe there are benefits to case conceptualization, many don't conscientiously incorporate conceptualization into their therapy practice. Others question the need for case conceptualization: "If there are evidence-based CBT manuals, why do we need case conceptualization? Isn't a diagnosis sufficient?" Even when therapists develop a case conceptualization, it is often applied in ways that limit its usefulness. As supervisors and consultants, we observe the following:

- The case conceptualization merely copies CBT theory with aspects of the client's presentation pasted into sections of the CBT model. Crucial aspects of the case are "cut off": the Procrustean approach.
- The case conceptualization integrates little or no CBT theory; instead it merely describes the person's experience.
- The therapist produces several different conceptualizations for each comorbid condition. These are difficult to link and would be incoherent and overwhelming if shared with clients.

- The conceptualization is so elaborate and complex it looks like an electrical circuit board.
- The level of conceptualization used does not match the phase of therapy. For example, the therapist develops an overly elaborate explanatory conceptualization very early in therapy before a simpler descriptive conceptualization has been derived.

In addition, when we observe audio or video recordings of CBT therapy sessions as part of supervision or consultation we often notice:

- Therapists conceptualizing unilaterally, not collaboratively.
- The content of CBT sessions seems unrelated to the case conceptualization.
- The therapist assumes he or she has understood something but does not pause to check whether this view is shared by the client.
- The client appears to be working from a different understanding than the therapist's. The therapist either does not detect this or does not seek a clarified agreement on the conceptualization.

All of these common case conceptualization missteps are easy for CBT therapists to make in everyday practice, but our new approach can help therapists avoid them. The model of case conceptualization we propose emerged from (1) our clinical experience as CBT therapists, supervisors, consultants, and instructors, and (2) our response to key findings in the empirical research on CBT case conceptualization summarized in the previous chapter.

GUIDING PRINCIPLES FOR CBT CASE CONCEPTUALIZATION

As introduced briefly in Chapter 1, we use the metaphor of a crucible to describe the process of case conceptualization. The crucible is where theory, research, and client experiences are integrated to form a new description and understanding of client issues. While grounded in evidence-based theory and research, the conceptualization formed in the crucible is original and unique to the client and reveals pathways to lasting change. There are several features that we consider key defining principles of CBT conceptualization. The three guiding principles are (1) levels of conceptualization, (2) collaborative empiricism, and (3) incorporation of client strengths (see Box 2.1). These principles enable a flexible yet systematic approach to conceptualization.

Box 2.1. Principles for Guiding CBT Case Conceptualization

1. Levels of conceptualization	Conceptualization moves from description of a client's presenting issues in CBT terms to providing explanatory frameworks that link triggers, maintenance cycles, and/or predisposing and protective factors.
2. Collaborative empiricism	Therapist and client work *together*, integrating the client's experience with appropriate theory and research in an unfolding process of generating and testing hypotheses.
3. Strengths focus	Conceptualization actively identifies and incorporates client strengths in order to apply existing client resources to presenting issues and to strengthen client awareness and use of strengths over time (i.e., building resilience).

Principle 1: Levels of Conceptualization

The process of conceptualization evolves over the course of CBT. The steam rising from the crucible in Figure 1.1 represents the different levels of descriptive and explanatory conceptualizations.

CBT case conceptualization necessarily begins by *describing* presenting issues in cognitive and behavioral terms. As clients recount what brought them to therapy, the therapist helps them describe the presenting issues in terms of thoughts, feelings, and behaviors. Often this level of conceptualization occurs during the early assessment phase of therapy. Typically, this is the crucible's first product.

Next, client and therapist begin to *explain* how current presenting issues are triggered and maintained using CBT theory. Typically this is the crucible's second product. Finally, a third level of conceptualization can be developed to *explain* how presenting issues originated. This level outlines predisposing historical and protective factors that explain clients' vulnerability and resilience in cognitive-behavioral terms. Typically, this third product is a longitudinal conceptualization that provides a historical context for understanding the presenting issues. In summary, CBT begins with descriptive levels of conceptualization, moves to explanations of triggers and maintenance, and then, when necessary, considers factors that predispose people to and protect them from presenting concerns. Not all cases require this third level. Conceptualization typically progresses through these three increasingly inferential levels of explanation as necessary to achieve client therapy goals. For some clients the first descriptive level will suffice. More often, descriptive conceptualizations followed by explanatory conceptualizations of triggers and maintenance are sufficient. For some clients, especially those with chronic difficulties, all three levels may be required.

Principle 2: Collaborative Empiricism

In a crucible, heat acts as a catalyst for the chemical reaction. In case conceptualization, collaborative empiricism is the catalyst that integrates CBT theory, research, and client experience. The hands in Figure 1.1 represent therapist and client working together using collaborative empiricism. For reasons elaborated below, our case conceptualization process will only be effective if it is developed collaboratively by the therapist and client; the client must be integrally and explicitly involved at every stage of the conceptualization process. The therapist and client each bring something important and different to the process: CBT therapists draw on the most relevant theories and research to describe and explain clients' concerns, while clients provide essential observations and feedback that keep a conceptualization on track. Empiricism is employed throughout the conceptualization process as a methodical check and balance among competing ideas and to encourage use of the best available evidence. Collaboration and empiricism work in tandem. Thus we call our second principle "collaborative empiricism." We regard collaborative empiricism as essential if case conceptualization is to achieve its functions (Box 1.1).

Principle 3: Incorporate Client Strengths

Most current CBT approaches are concerned either exclusively or largely with a client's problems, vulnerabilities, and history of adversity. We advocate for therapists to identify and work with client strengths at every stage of conceptualization. A strengths focus is often more engaging for clients and offers the advantages of harnessing client strengths in the change process to pave a way to lasting recovery. Within the case conceptualization crucible, client experience includes client strengths. CBT theories of resilience (Snyder & Lopez, 2005) are highlighted and elaborated during the conceptualization process along with CBT theories relevant to problems.

Why Use a Principle-Driven Approach to Conceptualization?

When topics are complex, expert decision making typically involves multiple choice points (Garb, 1998). At each choice point during conceptualization, therapists need to incorporate different types of information (client, theory, research) that are layered and complex. Information can be descriptive (e.g., a client's account of her fear of dogs), incorporate details about how presenting issues vary across situations (e.g., the fear is greater in some contexts than others), and encompass a historical perspective (e.g., how the fear originated and how it has changed over time). Moreover, conceptualizations are dynamic, evolving over the course of therapy. As such, therapists are likely to be helped by having key principles to follow. In the same way a sailor can use a compass to follow a course in most areas of the world and weather conditions, a therapist can use principles to stay on course when faced with considerable complexity and change.

The following sections provide theoretical and empirical rationales for our choice of levels of conceptualization, collaborative empiricism, and inclusion of client strengths as the three primary principles guiding case conceptualization.

LEVELS OF CONCEPTUALIZATION

Why View Conceptualizations as Evolving Levels?

Case conceptualization develops progressively over the course of therapy as aspects of the client's experience are brought forward. A given case conceptualization can only be as good as the current information available to client and therapist. New information is continually being gathered via observation, interview, and experiments. Thus case conceptualizations develop over time to provide the current "best fit." One client described it this way: "I don't think I'll ever have a complete understanding ... I keep finding things that link to how I am feeling now." A therapist put it this way: "What you do is change the conceptualization to fit the information the client gives rather than change the information to fit. The client's life will either support or disconfirm the conceptualization, and if it disconfirms the conceptualization, the conceptualization is wrong." Most revisions are incremental as we move from description to higher levels of explanation—observations are added, particular factors are emphasized or eliminated, and new connections are discovered among different parts of the client's experience.

As diagrammed in Figure 2.1, our approach progressively builds a case conceptualization from an initial description of the presenting issues to identification of triggers and the factors that maintain the current difficulties. Over time, we may build a longitudinal conceptualization in which clients' presenting issues can be understood in terms of their developmental history. As they become known, predisposing factors are incorporated into the case conceptualization along with protective fac-

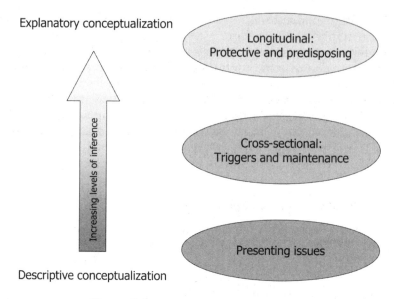

Figure 2.1. Levels of conceptualization.

tors that help the client cope in the face of difficulties. What is common to all these levels of conceptualization is the integration of CBT theory and research with client experience.

As therapy progresses the therapist is continually evaluating what CBT theory fits best with the client's experience. Initially, a simple disorder-specific model may appear to fit well, but as therapy progresses new client information may suggest the need for a different disorder-specific model or the use of the generic CBT model. For example, when working with clients with recurrent unipolar depression it is not unusual for evidence of hypomania to emerge, suggesting the need for therapists to consider CBT models of bipolar disorder (Newman et al., 2002). Alternatively, the focus of therapy may evolve so that a disorder-specific model no longer fits well with the client's presenting issue. For example, a client may initially request help with social anxiety, a problem for which a disorder-specific model exists, and later ask the therapist for help making a life choice that is unrelated to any particular diagnosis.

We view case conceptualization as an ongoing, layered activity. This suggests one reason why research on CBT conceptualization has yielded such disappointing results. To date, the research has failed to recognize that the level of conceptualization evolves as therapy proceeds. Research studies ask therapists to complete case conceptualizations unilaterally, immediately upon exposure to client information and without opportunities for hypothesis testing. Under these circumstances, we would expect therapists to be able to reliably describe problems but not agree on underlying mechanisms. This is exactly the pattern of findings in the research. The research also suggests that incorporating more inferential levels in a case conceptualization is a higher-order skill (Eells et al., 2005; Kendjelic & Eells, 2007; Kuyken, Fothergill, et al., 2005).

In later chapters of this book we show therapists in detail how to develop descriptive and explanatory accounts of clients' presenting issues during early, middle, and later phases of therapy using relevant CBT models. Here we briefly describe and illustrate the three levels.

Level 1: Descriptive Conceptualizations

During initial sessions, the client's presenting issues are described in cognitive and behavioral terms drawing on relevant CBT theory and research. These first conceptualizations connect individual client experiences with the descriptive language of CBT theory. For this stage of conceptualization, any number of CBT descriptive frameworks is available (Box 1.3). We argue that any evidence-based model is appropriate as long as it accomplishes the task of the first level of conceptualization. This task is to bring theory and client experience together to *describe* clients' presenting issues in cognitive and behavioral terms.

Ahmed: A Case Example

Ahmed came to therapy reporting symptoms of depression, generalized anxiety, and work difficulties. At the end of the intake interview, the therapist helped Ahmed form a descriptive conceptualization (see Figure 2.2) of his concerns using the five-part model (Padesky & Mooney, 1990):

THERAPIST: Thank you for patiently answering all these questions, Ahmed. In the time we have left today, I'd like to see if we can make some connections among the issues you've described to me. These connections might point us in a helpful direction so you can begin to feel better. Would that be OK?

AHMED: I don't know what you mean.

THERAPIST: Let me show you (*picking up a notepad and pen*). On this paper, let's write some of the main topics we discussed from today. For example, you began by telling me about your difficulties at work. You were put on notice by your boss that you need to perform better or you will lose your job. (*Writes at top of page:* "*My boss says I need to perform better or I will lose my job.*")

AHMED: Yes, that worries me a lot.

THERAPIST: OK. Let's write "Worries" over here. You told me some of the types of worries you have: you are worried about your job, worried about money. … Was there anything else?

AHMED: Yes. I worry about my future.

THERAPIST: (*Writes "job, money, future" under "Worries."*) Is your job the main thing in your life that makes you worry about your future?

AHMED: I also worry because I am Muslim and many people here hate Muslims.

THERAPIST: What experiences have you had that worry you?

AHMED: I hear hate in talk shows on the radio. People at the shopping center look at me oddly sometimes. At work I notice people stop talking about politics when I come in the room.

THERAPIST: So it seems some people might hold prejudice against you as a Muslim. Does this worry you because you are afraid someone might try to hurt you or your family?

AHMED: Definitely. And I pray about it too, asking Allah for strength and mercy toward these people who don't know me.

THERAPIST: So your faith in Allah offers you strength but also might put you at risk with some people.

AHMED: That's right.

THERAPIST: Let's put that on the chart under "My Life"—how your faith is both a source of strength and a risk. And let's add your worries about other people's prejudice here.

AHMED: OK.

THERAPIST: You told me your worries keep you awake at night.

AHMED: Yes, they do.

THERAPIST: I'm going to write that over here under "Physical reactions." Can you think of some other physical reactions you've had lately?

AHMED: I'm tired a lot.

THERAPIST: (*Writes "Tired."*)

AHMED: And I feel jumpy too.

THERAPIST: (*Writes "Feel jumpy."*) When you lie awake at night and then feel jumpy and tired during the day, what moods do you experience?

AHMED: Nervous … and sort of sad.

THERAPIST: And when you are nervous and sad and having all these worries and feeling tired, what changes have you noticed in your behavior?

AHMED: I put things off because I don't have confidence like I used to. Sometimes I just stare at the wall. No wonder my boss is upset. I'm just no good to anyone.

THERAPIST: I'm going to write that here under "Behavior": "I put things off. Stare at the wall." And I'm going to put this idea, "I'm no good to anyone," over here under "Thoughts." Do you think these lists capture the most important things you've told me today?

AHMED: Yes.

THERAPIST: The reason I've listed the things in these categories (*pointing to each*) is that these areas are each important in understanding difficulties. Your life (*pointing to large circle*) surrounds and affects these

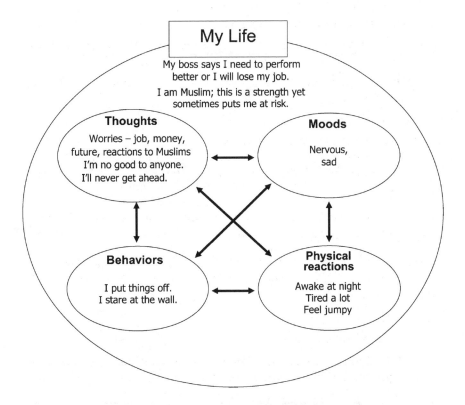

Figure 2.2. Descriptive conceptualization for Ahmed.

four parts of your experience—your thoughts, physical reactions, moods, and behavior.

AHMED: Uh-huh.

THERAPIST: I'm going to draw arrows between these four parts. Why do you think I'm doing that?

AHMED: Maybe to show they affect each other?

THERAPIST: Yes, usually they do. Can you think of a time this week when one of these four parts affected another part?

AHMED: (*thinking*) Well, when I lie awake at night I worry.

THERAPIST: OK (*tracing over arrow from "Physical reactions" to "Thoughts"*). When you lie awake you worry. And then, when you worry, does that connect with either of these moods here (*tracing over arrow between "Thoughts" and "Moods"*)?

AHMED: Yes, I feel nervous. And sometimes sad because I think I'll never get ahead.

THERAPIST: Good observation! So when you are sad (*tracing over arrow from "Moods" to "Thoughts"*) that also leads to another thought, "I'll never get ahead." Let's write that thought here under "Thoughts." (*Adds these words to model.*)

After some additional discussion of links between the five different parts of the model, the therapist introduces the following summary and treatment planning suggestion:

THERAPIST: As these arrows we've drawn show, each of these five parts affects the others. That helps explain how you got into such a tough spot, Ahmed. Small negative changes in our life can build up because each negative can lead to negatives in the other four areas. (*Points to relevant parts of five-part model during the following statements.*) You are worried and you don't sleep. When you don't sleep you get tired. When you are tired you don't feel like doing anything. When you don't do anything you start to think, "I'm no good to anyone." And around and around it goes. After a while, you can get into quite a hole, and things can even begin to look quite hopeless.

AHMED: Yes, that is how it looks to me right now.

THERAPIST: Fortunately, there is good news in this picture.

AHMED: There is? I don't really see it.

THERAPIST: Well, the good news is that small changes in one area can lead to small changes in the other areas. Just like small negative changes can eventually get you in a big hole, small positive changes in one area can lead to small positive changes in the other areas, and eventually these can help you out of the hole you are in. I see my job as helping you figure out the smallest changes you can make in any of these areas to lead to the biggest improvement possible in the whole picture. How does that sound to you?

AHMED: Well, that would be nice if it worked.

THERAPIST: Let's look at this picture together, Ahmed. If you were going to pick one of these areas in which to make a small change, where do you think you could start? What small change might help one or more of the other areas too?

AHMED: (*Looks at Figure 2.2 for a minute silently.*) Well, I think if I didn't put things off, I might feel better and that would help my job, too.

THERAPIST: That's an interesting idea, Ahmed. Can you tell me one small thing you have been putting off that you might be able to do this week as an experiment to see whether you are right?

As shown in this dialogue between Ahmed and his therapist, the descriptive five-part model helps clients begin to make connections between thoughts, moods, behavior, physical reactions, and life events. In addition, the five-part model provides a visual map to show how small changes can lead to big results. This notion is very helpful in the early stages of therapy, when client's struggles seem quite large relative to the client's perception of his or her capacity for change. Thus the five-part model often provides a good starting point for case conceptualization because it offers a clear description of presenting issues, demonstrates links among client experiences, and frequently engenders hope.

Throughout this book we illustrate how to use CBT models to describe clients' presenting issues. The actual CBT model selected to describe clients' presenting issues is not as important as the principle of describing client experience with an appropriate CBT model in the service of describing clients' presenting issues in cognitive and behavioral terms.

Level 2: Cross-Sectional Conceptualization—Understanding Triggers and Maintenance Factors

Cross-sectional explanatory conceptualizations link CBT theory and client experience at a higher level by identifying the key cognitive and behavioral mechanisms that underpin clients' presenting issues. CBT is "goal oriented" and "initially emphasizes the present" (J. S. Beck, 1995,

p. 6). At this level of conceptualization, therapists focus on the cross section of a client's life that captures the presenting issues. In what situations are the client's current presenting issues triggered and maintained? The task in this phase of conceptualization is to use CBT models to explain what triggers and maintains clients' presenting issues. Any one of a number of models can be used here, such as functional analysis (Hayes & Follette, 1992; Kohlenberg & Tsai, 1991), use of situation–thought–emotion–behavior sequences (Padesky & Greenberger, 1995), application of disorder-specific CBT models (see Box 1.3), or use of the generic CBT model of emotional disorders summarized in Chapter 1. These methods help develop conceptualizations that make sense of client behavioral patterns and emotional reactivity.

Sarah: A Case Example

Sarah presented with several interpersonal problems. At the beginning of session 3 she asked for help with a problem she was having with a good friend. Sarah had attended the funeral of her good friend's father, but she had been avoiding her friend since then and felt ashamed. She wasn't sure why she felt ashamed or why she had been avoiding her friend since the funeral. The therapist worked with Sarah to explore the links between the funeral and Sarah's subsequent behavior and feelings of shame. How can the therapist help Sarah make sense of her feelings and behavior?

THERAPIST: Sarah, what did you make of your friend not speaking to you at the funeral?

SARAH: (*Pauses to think.*) That I had offended her in some way.

THERAPIST: I am puzzled, how could you have offended her?

SARAH: Well, we were invited to bring a sunflower to the funeral to put on the coffin at the end of the service. I had come straight from dropping my kids off at school and the florist near the church had sold out so I arrived without a sunflower. She seemed to notice this.

THERAPIST: That's interesting. So you had the thought "She's noticed I didn't bring a sunflower"? (*Sarah nods.*) What do you suppose this meant to her?

SARAH: (*Reflects for a moment.*) That I don't care enough about her to remember to bring a flower. I felt she disapproved of me being there without a flower.

THERAPIST: OK, so let's write this down on this Thought Record. Write down what actually happened in the "Situation" column. (*Sarah writes it in.*) In the "Automatic Thoughts" column write the thoughts you just identified: "She thinks I don't care enough about her to remember to bring a flower" (*Sarah writes it in*) and "She disapproved of me being there without a flower." (*Pauses while Sarah writes.*) And the feeling was what?

SARAH: I felt ashamed. (*Writes "Ashamed" in the "Moods" column.*)

THERAPIST: So what we are trying to do here is better understand what led to your feelings and behavior ...

SARAH: (*interrupting*) It's interesting because in the heat of the situation my feelings of shame came very quickly, I hadn't really noticed the thought about her disapproving of me. (*After a pause.*) Funerals are often such emotional places.

This example illustrates how a cognitive-behavioral model is used to help a client understand what triggers the presenting issues in a single situation (Figure 2.3). For Sarah, the meaning she placed on her friend's distance at the funeral influenced her subsequent emotions and behavior. If examination of other situations can demonstrate to Sarah that the meanings she makes of events affects her behaviors and feelings, she and

THOUGHT RECORD

1. Situation	2. Moods (Rate 0–100%)	3. Automatic Thoughts (Images)	4. Behavior What did you do in this situation to help manage your feelings?
At my friend's father's funeral, I didn't bring a sunflower. She didn't speak to me at the funeral or afterward.	Ashamed (80%)	She thinks I don't care enough about her to remember to bring a flower. She disapproved of me being there without a flower.	Avoid my friend.

Figure 2.3. Using a Thought Record to derive a cognitive model of Sarah's automatic thoughts in an interpersonal situation.

her therapist have begun to form a working explanatory conceptualization of moods and behaviors that otherwise might perplex Sarah.

THERAPIST: It sounds like you have been able to make sense of why you have been avoiding your friend. (*Sarah nods.*) It can be helpful sometimes to begin to look for patterns in what triggers your moods so that we can begin to use these patterns to help you cope better with your relationships in the future.

SARAH: Yes, that would be helpful. I seem to get in a mess, always falling out with people. You know, after the funeral of my husband, John [who died several years ago], there were several people I fell out of contact with.

THERAPIST: Shall we use the Thought Record again to see if we can make sense of what happened to some of your relationships after John's funeral?

SARAH: OK. I feel most ashamed about John's parents. I don't see them anymore; we exchange Christmas cards, but that's it.

Sarah and her therapist work through another Thought Record (see Figure 2.4). Having completed the Thought Record, they reflect on Sarah's therapy goal of managing conflict with people better, so she doesn't always "fall out" with people.

THOUGHT RECORD

1. Situation	2. Moods (Rate 0–100%)	3. Automatic Thoughts (Images)	4. Behavior What did you do in this situation to help manage your feelings?
At John's funeral, which his parents organized.	Ashamed (90%)	They don't think I am capable of organizing the funeral. They think I wasn't a very good wife to John.	Avoid John's parents.

Figure 2.4. Using a second Thought Record to derive a cognitive model of Sarah's automatic thoughts in an interpersonal situation.

THERAPIST: Do you notice anything about these two Thought Records that suggests what might trigger you "falling out" with people?

SARAH: Apart from the fact that they both involve funerals? (*Therapist nods. After a pause Sarah continues.*) Well, in both cases I felt really disapproved of and then I felt ashamed. I hate that feeling!

THERAPIST: OK, and how did you handle that feeling?

SARAH: By avoiding them … and drifting apart.

The explanatory conceptualization that emerges from the dialogue above is a generic one (e.g., thoughts influence emotions and behaviors). Specifically, Sarah observes that perceived disapproval from others triggers feelings of shame, a feeling she manages by avoiding the people she thinks disapprove of her.

As CBT proceeds, conceptualizations often begin to incorporate factors that maintain clients' presenting issues. Many CBT therapists regard identification of triggers and maintenance factors as the "engine room" of conceptualization because it informs therapy within many disorder-specific models. Maintenance cycles specify how emotional, physical, and behavioral reactions to situational triggers help sustain client difficulties. These help clients understand why their problems aren't spontaneously recovering. An understanding of maintenance cycles also provides choice points for intervention. When clients step out of these cycles and try alternative cognitive or behavioral strategies they can evaluate the impact of such changes on the problem.

In Sarah's case, she and her therapist discovered that she frequently avoided people when she believed they disapproved of her. They began to hypothesize that Sarah's avoidance of conflict actually exacerbated and maintained many of her interpersonal difficulties. In Ahmed's case, the arrows in Figure 2.2 suggested several possible explanatory maintenance factors. For example, Ahmed's therapist noticed the thought "I'm no good to anyone" and wondered whether this thought might strengthen his behavior of putting things off. Therapists often form hypotheses regarding higher levels of conceptualization when working with clients at simpler levels of conceptualization. These hypotheses are shared with clients only when the therapist believes the client is ready to test them out and incorporate resulting ideas into therapy.

Level 3: Longitudinal Conceptualization— Understanding Predisposing and Protective Factors

The next level of conceptualization makes use of clients' developmental history to better understand their presenting issues. There are often reasons why particular people are vulnerable to specific problems. Predisposing factors describe any element that makes one person more likely to respond in a particular way to a life circumstance. Research shows that a range of factors, such as temperament and significant experience of adversity, predispose people to mental health problems (Rutter, 1999).

On the other hand, client strengths and positive experiences, such as good-enough parenting and good adolescent peer relationships, serve as protective factors. More than this, Rutter makes the important point that protective factors interact with predisposing factors in complex ways to affect vulnerability and resilience (Figure 2.5; Rutter, 1999). To illustrate this point, he offers the example of children exposed to extreme early privation who are able to recover fully in subsequent nurturing environments. He also describes how people at great risk have "turning points" in their lives. Rutter (1999) provides an example of how a young man at high risk for criminal activity joined the Army and changed his life trajectory in positive ways.

Although predisposing and protective factors are identified and incorporated into evolving models throughout the conceptualization process, they are especially emphasized in the later stages of therapy as clients prepare to manage independently. Skillful conceptualization of protective and predisposing factors can constructively improve clients'

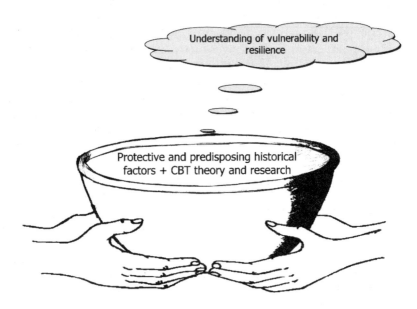

Understanding of vulnerability and resilience

Protective and predisposing historical factors + CBT theory and research

Figure 2.5. Longitudinal conceptualization of vulnerability and resilience incorporating predisposing and protective factors.

awareness and use of strengths and coping abilities. Later in therapy, Sarah and her therapist reviewed the probable origins of her presenting interpersonal problems. Sarah's marriage to John had been unhappy. He was possessive, jealous, and critical, and he criticized Sarah continually about her apparent shortcomings, which over several years undermined her self-confidence. Specifically, he would berate her for not being attentive enough to him, accusing her of attending more to her own family, colleagues, and friends. His typical refrain was, "You're so insensitive; you clearly don't care about other people. You're selfish."

During the relationship Sarah developed the underlying assumption, "If I don't constantly meet other people's needs, it means I'm selfish." This assumption was particularly upsetting for Sarah because duty was stressed as an important value in her family of origin. Her parents often said that it was important to "do your duty." When John died of leukemia at age 45, his parents arranged the funeral. The eulogies at the funeral portrayed John as someone very different from the person Sarah knew, a discrepancy she resolved by blaming herself for not having lived up to John's expectations. The beginning of the longitudinal conceptualization developed with Sarah using a generic CBT model (J. S. Beck, 1995) is shown in Figure 2.6. From this conceptualization we can understand how the funeral of her good friend triggered the underlying assumption, "If I don't constantly meet other people's needs, it means I'm selfish," that she learned during her unhappy marriage to John.

Longitudinal conceptualization is the highest level of inference and is used only when it is necessary to help work toward client goals. With Sarah it was necessary to move to this level of conceptualization because her interpersonal problems were maintained by a core belief about herself ("I'm selfish") and an underlying assumption about other people ("If I don't constantly meet other people's needs, it means I'm selfish") that were more understandable in historical context. We fully illustrate longitudinal conceptualization processes in Chapter 7.

Flexibility in the Level of Conceptualization

Using the appropriate level of conceptualization is a helpful guide for therapists. A sailor heading northwest uses the compass to follow a course, yet there are various choice points when landmasses, tides, and weather conditions indicate a need to change course to reach the destination. Working sequentially through levels of conceptualization in CBT is like following a compass course. These phases of conceptualization are the ways therapy might *normally* evolve. However, sometimes the process of conceptualization is influenced by the nature of the client's presentation, the strength of an appropriate evidence-based model,

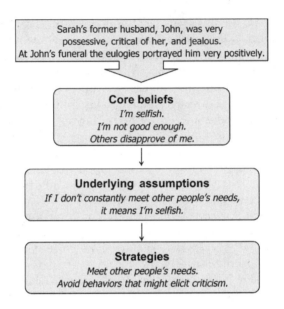

Figure 2.6. Longitudinal conceptualization of Sarah's interpersonal presenting issue.

and the client's goals. For example, if a client's presentation seems to
exactly fit an existing explanatory cognitive model that includes triggers,
maintenance factors, and predisposing factors, the therapist and client
might explore this model in opening therapy sessions without spending any time developing a purely descriptive model of presenting issues.
Similarly, if a client presents with an issue early in therapy that requires
a maintenance cycle, a CBT therapist might move more rapidly to map
one out. In these circumstances the therapist changes course to reach
the same destination of alleviating client distress and building resilience.
One therapist described this choice as: "I conceptualize in a way that is
sensitive to what suits the client at that time."

    Figure 2.7 shows some of the commonly used CBT models of con-
ceptualization. Many of these models can be used at each of these three
levels of conceptualization depending on whether the client content
explored is situation-specific, cross-sectional, or longitudinal.

    All of these conceptualization models are illustrated in this text. We
encourage readers to keep in mind that the actual models a therapist
chooses to use depend on what models best fit clients' presenting issues.
This often changes over the course of therapy. All these approaches
use the best available theory to understand how thoughts, beliefs, and
behaviors can describe and explain clients' presenting issues. However,

these elements are combined somewhat differently at each level of case conceptualization. Descriptive conceptualizations demonstrate links among thoughts, moods, and behaviors without necessarily weighting the importance of each. Explanatory conceptualizations look for patterns in these elemental links across situations and sometimes across presenting issues. Explanatory conceptualizations usually hypothesize about the relative importance of particular elements thought to function as triggers or maintenance factors. Higher-level longitudinal conceptualizations expand this cross-situational focus to look for patterns across an extended period of time, even a lifetime, to search for the origins of key beliefs, strategies, and situational determinants of presenting issues.

Greater flexibility and skill is required as a therapist moves to the higher levels of inference required to construct CBT models that explain triggers, maintenance cycles, and the developmental origins for presenting issues. As conceptualization proceeds to higher levels of inference, therapists are guided by appropriate CBT theory and client feedback. Sarah's shame was triggered by her perceptions of other people's behavior. These perceptions were shaped by Sarah's core beliefs and underlying assumptions. For clients with PTSD a visual cue may be a trigger for traumatic flashbacks. Excessive health anxiety can be triggered by somatic experiences and also by reading medical information on the Internet. Sometimes therapists and clients will wonder whether a particular experience is a trigger or a maintenance factor. Throughout this

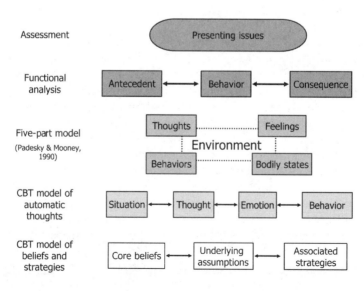

Figure 2.7. Models used at each level of conceptualization.

text we explore the flexibility and skill required to apply CBT models to understand triggers, maintenance cycles, and developmental origins.

It is important to regularly assess how therapy is proceeding toward therapy goals and whether improvements are occurring as would be expected. Typically, in CBT there is some form of outcome assessment during each therapy session with more detailed review points scheduled throughout therapy (e.g., J. S. Beck, 1995). If progress is not occurring at a rate comparable to that documented in outcome studies for similar clients and problems, a review of the conceptualization(s) can be critical to understanding why progress is slow. Sometimes a change in the level of conceptualization will get therapy back on track.

This first principle, levels of conceptualization, will be elaborated on further in Chapters 5 through 7, which follow an individual client, Mark, as he and his therapist proceed through the three levels of case conceptualization, from descriptive conceptualization (Chapter 5), to cross-sectional awareness of triggers and maintenance factors (Chapter 6), and, finally, to longitudinal identification of predisposing and protective factors (Chapter 7).

WHY COLLABORATIVE EMPIRICISM?

Our second principle recommends that therapists approach case conceptualization collaboratively with their clients, using an empirical approach. This section describes collaborative empiricism in more detail and provides a rationale for why it should be a principle that guides case conceptualization.

From its beginnings, cognitive therapy has advocated a process that is both collaborative and empirical (Beck et al., 1979). Therapists who embody a spirit of collaboration favor therapy methods that invite and encourage active client participation. An empirical framework values direct observation and data collection to evaluate beliefs, behaviors, and physiological and emotional responses. Consistent with these general processes within therapy sessions, cognitive therapists motivate clients to continue these processes outside of session via observational, written, and behavioral assignments. Thus the incorporation of collaboration and empiricism into case conceptualization is a natural extension of these processes that pervade so many CBT interventions.

Empiricism and Empirically Supported Therapy Protocols

Empiricism has a number of elements. The first involves therapists making the best available use of existing CBT theory, research, and therapy protocols. While this is a text on CBT case conceptualization, the studies reviewed in Chapter 1 that compare individualized and protocol-driven approaches are humbling. Given the research to date, we suggest that therapists follow evidence-supported protocols whenever possible, adopt relevant practice guidelines, and use the best available theory and research (Box 1.3). For example, when a client presents with panic as the primary presenting issue, our approach advocates turning to established panic models and treatment protocols as a first point of call (e.g., Clark, 1986; Craske & Barlow, 2001).

We propose that case conceptualization augments theory-driven CBT protocols. Conceptualization enters the foreground when clients' presentations are comorbid, especially complex, or do not fit any available evidence-based approach. At these times CBT offers transdiagnostic models like the generic CBT model outlined in Chapter 1. Throughout this book we hope to illustrate how a collaborative empirical model of case conceptualization enables CBT therapists to "stand on the shoulders of giants."

An Empirical Approach to Case Conceptualization

An empirical approach to case conceptualization also means that therapists and clients actively evaluate the conceptualizations derived in therapy. Case examples in Chapter 3 illustrate collaborative tests of the usefulness and accuracy of case conceptualizations. Further case illustrations in that chapter demonstrate how conceptualizations are used to generate explicit provisional hypotheses that can be tested via behavioral experiments conducted in and between therapy sessions. When observations from these experiments do not closely match client experience, the conceptualization is modified even if it was originally derived from an empirically supported CBT theory.

Empiricism as a Counterbalance to Common Decision-Making Errors

Case conceptualization is a complex process in which therapists integrate large amounts of information and adjust to new information as it becomes available. To manage this complex task, clinicians use heuristics that enable shortcuts in decision making based on "rules of thumb" (see, e.g., Kahneman, 2003). For example, during case conceptualization, therapists search for information that fits with a relevant theory, or they overlay a client's presenting issues onto mental templates derived from observations of clients who are intuited to be similar.

Decision-making processes have been mapped out and researched across many disciplines and settings (see, e.g., Kahneman, 2003). Most of the time decision-making heuristics (shortcuts) provide advantages over solutions that exhaustively use all available data because people do not have the resources or time to generate optimal solutions. Moreover, optimal solutions are not always that much better than good-enough solutions. Garb (1998) provides an excellent summary of clinical decision making in psychotherapy and points out that, while heuristics provide advantages, they are prone to significant errors. A few of the most common errors are described here because therapist awareness of these heuristic errors may support commitment to an empirical approach to case conceptualization.

Common Therapist Conceptualization Errors

One problematic heuristic is the tendency to overstate how representative a particular person is of a disorder, theoretical framework, or a pattern demonstrated by apparently similar clients. This is the Procrustean approach we described in Chapter 1, in which the client's experience is cut down to fit the theory. The following dialogue between Alan's therapist and a consulting therapist illustrates this point.

THERAPIST: I am expecting Alan will approach his therapy homework obsessively, losing sight of why we have agreed on a particular homework task.

CONSULTANT: That's an interesting hypothesis. What makes you think this? Has this happened?

THERAPIST: Not yet, no. But Alan reminds me of clients I have seen before with OCPD [obsessive–compulsive personality disorder] and the homework became part of the problem with them.

CONSULTANT: What's the evidence of this with Alan? How has he been getting on with the homework so far?

THERAPIST: Well, pretty good, actually. He says it has loosened some of his compulsive behavior that is driven by perfectionism. (*Laughs.*) Really, I don't have any evidence. I guess I need to check out my own negative thinking!

CONSULTANT: Perhaps. (*Smiles.*) Our experience with similar clients is really important, but we also need to check out our hypotheses with the evidence.

Another common cognitive error that can affect conceptualization is the tendency to overestimate the importance of the most readily available information. Information can become overvalued due to its frequency, recency, vividness, or apparent relevance. The client Ahmed (above and Figure 2.2) was particularly prone to talking about difficulties at work, which blinded his therapist to the importance of other aspects of his life. The following supervision dialogue that followed the assessment session illustrates this point:

THERAPIST: Ahmed's work is clearly at the heart of his problems, and I wonder whether he has some underlying assumptions and core beliefs about work that I need to draw out.

SUPERVISOR: This sounds like a good starting hypothesis to pursue. Let's also keep in mind that what Ahmed isn't talking about also may be important to understanding his difficulties. While you pursue your hypothesis about Ahmed's beliefs at work, are there other areas of his life that may be important but for whatever reason aren't getting much airtime?

Like all people, therapists tend to anchor information around a certain point, such as a favored hypothesis. This can lead to further errors in case conceptualization. For example, Ahmed and his therapist may draw out a conceptualization early in therapy and then anchor subsequent information around this conceptualization without being open to the possibility that it is incomplete or even wrong. Prior to a midtherapy review session, the therapist and supervisor pause to take stock:

THERAPIST: Ahmed and I are due to have a review session next week, and frankly we have not made as much progress as I would have expected.

SUPERVISOR: Let's have another look at the conceptualization and see whether it fits with what you know about Ahmed and also whether there is anything important you are missing. Maybe this will help you and Ahmed figure out in your review session why you have not made much progress so far.

His supervisor encouraged the therapist to collaboratively review the working conceptualization with Ahmed. While doing this, Ahmed articulated an underlying assumption, "To be a good family man I have to provide financially for my family," connected to a distressing prediction, "My family will end up destitute." It became clear that the thought elicited while developing a five-part model (Figure 2.2), "I am no good to anyone," resonated with Ahmed's underlying assumptions about his family life. To explore his underlying assumptions about the overarching importance of his financial contribution to the family, Ahmed agreed to invite his wife into therapy. She expressed her wish to spend more time with Ahmed and concern that his overwork was compromising both his health and the joy they used to share in their relationship. Ahmed was surprised to learn that a more relaxed atmosphere at home was more important to his wife than financial success.

Intuitive and Rational Systems

What guides therapists' decision making in these types of situations? Daniel Kahneman, a Nobel prize–winning psychologist, developed a model of heuristic decision making that is helpful for understanding how therapists conceptualize (Kahneman, 2003). Kahneman suggests that two relatively independent cognitive systems appear to underpin decision making: intuitive and rational systems. The intuitive system tends to be fast, automatic, and is often emotionally charged. The rational system is slower, more deliberate, and consciously monitored (see Figure 2.8). Due to their speed, intuitive processes are generally the first in operation during case conceptualization. The rational system is activated somewhat later as a check and balance for the intuitive system or when the intuitive system is unable to offer any hypotheses.

Thus a client may initially strike the therapist as "dependent" because frequent requests for help in session intuitively trigger this label. Later, when reflecting on the session while writing therapy notes, the therapist may entertain a competing hypothesis that the client lacks skills to do what the therapist is asking of him or her. There is evidence that the

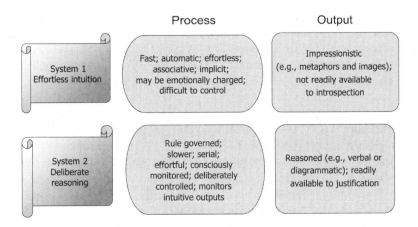

Figure 2.8. Clinical (heuristic) decision making: Process and output in two systems. After Kahneman (2003).

coordinating function of the rational system is enhanced by intelligence and training and impaired by time pressure, competing demands, and activated mood states (see Kahneman, 2003). These observations fit with the concept of therapist expertise (Eells et al., 2005) and, crucially, with the finding that training in case conceptualization leads to more elaborated, comprehensive, complex, and precise case conceptualizations (Kendjelic & Eells, 2007). Therapist expertise is the process of seeing larger patterns within complex case material, patterns geared toward comprehension and treatment planning. It is likely that therapists with expertise rely more on "intuitive" processes informed by prior experience, with the rational system providing a check and balance.

Therapist Commitment to Empiricism

These decision-making systems, as well as their inherent thinking errors, are familiar to CBT therapists. Unfortunately, familiarity does not prevent clinical errors. Heuristic errors in decision making may be one reason CBT therapists do not generate reliable case conceptualizations. We know therapists are prone to errors in conceptualization particularly when information is complex and ambiguous, or when therapists attempt to infer hypotheses without adequate information, work noncollaboratively, are less experienced, are under considerable time pressure, or have many competing demands for attention. We contend that if conceptualization is conducted in ways that counterbalance these heuristic errors, CBT case conceptualization can become reliable and reach evidence-based standards of validity. In the next sections we provide guidelines for how use of empiricism and collaboration can safeguard conceptualization from decision-making errors. Throughout the book we also emphasize the importance of these activities with text boxes labeled "Inside the Therapist's Head." These sections highlight ways a therapist can use collaborative empiricism to evaluate the client's presenting issues, plan therapy interventions, and review the process of therapy.

Guidelines for Following Empirical Principles in Conceptualization

Below and in Box 2.2 we identify a number of guidelines for "good-enough" case conceptualization practice consistent with an empirical approach.

• *Use the best available CBT theory and research.* Application of relevant theory and research to help describe and explain clients' presenting issues is at the heart of empiricism. Box 1.3 referenced some of the key theoretical and research bodies of knowledge that therapists can

---

Box 2.2. Evidence-Based Guidelines for Generating "Good-Enough" CBT Case Conceptualizations

1. Conceptualize using the best available CBT theory and research.
2. Use a hypothesis-testing approach.
3. Provide adequate tests for conceptualizations.
4. Counterbalance decision-making errors.
5. Make conceptualizations explicit.

---

use. CBT therapists who have a working knowledge of this relevant CBT theory and research will be better able to apply this knowledge to the conceptualization process.

• *Use hypothesis testing.* A commitment to empiricism also means using a hypothesis-testing approach. As a conceptualization develops, the client and therapist work together to continually formulate hypotheses that help make sense of the presenting issues. During this process, it is important for therapists to keep alternative hypotheses in mind to avoid premature commitment to a single conceptual frame. This way if a hypothesis is not supported, an alternative hypothesis can more easily be developed and tested. The consultation excerpt above with Alan's therapist is a good example of the therapist needing to hold two hypotheses in mind: either Alan's obsessive traits manifest across all situations (including homework) or, alternatively, his obsessive traits are manifest only in certain roles. Once the therapist became curious as to why Alan was not obsessive regarding homework, she learned that Alan's obsessive traits were relationship based. He held the underlying assumption, "If I inconvenience other people then they will regard me as irresponsible." This underlying assumption was linked to a core belief, "I am irresponsible."

• *Provide adequate tests.* Hypothesis testing necessarily involves providing adequate tests of each hypothesis. There are many ways of testing hypotheses in CBT (J. S. Beck, 1995). Behavioral experiments are often chosen during case conceptualization because they offer a classic approach for developing and testing hypotheses (Bennett-Levy et al., 2004). Other CBT "tools" for testing hypotheses include the process of Socratic questioning (Padesky & Greenberger, 1995), forms such as the Dysfunctional Thought Record (see Beck et al., 1979) or Automatic Thought Record (Greenberger & Padesky, 1995), standardized measures such as the Dysfunctional Attitude Scale (Beck, Brown, Steer, & Weissman, 1991; Weissman & Beck, 1978), and corroboration with other key people in the client's network (e.g., a partner).

As described earlier, Ahmed's partner was invited to attend a review session. Her presence led Ahmed to highlight more clearly the importance of a central underlying assumption ("To be a good family man I have to provide financially for my family") and dire prediction ("My family will end up destitute") that maintained his difficulties. Ahmed had escaped a famine in an African country by moving to Europe. This session enabled both his partner and the therapist to fully understand the realities behind the fear of hunger and poverty common among people in Ahmed's home country. A therapist who seeks multiple sources of information from different perspectives to form a conceptualization is more likely to see the big picture as well as important details within the picture that might otherwise have been missed.

• *Counterbalance decision-making errors.* As discussed earlier, heuristic errors that affect clinical decision making can lead to erroneous conceptualizations. These become more likely when problems are particularly complex, therapists are inexperienced, and there are competing demands (Garb, 1998). Reflective practice in therapy and supervision can boost awareness of these factors and help avoid problems. For example, therapists benefit from explicitly developing written case conceptualizations and sharing these with clients and supervisors/consultants, a process that necessarily engages the rational decision-making system that is a counterbalance to intuitive decision making (Figure 2.8; Kahneman, 2003). Given the preliminary evidence that experience enables higher quality case conceptualization, novice therapists can expect to work hard to develop case conceptualization skills. Training and supervision are central to this learning process (see Chapter 8).

• *Make conceptualizations explicit.* Writing case conceptualizations in session, in therapy case notes, and for consultation encourages a therapist to make intuitive processes explicit. The process of writing out the conceptualization often puts a spotlight on gaps in understanding or inconsistencies in thinking. As already stated, this is especially important if therapy is not proceeding as planned or expected. At these times, taking time to formulate can actually enhance outcomes (see Lambert et al., 2003).

In summary, empiricism involves making full use of the CBT evidence base to inform case conceptualization. In addition, the therapist adopts an empirical stance throughout therapy in which conceptual hypotheses are developed and tested via clinical observations and experiments. Heuristics are an essential part of clinical decision making, yet it is important to identify and remedy problematic heuristics to improve the reliability and validity of case conceptualization. The proposed guidelines for empiricism in case conceptualization are summarized in Box 2.2.

Collaboration: Two Heads Are Better Than One

Case conceptualization is often depicted as an activity that takes place in the therapist's head during or between therapy sessions. Many cognitive therapy texts describe case conceptualization as a formulation of problems, precipitating factors, and maintenance factors presented to the client by the therapist after clinical information is gathered and organized (e.g., Persons, 1989; J. S. Beck, 1995). Most of the research reviewed earlier in this chapter assumes that case conceptualizations are constructed primarily by therapists. In some studies the case conceptualization is presented to clients in a fairly comprehensive form at a particular point in therapy (e.g., Chadwick et al., 2003; Evans & Parry, 1996). The research suggests that when clients are presented with clinician-derived case conceptualizations, the impact on clients can be neutral and sometimes negative (cf. Chadwick et al., 2003; Evans & Parry, 1996).

Our case conceptualization model advocates that the therapist and client *collaboratively* develop every level of conceptualization. This approach transforms how we think about the reliability and validity of a case conceptualization. Reliability of case conceptualization can be thought of as tracking the dialogue between therapist and client and asking, "Have the therapist and client agreed on the working conceptualization?" The therapist and client co-create and continually check out their evolving conceptualization with each other so that there is not a unilateral therapist conceptualization or a client understanding that differs from the therapist's. In early phases of therapy the therapist may structure this interaction and, as therapy progresses, the client increasingly takes the initiative. One client described her experience of this process:

> "When the therapist was summing something up she would stop short of the crucial point and I took that as a cue to jump in and say ah-ha! (*laughing*), but I thought that was very clever as well. And then she would reinforce it by asking me to repeat it."

Validity of case conceptualization is considered in terms of its role within a course of therapy, not in absolute terms. For example, does the case conceptualization correctly predict outcomes of experiments? Do treatment methods suggested by the conceptualization lead to the expected outcome? Conceptualizations derived within the therapy hour and based on clients' active input are likely to offer face validity to the client. This face validity is enhanced if the therapist–client duo willingly edits the conceptualization over time to accommodate client experiences in and outside therapy. As client and therapist work together to formulate and test hypotheses, observational data or independent measures may indicate that a particular conceptualization has predictive or construct validity as well. Under these circumstances we can ask whether the case conceptualization matches the client's experience, any standardized measures, the therapist's clinical impressions, and a clinical supervisor's or consultant's impressions. These issues are largely unexamined in research. To study this perspective on the validity of case conceptualization, client and therapist views of conceptualizations need to be assessed and compared. To date, studies on case conceptualization have asked evaluators to rate therapist-derived conceptualizations without assessing the client's perspective.

Collaboration between therapist and client decreases the likelihood that cognitive errors will blur the conceptualization picture. Although the client is subject to the same cognitive processes and biases as the therapist, collaboration increases the likelihood of corrective feedback because the therapist and client inevitably approach conceptualization from different perspectives. The client and therapist each add different relevant information to the conceptualization crucible. The client contributes historical information, current observations about overt and covert events, and therapy goals, while the therapist mixes in ideas based on empirical research, psychological models, and past experience with similar client issues.

Yet the confluence of all this information is no guarantee that a meaningful conceptualization will emerge. A collaborative approach between therapist and client is essential if a meaningful conceptualization is to emerge.

PETE: I don't really know why I procrastinate so much.

THERAPIST: Some research links procrastination to perfectionism. As long as people don't finish something, they don't have to deal with anxiety about errors or criticism. If they do it at the last minute, then any criticism they receive is not so stinging, because they think they could have done better with more time. Is there any possibility something related to this idea is going on for you?

PETE: (*long pause*) I don't know. I think it is more a matter of I don't like to push myself to tackle big projects.

THERAPIST: Because if you push yourself to tackle big projects, then ... ?

PETE: Then I'll never get to do anything fun in my life. (*Looks thoughtful.*) I'll be with it all day without a chance to play. Is that a funny thing to say?

THERAPIST: Do any images or memories come to mind when you say that?

PETE: Yes. I see my father when I was about 8 years old. If I started anything, he said I needed to finish it before I could do something else. He had a big rule about finishing whatever you started. Once I started to build a playhouse, and when I got tired and wanted to go play with my friends, he said I needed to keep working on it with him until it was finished.

In this case, the therapist begins with a conceptual model that procrastination is fueled by perfectionism and fear of criticism. By explicitly stating this model to the client and asking for feedback, the therapist gives the client an opportunity to either confirm or correct the therapist's hypothesis before the therapy proceeds down this track. In addition, they may agree on a homework assignment to check out these ideas in the context of Pete's day-to-day experience. The therapist signals true collaboration by dropping the perfectionism model in order to explore the client's report of relevant thoughts and images.

Therapists' hypotheses are not necessarily shared in full with the client at every point in time. Imagine the client is driving a car and the therapist is reading a map. Sharing the whole map at a particular point in the journey is unlikely to help the driver. It is more helpful to share information sparingly at key points (e.g., Driver: "We are coming up to a T-junction, what do I do here?" Map reader: "You need to turn right."). In the same way, a therapist may not share conceptualization hypotheses that are far down the "road" of therapy when more basic conceptual agreement has yet to be achieved. For example, a client who sees her depression as "completely biological" is unlikely to benefit from examining hypotheses regarding underlying assumptions that predispose her to depression. Examining the hypothesis that behaviors and thoughts might sometimes contribute to her mood is much more likely to be helpful.

In summary, we regard collaborative empiricism as essential if conceptualization is to serve the functions for case conceptualization set out in Chapter 1 (Box 1.1). We also believe that a collaborative case conceptualization approach resolves many of the challenges presented by research studies.

WHY INCORPORATE CLIENT STRENGTHS?

Finally, we advocate a strengths-focused approach in case conceptualization. A conceptualization that includes "all that is right with a person" builds on existing resources and broadens the field of possible interventions (Mooney & Padesky, 2002; Padesky & Mooney, 2006; Mooney, 2006). Once strengths are identified, clients often are able to transfer skills from areas of strength to help manage areas of difficulty with greater ease. A primary purpose of case conceptualization is building client resilience. Incorporation of strengths in case conceptualization reveals broader avenues for intervention that can build client resilience. Resilience is a broad concept that refers to how people negotiate adversity. It describes the processes of psychological adaptation through which people draw on their strengths to adapt to challenges so that their well-being is maintained. The crucible once again is an apt metaphor for understanding how to conceptualize an individual's resilience (Figure 1.1). Appropriate theory can be integrated with the particularities of an individual case using the heat of collaborative empiricism. Because resilience is a broad, multidimensional concept, therapists can either adapt existing theories of psychological disorders (see Box 1.3) or draw from a large array of theoretical ideas in positive psychology (see, e.g., Snyder & Lopez, 2005).

Our emphasis on building resilience as a therapy goal is not new in CBT. The first CBT treatment manual written by Aaron T. Beck and colleagues states:

> The patient needs to acquire specialized knowledge, experience, and skill in dealing with certain types of problems; therapy is a training period in which the patient will learn more effective ways to handle these problems. The patient is not asked or expected to gain complete mastery or skills in therapy: *The emphasis instead is on growth and development.* The patient will have ample time after therapy to improve on these cognitive and behavioral coping skills. (Beck et al., 1979, pp. 317–318; emphasis added)

CBT has always stressed the importance of working with clients so they become their own therapists, able to apply cognitive and behavioral skills as needed. These processes described in original CBT texts (Beck, 1976; Beck et al., 1979, 1985) can be even more effective when client strengths are explicitly linked to resilience. In recent years CBT models have begun to emerge that integrate identification of client strengths and resilience seamlessly within mainstream CBT practice (e.g., Mooney & Padesky, 2002; Padesky, 2005; Padesky & Mooney, 2006).

It is possible that the research examining the impact of conceptualization on therapy process and outcome might be more compelling if conceptualization included more of a focus on client strengths. For example, we propose that clients are less likely to find conceptualization overwhelming and distressing when conceptualization is as much about what is right with them as it is about what led them to seek help. Moreover, client strengths offer natural pathways to reaching clients' goals. Cognitive and behavioral processes that have proven helpful for clients in the past are likely to prove helpful again.

Identifying and working with clients' strengths begins at assessment and continues at each level of conceptualization. As clients articulate presenting issues, therapists can inquire about times when clients were able to cope successfully. Chapter 5 demonstrates how to attend to clients' personal and social resources during broader psychosocial assessment. Conceptualization of triggers and maintenance factors includes identification of client resources that have prevented the difficulties from worsening (Chapter 6). As conceptualization becomes more longitudinal, factors that have predisposed *and protected* the client are drawn out (Chapter 7). Throughout therapy, we advocate that therapists elicit client values, longer-term goals, and positive qualities that can serve as a foundation to build toward long-term recovery and full participation in life (Chapter 4).

Although the CBT literature has only sparsely included strengths in cognitive models, a number of CBT innovators have begun to do so (see, e.g., Seligman & Csikszentmihalyi, 2000; Snyder & Lopez, 2005), and in Chapter 4 we review how this literature can inform CBT case conceptualization. By demonstrating throughout this book how strengths can be assessed and incorporated into case conceptualizations, we hope to support these developments.

TOWARD MORE EFFECTIVE CASE CONCEPTUALIZATION

Our review of the relevant CBT theory and evidence poses both an opportunity and a challenge. The evidence base for CBT theory and practice is compelling. The opportunity is for CBT therapists to make maximal use of the extensive cognitive-behavioral theory and research to individualize therapy for a range of emotional disorders. The challenge is that current approaches to case conceptualization are not realizing this opportunity. Why do therapists appear to be unable to agree about the explanatory aspects of client conceptualizations? Why does conceptualization not appear to affect the process and outcome of CBT?

A classic Sufi story of the "wise fool" Nasruddin provides a metaphorical answer to this challenge. In the story Nasruddin is seen by his neighbor one night under the street lamp searching for something. The neighbor goes out to speak with Nasruddin:

> NEIGHBOR: Good evening, Nasruddin. What are you looking for under the street lamp?
>
> NASRUDDIN: My keys, I have lost my keys.
>
> (*They search together for a while, to no avail. Then it occurs to the neighbor to ask:*)

NEIGHBOR: Nasruddin, where did you lose the keys?

NASRUDDIN: Over there, by the house.

NEIGHBOR: (*puzzled*) So why are you searching under the lamp?

NASRUDDIN: Because it is light here!

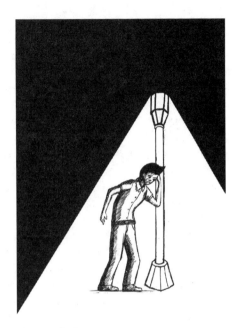

Rather like the neighbor's realization at the end of this story, we argue that current approaches to case conceptualization focus their search in the wrong places (because there is light). In order for case conceptualization to fulfill its promise, we believe it should be practiced and researched in the context of active collaboration between a therapist and client, using

Figure 2.9. Nasruddin looking for his keys.

empirical methods. Research on case conceptualization must take into account that conceptualizations develop over time and often evolve from descriptive to explanatory levels of understanding. Furthermore, we suggest the best conceptualizations are likely to incorporate client strengths. Identification of positive client resources helps form a holistic understanding of client concerns and can provide a basis for building resilience and lasting change. While there is currently less empirical light shed on these issues than is ideal, we make the case that the three principles of case conceptualization described in this chapter may be the keys we are looking for.

Chapter 2 Summary

This chapter presents a new model of conceptualization that responds to research and therapist practice challenges. We use a crucible metaphor to describe key features:

- Client experience, theory, and research are synthesized to yield a unique description and explanation of client-presenting issues.

- The crucible is heated through collaborative empiricism, essential to form a unique description and explanation with face validity for both client and therapist.
- Conceptualization develops from descriptive to explanatory levels over the course of therapy.
- Client strengths are incorporated in each level of conceptualization in order to reveal positive pathways to change and build resilience.

Chapter 3

Two Heads Are Better Than One
Collaborative Empiricism

PAUL: The voices tell me things that scare me.

THERAPIST: What sort of things do the voices tell you?

PAUL: They tell me to hurt myself and to hurt other people.

THERAPIST: Would you be willing to talk to me about the voices today? Maybe we can figure out a way to help you handle them.

PAUL: (*Appears cautious.*) Yes.

THERAPIST: Who do you think the voices are?

PAUL: I think they are angels ... or devils.

THERAPIST: Does that mean they are powerful?

PAUL: Yes, of course. That is what scares me so much. I'm afraid they will force me to do bad things.

THERAPIST: Have you done any bad things so far?

PAUL: Not so bad.

THERAPIST: How have you managed to stop yourself when the voices tell you to do bad things?

PAUL: I say prayers. And I play loud music so I don't have to listen. And I stay away from people I might hurt.

THERAPIST: It sounds like you have used your faith and problem solving to figure out some ways to protect yourself and others.

PAUL: Yes. But I don't know how long I can outsmart them.

THERAPIST: Maybe we can learn some more things about the voices today that will help. I have a theory I'd like to tell you about that might help.

PAUL: What is it?

THERAPIST: These voices could be angels or devils. Or it is possible that they are thoughts in your head that scare you and that they really don't have much power. I think it is important that we try to figure out just who the voices are and how much power they have. Do you think learning more about the voices will help you?

PAUL: Yes, but I am pretty sure they are not just in my head.

THERAPIST: OK. So maybe that is something we should test out.

Paul's therapist is beginning to help him conceptualize the voices he hears. Notice how the three elements in the crucible of case conceptualization described in Chapter 2—theory, research, and the client's individual details—are collaboratively woven together in this exchange. The therapist has her own theory about the voices Paul hears, informed by clinical experience and research on psychosis (Kingdon & Turkington, 2002; Morrison, 2002). Even so, she is respectful of Paul's theory and invites him to collaboratively examine his experiences with voices to see what can be learned. As the session proceeds, the therapist will encourage Paul to take an empirical approach, conducting experiments in and outside of session to help him evaluate various theories about the voices.

At this early stage of discussions, the conceptualizations are quite simple: angels/devils, or thoughts in Paul's head. As therapy proceeds, these conceptualizations will become elaborated. As higher levels of conceptualization are explored, Paul and his therapist will move from a descriptive understanding of the voices to explanatory identification of triggers, maintenance factors, and predisposing and protective factors. Throughout this conceptualization process, the therapist inquires about and expresses interest in Paul's strengths. She will include these in the conceptualizations and use them to foster Paul's resilience.

Most readers with case conceptualization experience are familiar to some degree with every part of the conceptualization process described in the preceding paragraphs. However, even advanced CBT therapists often lack experience or skill in one or more of these areas. Therapists sometimes forget to empirically test the case conceptualization with the client. Client strengths might occasionally be assessed but not routinely incorporated into conceptual models. Because we want case conceptualization to serve as an active crucible for change, we think it is important to integrate theory, research, and individual aspects of a case as fully as possible throughout therapy. In addition, we think it is paramount that every step of this integration be done collaboratively with the client with empirical evaluation of ideas discussed.

In this chapter we focus on how collaborative empiricism works in practice. Diverse case examples illustrate how it creates a synthesis from the three elements of theory, research, and client experience.

COLLABORATION IN ACTION

A collaborative therapy relationship is one in which therapist and client respect each other's ideas and work as a team in therapy to achieve the client's goals. Unlike some therapy models in which the therapist is the expert working on a "patient" who waits to receive expert advice, cognitive therapists foster relationships in which all participants equally contribute to the therapy process. Equal contribution does not mean that therapist and client(s) contribute the same skills and knowledge to the process. The therapist brings his or her educational, personal, and professional experience, which ideally includes an empirical knowledge base. Each client brings a unique understanding and awareness of his or her own personal and interpersonal experience, as well as the potential to observe and report internal and external reactions to change efforts.

Collaboration describes the process by which the strengths of both therapist and client are joined to the client's best advantage. In CBT, collaborative therapy relationships are achieved and maintained via explicit discussion, use of a collaborative framework within the therapy session, a positive therapy alliance, therapy structure, and optimal balancing of alliance and structure throughout the course of therapy.

Explicit Discussion

Usually, cognitive therapists directly discuss the importance of collaboration in the first therapy session. A simple explanation is often all that is required if it is followed by collaboration in action:

THERAPIST: (*at the beginning of the first session*) Let's take a few minutes and discuss how we can work together. I like to work together as a team. I know quite a bit about helping people with moods and worries and have helped many people manage them better. But you are the expert on your own mood and worry experiences. If you tell me what you experience and I tell you what I know, it is likely we will be able to come up with a plan that can help you. How does that sound?

ELLEN: OK, I guess.

THERAPIST: For example, today I'd like to ask you some questions about what brought you here and other questions to learn more about your struggles and strengths. As we go along, I will give you information about things that I think might help you. But it will be up to you to let me know whether these ideas are helpful. Would you be willing to tell me about yourself and also give me feedback on whether what I say to you is helpful or not?

ELLEN: Sure.

THERAPIST: And since we are working together, if you think of something that is important to tell me and I haven't asked about it, I want you to bring it up. OK?

ELLEN: OK. That sounds good.

THERAPIST: Let's begin by making a quick list of all the things we want to be sure to talk about today. This will help make sure that we spend our time in the ways that are most helpful to you. As I said, I want to find out what brought you here and learn a bit about you, especially what helps you get through the hard times. (*Writes on paper or whiteboard so Ellen can see what is being written: "what brought me here," "what gets me through hard times."*) Is there anything you want to make sure we talk about?

ELLEN: I had to take off work early to get here today. I was wondering whether we could find a different time to meet.

THERAPIST: Thanks for bringing that up. Let me write that on our list. (*Writes "New time?"*) Anything else?

ELLEN: My doctor put me on some medication, and it makes me jittery. Is there a different medication I could take?

THERAPIST: OK. I'll put medication on the list. (*Writes "Medication."*) Oh, that reminds me. I'd like to talk to you about the results of these mood questionnaires you filled out when you arrived today. Would you like me to do that today or next time?

ELLEN: Today! (*Therapist writes "Mood scores."*)

THERAPIST: Anything else?

ELLEN: (*Shakes head no.*)

THERAPIST: OK. (*pause*) I'd like to add two more things to our list, which is to give you a chance to ask me some questions if you want and also to give me feedback at the end of today about whether this session was helpful or not. Is that OK with you? (*Ellen nods; therapist adds these two items and then reads from list.*) We want to talk about what brought you here, what gets you through hard times, a new time to meet, medication, your responses on the mood question- naires, any questions you have for me, and your feedback to me on today's session. Let's take two more minutes and decide what order to talk about these things and how much time we think each topic will take.

Use of a Collaborative Framework

As the preceding dialogue demonstrates, explicit discussion of the desir- ability of collaboration is followed immediately by an experience of active collaboration. By inviting Ellen to help plan and structure the first therapy session, she has an opportunity to learn directly what the therapist means by collaboration. As the session proceeds, the therapist continually frames interactions as collaborative. If the therapist does not do this, therapy may inadvertently shift to an expert–patient dynamic. Here are a few examples of common session events that highlight a col- laborative framework:

- *Frequent checks on client understanding*

  "Does that make sense to you? Can you give me an example from your own experience where this idea seems to fit? Any examples of where it doesn't fit?"

- *Negotiation of changes in the session agenda*

  "I notice we only have 15 minutes left. I can tell what we are talk- ing about is important to you. I also remember that you wanted to talk about medication and changing our meeting time, and I wanted some feedback on today's session. Shall we continue talking about [current topic] and talk about these other things next time, or do you want to shift to these other topics soon?"

- *Collaborative design of homework assignments*

  "Today you've made some important observations about the links between your thoughts and moods. Let's talk about what you might do this week to use this information to help yourself. (*pause*) Sometimes I ask people to write down some thoughts when their mood gets activated. This might help you become more aware of your thoughts as a first step toward testing out your beliefs. Do you think this would be helpful for you, or do you have another idea?"

- *Asking client's opinion regarding therapy choice points*

"As you describe your difficulties, it sounds like you struggle with both depression and panic attacks. There are good treatments for both of these concerns, but it may be more helpful to work on one at a time. Would you be willing to work on one problem at a time? [If so] which one would you like to tackle first? Why do you think this would be best?"

Regular use of a collaborative frame helps minimize clients' tendency to defer to the therapist's judgment. It also can reduce unnecessary therapy struggles that result when therapist and client inadvertently begin pursuing different goals or operating under different expectations. When clients refrain from expressing opinions despite the therapist's efforts, the therapist will directly ask about this stance. Sometimes clients have limited experience with other people showing interest in their opinions and so they have never learned to pay attention to personal preferences. This is a skills issue that can be addressed by asking the client to spend time before each session thinking about possible agenda items and giving the client time in session to think about his or her preferences. If clients do not express themselves because beliefs interfere, the therapist can help the client identify and test these beliefs.

A collaborative framework does not mean the therapist always does what the client wants in therapy. If a client's choices seem off target, the therapist expresses his or her own opinion, ideally grounded in empirical evidence or professional experience that is communicated effectively to the client. For example, if a client persistently chooses topics that avoid addressing central concerns, the therapist will point this out and ask the client what thoughts or fears might be preventing the client from working on a particular issue. Or if the client requests a form of treatment that is contraindicated by empirical evidence (e.g., a client with health worries who wants to spend each session getting reassurance from the therapist that particular symptoms are not serious), the therapist helps the client understand why this preferred treatment approach is unlikely to help (Warwick, Clark, Cobb, & Salkovskis, 1996). It is much easier for the therapist and client to sort out such disagreements collaboratively when there is a positive therapy alliance.

Therapy Alliance

The effectiveness of CBT is enhanced when therapists maintain a positive therapy alliance within a structured therapy format (Beck et al., 1979; J. S. Beck, 1995; Padesky & Greenberger, 1995; Raue &

Goldfried, 1994). A positive therapy alliance is correlated with positive outcome in psychotherapy (Horvath & Greenberg, 1994), including cognitive-behavioral therapy (Raue & Goldfried, 1994). However, cognitive therapists do not believe a positive therapy alliance by itself ensures the best therapy outcome. Cognitive therapists strive to use empirically supported therapy methods in the context of a positive therapy alliance.

Both positive therapy alliance and empirically supported treatment methods enhance therapy outcome. There is evidence that positive therapy alliance potentiates the effectiveness of empirically supported methods (Raue & Goldfried, 1994) and also evidence that using effective therapy approaches leads to a more positive therapy alliance (DeRubeis, Brotman, & Gibbons, 2005; Tang & DeRubeis, 1999).

Measures of therapy alliance such as the Working Alliance Inventory (Horvath, 1994) assess three aspects of alliance: (1) positive bond, (2) agreement on therapy tasks, and (3) agreement on therapy goals. Each of these alliance markers is consistent with the basic principles of CBT practice (Beck et al., 1979). Collaborative resolution of disagreements regarding therapy tasks or goals helps maintain or restore a positive alliance and can therefore enhance therapy outcomes.

Therapy Structure

Therapy sessions are structured in CBT to maximize the impact of each therapy session. A typical CBT session will have the following components: agenda setting, review of client learning since the previous session (e.g., homework assignments and life events relevant to therapy focus), introduction of new learning and skills, application of new ideas to current client issues, development of learning assignments (i.e., homework) for the following week(s), and feedback from the client on the session (J. S. Beck, 1995; Padesky & Greenberger, 1995). Collaboration helps maintain therapy structure, especially when the client understands the advantages of structure. Although the client takes the lead in agenda setting, the therapist also contributes ideas and suggestions for session topics. Generally, most of the session time is spent debriefing client learning from homework assignments, testing beliefs, teaching skills, and devising ways to test beliefs and practice skills outside therapy sessions.

Just as therapy sessions are structured within the hour, there is a general structure to CBT across therapy sessions. Initial sessions generally identify and conceptualize presenting issues as illustrated in Chapter 5. As treatment plans are devised, middle therapy sessions systematically address the automatic thoughts, underlying assumptions, and behaviors that maintain client difficulties, teach the clients relevant new skills, and help the client apply new skills and beliefs to increasingly challenging life circumstances. Later sessions explore how the client can use newly acquired skills and beliefs in tandem with existing strengths to reduce relapse and become more resilient over time.

Optimal Balance between Structure and Alliance

Many therapists believe that a structured approach weakens the therapy alliance or leads to therapist control of session content. This belief is not supported by research. Decades ago, Truax (1966) studied the relative influence of therapist and client in client-centered therapy as conducted by Carl Rogers, founder of the approach. Rogers closely followed client verbal expressions, making reflective comments rather than directive interventions. Surprisingly, the study found that the therapist, not the clients, controlled the content of the therapy hour, even with interventions intended to be highly nondirective. Truax discovered that clients were so attuned to minor therapist reflections and nonverbal expressions that clients spoke in more detail about topics that received positive therapist attention or reaction. Thus even attempts at nondirective therapy prove unwittingly to be very directive.

Of course, structured therapy can also be highly directive and reflect only the therapist's frame of reference. It is impossible to remove the influence of the therapist during the therapy session. And given that a therapist is hired for professional knowledge and expertise, it does not make sense to remove the therapist's influence. However, CBT therapists believe it is desirable for clients to share control over the content and course of their therapy. Thus CBT has always advocated that the ideal therapy relationship entails active teamwork between therapist and client (Beck et al., 1979, p. 54).

A *collaboratively structured* approach to therapy may be the best way to ensure that the client and therapist share influence over the therapy session. As we learn from Truax's (1966) research, with or without explicit structure, the therapist controls the direction of the session by choosing which parts of client comments to question, reflect, or interpret. When clients are asked to set the agenda, prioritize topics, and make decisions about choices within the session, clients exert greater influence over their own therapy. Greater client participation can increase therapy alliance and may partly account for the high alliance ratings clients give cognitive-behavioral therapists (Raue & Goldfried, 1994). One study examined why deviations from treatment structure sometimes compromised therapy outcomes (Schulte & Eifert, 2002). They found that therapists tend to move from therapy methods (e.g., exposure) to therapy process (e.g., addressing patients' motivation) too soon, too often, and sometimes for the wrong reasons.

Can cognitive therapy be too structured? Structure and relationship factors should be balanced to maximize each:

> The therapist must carefully time when to talk and when to listen. If the therapist interrupts too frequently or in a tactless or curt manner, the patient may feel cut off, and rapport will suffer. If the therapist allows long silences or simply allows the patient to ramble without apparent purpose, the patient may become excessively anxious and rapport will diminish. (Beck et al., 1979, p. 53)

Because research finds a positive correlation between therapy structure and outcome in CBT (Shaw et. al., 1999) the optimal balance of structure and relationship factors is probably the most structure possible that does not damage the therapy alliance. Of course, the degree and nature of structure vary with the therapy task. There may be more structure when setting up a specific learning assignment and less when client and therapist are exploring a new topic. As highlighted in the quote above, greater structure is likely to be tolerated better within a warm, responsive relationship. In addition, collaboration and alliance are enhanced when the purposes of the structure are made clear to the client as in the following sample statements:

Therapist Statements That Provide a Context for Therapy Structure

- "I want to make sure you get the most out of each meeting, so we will take some time at the start of each session to discuss what is most important to accomplish that day. Then we will plan our session and check in periodically to make sure we are on track and you feel we are making progress."
- "There are some methods for helping [this problem] that I think might help you. Would you be willing to spend the next few sessions trying out this step-by-step approach? I'll want you to give me feedback as we go along for how helpful it seems to you."
- (*in response to a client who tells numerous lengthy anecdotes*) "I can tell it is important to you to fill me in on the details. At the same time, I worry that you are not getting the best help I can offer. When most of our time together is spent with you describing your concerns, we don't have much time left to talk about options for helping you. How would you feel if I interrupted you at times and asked you to give me the main ideas rather than all the details—so we can have more time to talk about how to help you with these issues?"

The preceding pages illustrate qualities that typify the collaborative relationship in CBT. Collaboration is a fundamental process that pervades all aspects of CBT and is also a natural component of case conceptualization. Just as a collaborative stance in therapy elicits greater client participation, the next section shows how cognitive theory and an empirical approach positively guide the nature of that participation.

EMPIRICISM IN ACTION

The word *empiricism* encompasses several aspects of CBT practice: therapist knowledge of cognitive theory and research, the use of scientific methods within the therapy session, and a preference for evidence-based practice methods. Without empiricism, all ideas in the crucible have equal weight.

First, the therapist's knowledge base includes familiarity with evidence-based theories and conceptual models for particular problems as well as empirically supported treatments (see Box 1.3). These are the scaffolding within which we build CBT case conceptualizations with our clients. Such knowledge can help the therapist to distinguish among similar disorders; to know what links commonly occur among thoughts, behaviors, emotions, and physiological responses in particular disorders; and to choose treatment options that are most likely to be effective. The more therapists are thoroughly familiar with theory, the more naturally they can synthesize client experience and theory collaboratively in the case conceptualization crucible.

A second aspect of empiricism is the use of scientific methods within the session. This encourages empiricism in clients. Therapist and client base their conceptual understanding of client difficulties on data drawn from the client's life. Empirical evidence with a particular client often points to the centrality of particular beliefs, behaviors, environmental contexts, and physical and emotional responses in the maintenance of his or her problems. Thus an empirical frame increases the odds that therapy time will be spent fruitfully exploring the client's most central issues. If the therapist has a cognitive model that seems to fit the client's experience, this is introduced by guiding the client's awareness to his or her personal experiences that illustrate the model. If there is no existing model that fits the client's experience, the therapist and client carefully observe links between aspects of the client's experience and develop a model based on these observations. In either case, a conceptual model is empirically tested by seeing whether it maps onto client experience and makes reliable predictions about subsequent client experience.

Third, a CBT therapist considers evidence-based theories of a particular problem first. Only if such a model is nonexistent or does not match the client experience does the therapist turn to a generic CBT framework or some other model. Whatever the original source of a conceptualization model, it will be compared with data from the client's life to see if it meets the criterion of being evidence based for the individual client. Collaborative examination of evidence-based models leads to the most efficient and effective case conceptualizations. Furthermore, evidence-based conceptualizations offer the greatest hope for transforming problems into positive development.

Empirical Conceptualization Processes in Session

The exploration of whether evidence-based models are well matched to a client's presenting issues is usually accomplished through use of (1) observation, (2) Socratic dialogue, and (3) behavioral experiments. Curiosity is fundamental to each of these three methods.

Curiosity

Therapist curiosity is the face of empiricism to the client. Rather than didactically expounding on cognitive theory, adept CBT therapists express frequent and genuine interest in the client's opinions, insights, observations, and choices because they want to understand how clients make meaning from their experience. Therapist curiosity not only prompts clients to become more accustomed to self-observation and self-expression, it also sparks greater client curiosity. Curiosity activates clients and helps them overcome the natural avoidance often elicited by feelings of shame or embarrassment.

For example, a client named Gabriel tried to hide his problems from colleagues at work and most of his friends. When his therapist expressed curiosity about how problem behaviors might be connected to thoughts and feelings, Gabriel began to observe his thoughts and feelings with interest rather than aversion. Without an atmosphere of curiosity, Gabriel might have found it difficult to report thoughts and feelings that, although central to his difficulties, seemed "foolish" to him when he was not currently in a problematic situation.

Curiosity powers empiricism. Due to the risks of decision-making errors described in Chapter 2, therapists must remain open to disconfirmation of a hypothesis. This is especially true when there is an existing evidence-based model that the therapist believes fits the client's experience. In this instance, it is important that the therapist be equally attentive and curious regarding client observations that fit and do not fit the model. Otherwise, expressed curiosity is a thinly veiled method for convincing the client of a therapist's belief (Padesky, 1993)—the Procrustean approach described in Chapter 1. The following case example illustrates the importance of therapist curiosity when client observations do not fit a chosen conceptual model.

Katherine: A Case Example

Katherine was referred for cognitive-behavioral therapy for panic disorder by a neurologist who had ruled out any physical problems. Katherine was an older woman, age 72, who reported symptoms of lightheadedness and unsteadiness when walking. She insisted on using a wheeled walker because she was afraid of fainting and hitting her head on the sidewalk. Her anxious imagery included a vivid picture of her skull split open followed by brain hemorrhage and death. Based on the physician's assurance there were no organic explanations for her symptoms, the therapist began CBT for panic disorder. According to CBT theory, panic disorder results from catastrophic misinterpretation of physical and mental sensations and is maintained by both safety behaviors and increased focus on the sensations that concern the individual (Clark, 1997).

Katherine entered therapy still believing that she had a physical problem that left her vulnerable to fainting and falling. Her therapist explored with Katherine an alternative explanation that her fears led to reliance on a walker as a safety behavior; use of the walker had reduced her leg strength and contributed to muscle weakening and greater unsteadiness. In addition, through induction experiments recommended by the panic treatment protocol (Clark, 1997), the therapist helped Katherine understand that her lightheadedness could be a symptom of anxiety rather than an indicator of a physical problem.

To test and compare Katherine's and the therapist's explanatory hypotheses, Katherine began a series of behavioral experiments both in therapy and outside of therapy. She began to strengthen her leg muscles through exercises prescribed by a physical therapist. In addition, she walked increasing distances without the assistance of her walker. After 4 weeks of treatment, Katherine reported somewhat steadier walking although she still reported occasional bouts of lightheadedness. Both therapist and client confidence grew in the cognitive model of panic disorder as explanation for her symptoms.

In the fifth week, Katherine was walking unassisted next to her husband when she fainted. Although fear of fainting is consistent with the cognitive model for panic disorder, actual fainting is not. The therapist maintained a curious stance and inquired whether Katherine was overheated or hungry when she fainted, two physical conditions that could help explain fainting in an older woman. When both Katherine and her husband assured the therapist that it was cool and she had eaten a normal lunch an hour earlier, the therapist began to doubt the earlier hypothesis that Katherine's lightheadedness was related to anxiety. Furthermore, Katherine assured the therapist she was not anxious in the least when she fainted; she was walking, felt momentarily dizzy, and then blacked out.

Actual fainting is more consistent with an organic cause than with panic disorder. Thus the therapist referred Katherine back to the neurologist for further tests. More detailed brain scans revealed a small tumor in Katherine's brain that was pressing on a nerve and causing her symptoms. Surgery was required to resolve her presenting issues.

Katherine's therapist demonstrated good empiricism throughout treatment. As discussed in Chapter 2, there are many ways that therapists can use decision-making heuristics in problematic ways (e.g., seeking only confirmatory evidence for hypotheses; Garb, 1998). Once the initial physician's report ruled out an organic cause for her symptoms, the therapist chose an evidence-based psychological model for understanding Katherine's experiences. The therapist set up a series of experiments to evaluate the applicability of the CBT model for panic disorder to her symptoms. Initially, results of these experiments supported this model; Katherine gained leg strength and was able to walk more steadily. However, when Katherine fainted the therapist gave full attention to this experience, which contradicted predictions of the cognitive model of panic. The therapist can be credited with advocating renewed curiosity regarding an organic explanation when the psychological explanation was not a good match for client experience. In this example, the therapist continually and collaboratively evaluated hypotheses with Katherine, remaining open to novel and unexpected outcomes.

Katherine's case is atypical. Usually when organic difficulties have been ruled out and a client's presenting issues are well matched to existing evidence-based conceptual models, client data collected over time remain consistent with a psychological explanation. The next section describes how a therapist can follow principles of collaboration and empiricism to engage a client in exploration of an evidence-based conceptual model.

Empiricism in Using Existing Evidence-Based Conceptual Models

After an initial interview, a CBT therapist often recognizes that one or more evidence-based conceptual models have helpful explanatory value for understanding client experiences. Rather than simply telling the client, "You seem to be depressed and anxious, let me tell you how depression and anxiety operate," a therapist employing collaborative empiricism asks questions to gather client observations that can be used to derive these models from the client's own experience. For example, in a filmed demonstration, Padesky (1994b) collaboratively derives a case conceptualization with a client, Mary, who panics whenever her heart starts beating rapidly.

At the beginning of this session, Padesky asks Mary to identify her sensations, thoughts, feelings, and behaviors during a recent panic attack. Mary's responses, written down so both she and the therapist can look for connections among them, form the first level of empirical data— observation of the client's naturally occurring experiences. Padesky helps Mary identify the sensations that most frightened her during a recent panic attack and then asks, "When you were experiencing [these sensations], what went through your mind?" After asking Mary to link particular physical sensations with catastrophic thoughts and images (e.g., "[These symptoms convinced me I was having] a heart attack," "I [was] watching my funeral"), Padesky shows her a CBT model of panic disorder (Clark, 1997) that closely matches Mary's reported experience.

Next, Padesky initiates an in-session behavioral experiment with Mary, suggesting they both hyperventilate and observe the resulting sensations and thoughts. After the hyperventilation experiment, Padesky enlists Mary's collaboration in writing down this second level of empirical data—observation of experiences during an experiment designed to test beliefs. In this case, Mary's belief that she is having a heart attack when her heart races, chest becomes heavy, and fingers begin to tingle is evaluated in the context of similar symptoms induced by less than a minute of hyperventilation.

The comparison of observations made during the client's naturally occurring panic attack with those made during the experimental hyperventilation allow Padesky to help the client compare two possible conceptualizations of her experiences: (1) her physical symptoms signal a heart attack, or (2) her physical symptoms are not dangerous but are common to both hyperventilation and anxiety. Rather than directing the client to adopt the second conceptualization, the following excerpts (Padesky, 1994b) show how Padesky employs Socratic dialogue to guide the client in her analysis of her experiences:

PADESKY: (*immediately after hyperventilation*) What are the sensations that you are experiencing?

MARY: I'm really lightheaded.

PADESKY: Very lightheaded. Do you feel at all dizzy or like you are about to pass out?

MARY: Yes. Yes … I'm really clammy …

PADESKY: What other symptoms?

MARY: I can feel my heart beating in my ears.

PADESKY: Is your heart pounding pretty hard?

MARY: Yes.

PADESKY: How about that sense of suffocating?

MARY: Yes.

PADESKY: So you have all the symptoms?

MARY: Yes.

PADESKY: What sorts of thoughts and images do you have?

MARY: I remembered there were a couple of MDs [physicians] who checked in [to view this clinical demonstration].

PADESKY: And what were you thinking we might need the MDs for?

MARY: I might have a heart attack.

PADESKY: So it is very credible to you that you might have a heart attack right now?

MARY: It feels very real …

(*a minute later in the interview*)

PADESKY: What does hyperventilation do in terms of … physical sensations?

MARY: (*writing*) "Hyperventilation causes rapid breathing, increases heart rate, can cause dizziness."

PADESKY: So hyperventilation can cause all of those symptoms. Can it cause heaviness in the chest?

MARY: I don't know. I didn't get that feeling.

PADESKY: How about when you said "an elephant's sitting on my chest"?

MARY: I just got very scared and then I felt that. I felt that before I started breathing fast.

PADESKY: So being anxious can cause a heaviness in the chest? It can cause an "elephant on the chest" feeling?

MARY: Yes.

PADESKY: Why don't you write that down?

(*after Mary writes a few more observations*)

PADESKY: How many symptoms are you experiencing right now?

MARY: I feel much better right now.

PADESKY: How do you explain that? A few minutes ago you had all these symptoms and now you feel better?

MARY: As I'm writing I feel less anxious.

(After a few more interchanges regarding this observation, Mary writes a summary of her observations and rates her confidence in each statement highly from 95 to 100%.)

PADESKY: Now read each of these statements aloud and think about them.

MARY: *(reading her summary)* "Hyperventilation causes rapid breathing, increases heart rate, can cause dizziness and shallow breathing. Anxiety can cause heaviness in chest and a suffocating feeling. When I'm not focusing on these sensations they diminish. When I focus on these sensations they increase."

PADESKY: Do these sentences as a group help you understand the panic attacks you've been having?

MARY: Yes.

PADESKY: Can you say in your own words what these sentences suggest?

MARY: Well, I think as soon as I noticed something [a symptom], I increased it because I paid a lot of attention to it and judged it and checked it out and diagnosed it and each symptom that I checked increased.

(A few minutes later Padesky summarizes.)

PADESKY: So we have two hypotheses to test out. One hypothesis is *(writing)* "When I have these symptoms it means I'm having a heart attack." The second hypothesis is "When I have these symptoms it means I'm anxious and there's no real danger and, in fact, the symptoms might be caused by even small amounts of breathing shallowly or quickly." Even a very small amount can lead to sensations. For instance, when we started, how many seconds did it take before you started having sensations?

MARY: Almost immediately.

PADESKY: *(writing)* "Even a few breaths can lead to these kinds of sensations."

As this demonstration session illustrates, when a case conceptualization is based on existing evidence-based models it is still possible to derive this conceptualization collaboratively with the client. Therapist probes ensure that relevant client observations are added to the crucible so therapist and client can evaluate whether the theory-based conceptualization maps onto client experience. Behavioral experiments rely on empirical reasoning by manipulating relevant variables so the client can weigh competing explanations. Socratic dialogue is used to guide the client to notice and evaluate key aspects of a conceptual model as embodied in personal experiences. Client observations, behavioral experiments, and Socratic dialogue are three common empirical methods the cognitive-behavioral therapist employs to provide "heat" in the crucible so the client can evaluate whether a generic evidence-based case conceptualization provides a good explanatory fit for the client's personal experience.

Empiricism in Generating an Idiosyncratic Conceptual Model

Client experiences often do not closely match an existing evidence-based conceptual model. Clients frequently present with multiple diagnoses, and the therapist may find several relevant evidence-based models, each of which apply to different portions of the client's concerns. Some clients report problems that appear quite idiosyncratic. In these cases, therapists can draw on elements of the basic CBT conceptual model (e.g., thoughts, emotions, behaviors, and physical reactions mutually interact; beliefs often guide behavior and help make sense of emotional responses). In collaboration with the client, the basic CBT model can form the foundation for an individualized conceptualization that accounts for the client's presenting issues. For acute problems, therapists and clients identify automatic thoughts, emotions, and physical and behavioral responses that connect to one another in target situations. For long-standing issues, core beliefs, underlying assumptions, and associated behavioral strategies are identified to help understand the origins and maintenance of presenting issues. Individualized conceptualizations are derived through the same therapeutic processes outlined above: client observation, behavioral experiments, and Socratic dialogue.

Rose: A Case Example

Rose is a 31-year-old computer programmer seeking therapy for insomnia, anxiety at work, and recent conflict with her family of origin, especially her two youngest sisters. Her initial description of her presenting issues led her therapist to speculate that Rose might be experiencing social anxiety, problems related to discrimination, and/or stress-related difficulties linked to her very demanding job. As an additional dimension, the therapist wondered how her cultural experiences might play a role in her difficulties. Rose is Hispanic (third generation Mexican American living in the United States), Roman Catholic (no longer attending church), lesbian (in a happy, committed relationship for the past 5 years), the eldest of seven children, the first college graduate in her extended family, and a self-supporting woman in a predominately male field. The therapist considered each of these four factors (social anxiety, social discrimination, work stress, culture) in the course of case conceptualization, as well as remaining open to unforeseen elements that might prove important.

Rose and her therapist actively collaborated over the course of the first three therapy sessions to reach an initial understanding of her central struggles. At intake Rose was much more aware of her physical state (sore neck, restless energy, agitation, fatigue) and emotions (nervous, irritated) than she was of her thought processes. Therefore the therapist encouraged Rose to observe what was going through her mind as she lay in bed sleepless at night, when she noticed increases in neck tension at work, and as she quarreled with her siblings.

Client Observations. In the second session, Rose's observations led to essential information for understanding her presenting issues. She reported lying awake at night thinking about two main topics: (1) unfinished work projects and (2) her frustration that people did not listen to or respect her. Rose was hurt that her younger sisters no longer listened to her. When they were children, Rose raised them while their mother worked. Now that they were adults, Rose thought they criticized her, discounted her opinions, and disapproved of her lesbian identity.

She also believed her male colleagues in the work team ignored her quiet reports of "bugs" in the software they were writing. She worried she would be blamed for software problems when these flaws emerged in the testing phase of her company's products. Yet she felt it was dangerous to speak out assertively about her fears. A few months earlier she was added to this work group because they were behind schedule. Rose recalled that she felt marginalized from her first day on this new team. On her first day, one member of the formerly all-male group made pointed "jokes" about her ("We'll see if a woman can be a team player. Did you play any sports in school?").

Socratic Dialogue. To evaluate the hypothesis that Rose's anxiety was linked to stress or discrimination and not social anxiety, the therapist asked Rose a series of questions.

THERAPIST: Rose, when you feel anxious thinking about reporting the software problems, what is your biggest concern?

ROSE: If I am not a team player then I'm in trouble.

THERAPIST: What's the worst that might happen?

ROSE: They might withhold important code from me to interfere with my work on the software.

THERAPIST: So is it fair to say you are more concerned with their retaliation than their criticism?

ROSE: Exactly. I don't care if they like me or not. But I want to do a good job so I can get promoted. If I don't follow their "team rules," they can make my job very difficult.

INSIDE THE THERAPIST'S HEAD

Cognitive specificity theory (Beck, 1976) links particular types of thoughts with each emotion. Rose's self-report of thoughts suggests she may be experiencing anxiety and/or anger as primary emotions. Anxiety is marked by "what if" worries and concerns about threats and danger. Rose's worries about receiving the blame for software problems and sensitivity to the dangers of speaking out suggest anxiety. Anger is associated with thoughts of unfairness, lack of respect, and violation of rules. Rose's irritation that people do not respect or listen to her match up well with anger. Based on Rose's recounting of her thoughts, the therapist thought Rose's anxiety was more related to stress or discrimination than to social anxiety. This is because her danger worries did not center on social rejection as one would expect for social anxiety.

To completely rule out social anxiety, the therapist made the following inquiry:

THERAPIST: Are there any situations in your life where you do get anxious that other people will criticize you?

ROSE: Well, I don't like my sisters criticizing me. But it doesn't make me anxious. It makes me mad because I think they don't appreciate all I did for them when they were young. It wasn't always easy giving up my social life to take care of them.

These interchanges ruled out social anxiety, because social anxiety is characterized by fears of criticism and social rejection (Clark & Wells, 1995). Rose's underlying assumption, "If I'm not a team player, then they can make my job very difficult," did not fit the pattern of social anxiety or any other specific anxiety diagnosis. Thus there were no specific evidence-based conceptualization models to draw on. As a result, the therapist collaborated with Rose to formulate an individualized conceptualization of her work and family difficulties. Rose expressed a preference for understanding work concerns because these were a daily source of stress for her. She insisted that the heavy workload was not the cause of her distress because she had worked under similar conditions for the past 3 years without problems. She reported she felt at ease working as the only female on a team because this had been the norm in her work history and had never been a problem before. Discussion of her workplace concerns narrowed the focus to evidence of gender bias in certain members of her current work team.

Before settling on gender-biased responses from work colleagues as the prime trigger for her distress, Rose's therapist probed for evidence of discrimination due to her sexual orientation or ethnicity. Rose did not think coworkers knew she was lesbian and did not believe her sexual orientation played a role in their treatment of her. She felt comfortable with her decision not to discuss her lesbian identity at work, especially because she had no desire to socialize with work colleagues. She had been openly lesbian with her family and friends for 7 years and felt happy with her sexual orientation. Rose was less sure whether being Mexican American influenced coworkers' treatment of her. She could not recall direct comments about her Latina heritage and, after some discussion, concluded her gender was the main source of discomfort in her male colleagues.

Once Rose identified potential gender bias in coworkers, her therapist began to explore whether Rose's personal cultural history influenced her reactions to these workplace issues.

THERAPIST: We've talked about the many cultures that enrich your life, Rose. I wonder if these cultures have any influence on how you react to the men on your work team when they marginalize you as a woman.

ROSE: I'm not really sure. What do you think?

THERAPIST: I don't know. Maybe if I ask some questions we can figure this out together. When some of the men make jokes about having a woman on the team, how do you react?

ROSE: Inside sometimes I feel angry and sometimes I just think they are being stupid. Outside, I act like it doesn't bother me. Or I roll my eyes and walk away.

THERAPIST: Does your reaction fit with any of your cultures that we've talked about? Female–Mexican American–lesbian–Catholic–oldest sister?

ROSE: Well, that's definitely how I was raised. Women in our family are quiet in public when men criticize them. It may be different at home with your husband or other male relatives, but the women in my family don't pick fights with men outside the family. I remember men whistling at my mother at the bus stop—she would just hold her head high and look straight ahead. But she would never say anything.

THERAPIST: Would you respond differently if it was a woman putting you down?

ROSE: Definitely. I would stand up for myself with a woman. It doesn't seem so dangerous.

THERAPIST: And if you were a Mexican American man and the men at work made racist comments, how would you respond?

ROSE: I would quietly answer them.

THERAPIST: For example?

ROSE: Well, if they joked about me being a "lazy Mexican," I would say, "I'm working as hard as you. When you work harder than me, then you can make comments about me being lazy."

THERAPIST: Wouldn't it seem dangerous to speak back like that?

ROSE: No, because that is how men talk to each other. I guess it would be dangerous if I said it with aggression. But the Mexican way is to speak softly and firmly with prejudiced people.

THERAPIST: How do you think it would sound if a Mexican American woman quietly answered the men's criticism?

ROSE: I'm not sure.

THERAPIST: Have you ever seen any other women at your company get these comments from any of the men?

ROSE: Yes. Most of the men work fine with women, but there are a few in every department who make sexist comments.

THERAPIST: How do the other women handle it?

ROSE: I'm not sure. Some say things back or make a joke. I remember one woman saying, "You better watch it or you'll be needing to take one of those diversity classes on your way out the door." But I can't imagine saying that myself.

THERAPIST: What happens when the women react to those men in that way?

ROSE: I can't remember.

Following a bit more discussion, Rose and her therapist drew the case conceptualization in Figure 3.1. In essence, they conceptualized Rose's work stress as the by-product of gender bias in coworkers inter-

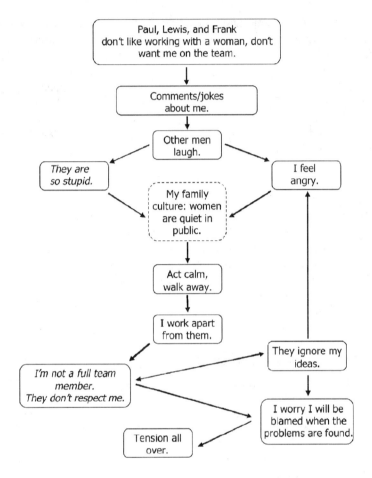

Figure 3.1. Rose's case conceptualization.

secting with her own cultural rules about gender-appropriate behavior. When angry, instead of perceiving options for expressing her feelings or negotiation, Rose quietly walks away because this is her cultural mandate. While she feels good about this choice in the moment, the consequences are isolation from the work team, ongoing anger, worries, and tension. For Rose, this individualized conceptualization made sense to her and linked culturally embedded beliefs and behaviors with her emotional and physical responses to coworkers' taunts.

Behavioral Experiments. To test the "fit" of this case conceptualization, Rose and her therapist agreed she would do an observational experiment. They constructed a written chart so that, during the next week, Rose could record any incidents in which coworkers made gender-biased comments about her. She would observe and write down (1) automatic thoughts and images about herself and her coworker, (2) her behavioral reactions, and (3) ratings of her physical tension immediately following the incident. In addition, because she and her therapist were curious about how other women handled similar incidents in this company, Rose agreed to fill out the same chart for an incident involving another woman. When Rose observed another woman responding to gender-biased comments, she agreed to record that woman's behavioral responses, the man's responses to that woman, and Rose's own automatic thoughts and physical reaction.

As Figure 3.2 shows, Rose's own experiences provided support for the conceptual model that Rose and her therapist had devised. Rose felt anger in response to sexist comments and had many automatic thoughts related to anger, but her behavior was very calm and quiet. Her behavior matched the image she reported of her mother's quiet reactions to men's laughter. Yet her physical tension was more in sync with her angry automatic thoughts. These observations helped Rose understand that her physical tension was probably linked to the anger she felt but did not think she should express.

Her observations of another woman, shown in Figure 3.3, led to information Rose and the therapist could discuss to consider alterna-

Situation	Automatic Thoughts (Images)	My Behavior	Rate Physical Tension (%)
Lewis says if I were a man I'd understand his changes to the code.	*What a jerk.* *His code is inefficient.* *He's just trying to put me down because I made a correction.*	*I ask him to run the new code and see what he thinks.* *I go back to my desk.*	*90%*
Frank tells a joke about women and then says, "I suppose I shouldn't say that in front of you, Rose." All the men chuckle.	*The joke was offensive but it's not like I haven't heard worse.* *He's like a little boy—trying to get away with being naughty.* *Image: My mother holding her head proudly when men laughed at her.*	*I say, "It doesn't bother me."*	*50%*

Figure 3.2. Rose's observations about her experiences.

Situation	Her Behavior	His Response	My Automatic Thoughts	Rate Physical Tension (%)
One of the men commented that Beth was "too pretty to be a computer programmer."	She asked, "What do you mean by that?" Next she said, "It's not a compliment if you are saying women can't be smart."	He said, "I'm just complimenting you." He said, "Geez, you're so sensitive."	He's putting her down. She's going to get in trouble.	
	She said, "You are pretty dense if you don't see the problem with what you said."	"Look, I didn't mean to offend you."	She did not act overly angry, and I think she handled herself well.	At first, 70%
	"I'll accept that as an apology."	"Fine." Then he shook his head and walked away.	I wonder if he will be angry with her and talk behind her back.	A few minutes later, only 20%

Figure 3.3. Rose's observations of another woman at work.

tive behaviors for future experiments. One of the values of an observational experiment is that, in the observer role, Rose's tension levels were lower and quickly dissipated. Lower tension affords greater objectivity in discussions. Thus case conceptualizations sometimes benefit from comparison observations of others in similar circumstances. Observations of others often reveal the diverse ways in which people respond to similar circumstances. Rose, of course, needed to evaluate what types of responses would be compatible with her own values.

Empirical Tests of Conceptualizations Outside of Sessions

As illustrated in Rose's case, conceptualizations collaboratively derived in session are tested empirically outside of session. Client observations and behavioral experiments conducted between therapy sessions provide evidence that either support or lead to modifications of the case conceptualization. Just as therapist and client do in session, the client is asked to identify thoughts, feelings, behaviors, and physical responses in particular situations outside of session. These observations are examined through the Socratic dialogue process so the therapist and client can see whether the current conceptual understanding is supported. Behavioral experiments are also conducted outside of session to test out conceptual ideas and evaluate pathways for change (cf. Bennett-Levy et al., 2004).

CLIENT SPECIFICS IN THE CRUCIBLE

In order to capture the diverse aspects of a person's life related to current presenting issues, Padesky and Mooney (1990) developed a five-part model for descriptive case conceptualization. Their five-part model helps clients link thoughts, feelings, behaviors, physical reactions, and broader life experiences. The case example of Ahmed in Chapter 2 illustrated how cultural issues can be assessed and recorded in appropriate places on the five-part model. This five-part model was incorporated in the CBT self-help book *Mind Over Mood* (Greenberger & Padesky, 1995) because it is simple enough for clients to apply in a self-help context. The ease with which this descriptive five-part model can be used collaboratively with clients in the first session(s) of therapy combined with its flexible inclusion of all aspects of a client's presenting issues make it an ideal starting point for case conceptualization (see Chapter 5).

The five-part model is only one of several broad frameworks for CBT conceptualization (J. S. Beck, 1995; Padesky & Greenberger, 1995; Persons, 1989). Rather than advocate one approach, we view the principles that therapists follow as more important in case conceptualization; these principles dictate the types of generic or disorder-specific frameworks therapists choose. It is through the principle of collaborative empiricism that the specifics of client experience are identified for the case conceptualization crucible.

As illustrated in all the case examples in this chapter, it is best if therapists use the client's own words, metaphors, and images when reflecting and summarizing the issues discussed. Use of client language in a case conceptualization personalizes the model and increases the likelihood that clients will understand and be able to apply the model outside of therapy sessions. Often clients will copy down conceptualizations in a therapy notebook. A conceptualization written in the client's own language, and even handwriting, is likely to resonate more strongly for the client.

Therapists usually need to ask direct questions to draw out the specifics related to presenting issues. People have differential awareness of thoughts, behaviors, emotions, physical responses, and environmental contexts. Whereas one client might readily volunteer beliefs associated with behaviors, another might only report emotional responses to events. Therapist questions are likely to be well received as long as they are asked in a context of curiosity and concern for the client.

Strengths and Resources

While it is natural for clients to describe problems when they begin therapy, it is important the therapist notices and inquires about client strengths and includes these in the case conceptualization, as will be elaborated on in Chapter 4. Clients are often relieved when the therapist shows an interest in their strengths. Awareness of internal and external resources is often poor during times of distress, and therapist queries can help the client remember and harness helpful skills and supports. Furthermore, strengths often provide a solid foundation for initial therapy interventions.

Cultural Factors and Broader Life Experiences

This chapter's extended case example of Rose illustrates how the inclusion of cultural factors can strengthen some case conceptualizations (Hays & Iwamasa, 2006). A conceptualization could have been formulated with Rose that did not include the cultural context. However, if her therapist had not inquired directly about the cultural bases of Rose's reactions, important information would have been missed. In addition, a cultural framework helped Rose see her coworkers' taunts as a form of posturing within their own cultural system. This perspective lessened Rose's personalization of the comments and speeded her progress in therapy. Furthermore, when Rose later explored her relationships with her sisters, it occurred to her that she and her sisters had experienced divergent cultures in recent years. Rose was able to use this insight to develop responses to her sisters that were more constructive and helped repair their frayed relationship. Ultimately, this conceptualization helped Rose use cultural awareness as a source of power, strength, and mental health.

Life events are often filtered through cultural frames of reference. All clients are immersed in diverse cultures that influence individual and group experiences. Gender, race, ethnicity, socioeconomic status, religious/spiritual beliefs, sexual orientation, education, political and moral values, neighborhood, and nationality are but a few aspects of one's culture that influence meaning structures, interpersonal patterns, and emotional expressions. With the case example of Ahmed in Chapter 2, it was only when the therapist explored Ahmed's experience of impending famine in his African homeland that the triggers for his anxiety made sense. Moreover, Ahmed's attempts to respond to his automatic thought

"I am no good to anyone" did not reduce his anxiety until the underlying assumption, "To be a good family man I have to provide financially for my family," was addressed. Cultural identities can shift over a lifetime, across circumstances and relationships, and in different social contexts. The role of culture has only recently been explored in any depth in the CBT literature (Hays & Iwamasa, 2006), although various CBT writers in the past have highlighted the importance of cultural considerations in both conceptualization and treatment (Davis & Padesky, 1989; Hays, 1995; Lewis, 1994; Martell, Safran, & Prince, 2004; Padesky & Greenberger, 1995).

CBT case conceptualizations are strengthened when they include relevant life events. Traumatic events are often cited as important precursors of client difficulties, yet positive life events can also play a pivotal role. Someone who grows up in a safe and loving community environment may respond more strongly to betrayal than someone who grows up in a somewhat untrustworthy environment.

Physical Factors

It is important that cognitive-behavioral therapists avoid a narrow view of only cognitive, behavioral, and emotional aspects of a client's life. A client's internal experiences can be understood in terms of links among cognitions, emotions, behaviors, and physical reactions. Yet these internal experiences do not exist in a vacuum. The role of genetics and the effects of nutrition and other chemicals on brain functioning are only vaguely understood in connection with many human experiences, and yet may prove to be primary causes of some difficulties. For example, anxiety can be linked to caffeine consumption rather than predisposing thought patterns. A person with caffeine-induced anxiety symptoms will show anxious cognitive thought patterns, yet the caffeine may be the primary problem. Thus therapists and clients who ignore physical, nutritional, and chemical inputs can develop erroneous conceptualizations.

Cognitive, Emotional, and Behavioral Factors

As higher-order conceptualizations are formed, each of the elements of the five-part model are more specifically defined. Emotions and physical reactions are rated for intensity, and behaviors are specified in terms of frequency, context, and impact, with special attention paid to whether behaviors trigger or maintain presenting issues. As defined in Chapter 1, thoughts are identified at three levels: automatic thoughts, underlying assumptions, and core beliefs. In the following sections we offer succinct guidelines for identifying cognitions at each of these three levels.

Identifying Automatic Thoughts

Recall that automatic thoughts describe the thoughts, images, and memories that occur spontaneously in one's mind throughout the day. These are different from consciously directed thoughts (e.g., "I'm going to make a list of what I need to buy at the grocery store"). Automatic thoughts pop into one's mind effortlessly while we go about the day's activities (e.g., "I feel so fat"). During conceptualization, therapists ask clients to identify automatic thoughts connected to presenting issues. Common prompts include:

- "What was going through your mind just then?" [in a particular situation the client describes or in session when the therapist notices an affect shift]
- "What does that mean to you?"
- "What does that say about you/others?"
- "Notice what goes through your mind [when you start to feel/act in a certain way]."
- "Are there any pictures or images that come to mind when you think/feel [insert belief or emotion]?"
- "Are there any memories or stories that come to mind when you think/feel [insert belief or emotion]?"
- "Were there any images in your mind? Try and imagine it as if it were happening right now. What do you see? Hear? Taste? Smell? Feel?"

For example, when Rose is heckled by men in her work group, an image flashes through her mind of her mother proudly and silently walking across the street while being heckled. This image helps make sense of Rose's quiet behavior, which contrasts sharply with the intense anger she feels.

Automatic thoughts reveal the meanings people make of situations and experiences. At the beginning of this chapter, Paul tells his therapist he hears voices. Without knowing his automatic thoughts, it is hard to predict what this means to Paul or how he might react. If someone thinks hearing voices means they have been chosen as a special prophet and this is a welcome honor, this person might be thrilled and eagerly listen for the voices. Paul's automatic thoughts are that the voices he hears are angels or devils who will force him to do bad things. These automatic thoughts help make sense of Paul's behavior, which is designed to prevent him from harming himself or others at the behest of these voices. Inclusion of these automatic thoughts in an initial descriptive conceptualization provides a more complete understanding of Paul's reactions.

Some automatic thoughts are more important to a case conceptualization than others. Therapists and clients are often able to identify recurring themes in situations representative of the presenting issue(s). For example, a particular automatic thought sometimes recurs over and over again on Thought Records. In searching for central themes, therapists can consider:

- Do the same thoughts occur in different types of situations or domains (home, work, friendships, social activities)?
- How frequently are thoughts experienced?
- To what degree do clients believe these thoughts (0–100%)?
- How often are these thoughts associated with distressing emotions (0–100%)?

More enduring, strongly endorsed or pervasive beliefs and strategies are more likely to be central in a conceptualization and provide a useful therapy focus. A search for common themes can also help identify automatic thoughts linked to important strengths.

Identifying Underlying Assumptions

Underlying assumptions encompass predictions about how the world operates as well as cross-situational rules for living. Some underlying assumptions are generally helpful, such as, "If I keep trying, then I can make progress." Other underlying assumptions are generally unhelpful, such as, "If something is not perfect, then it is has no value at all." When someone persistently uses a behavioral strategy even when it seems self-defeating to do so, there probably is an underlying assumption driving it. Therefore, to fully understand presenting issues, it is often necessary to identify underlying assumptions and include these in conceptualizations.

Identification of relevant underlying assumptions does more than offer explanatory power. Once clients are aware of the assumptions that underpin issues, they are often more willing to conduct behavioral experiments to try out alternative responses. For example, Rose identified the following underlying assumption guiding her behavior, "If a man criticizes me, then it is dangerous to speak back to him." Once this assumption was highlighted, she realized that the dangers she faced in her office were quite different than the dangers her mother faced on the street. She also considered new assumptions such as, "If I don't speak back, then the harassment may get worse." Until Rose became aware of her underlying assumptions, she was too anxious to experiment with other responses to the men on her work team.

As described in Chapter 1, when underlying assumptions are stated in an "if ... then ..." format they can be used to understand a client's predictions about what outcomes they expect from particular behaviors. Also, assumptions stated in an "if ... then ..." format can be tested more readily via behavioral experiments (Padesky & Greenberger, 1995). To identify underlying assumptions in this format, clients can be asked to complete sentences such as:

- "If [*insert relevant concept*] then. ..."
- "If [*insert relevant concept*] is not true then. ..."
- "If I [*insert relevant behavior, emotion, thought or physical sensation*] then. ..."
- "If I don't [*insert relevant behavior, emotion, thought, or physical sensation*] then. ..."
- "If someone else [*insert relevant behavior, emotion, thought, or physical sensation*] then. ..."
- "If someone else doesn't [*insert relevant behavior, emotion, thought, or physical sensation*] then. ..."

For each assumption, there can be further discussion to explore what goes through the client's mind in relation to this assumption. What does the client think will happen? What meaning does this hold for the client? What is the client likely to feel if this is or is not true?

Identifying Core Beliefs

Situations that are consistently troublesome or associated with frequent and pervasive negative emotion are opportunities to identify deeper core beliefs. Recall that core beliefs are central, absolute beliefs about self, others, and the world. People develop both positive and negative beliefs about themselves (e.g., "I'm a 'can-do' person" vs. "I'm useless"), other people (e.g., "People are trustworthy" vs. "People are manipulative"), and the world (e.g., "The world is miraculous" vs. "The world is frightening"). The automatic thoughts and underlying assumptions already identified guide the therapist and client toward relevant core beliefs that protect and predispose clients to their presenting issues.

Although core beliefs are the deepest level of belief, they can be accessed easily via direct questions. The downward arrow technique is one way to identify beliefs that underpin strong reactions to a situation. To use the downward arrow technique the therapist asks, "What does this say about you/mean to you?" and then repeats these same questions in response to each subsequent answer the client provides. Padesky (1994a) recommends that therapists identify core beliefs by asking clients to complete sentences such as:

"I am. ..."
"Others are. ..."
"The world is. ..."
"The future is. ..."

These sentence stems can be introduced in the context of a relevant central issue. For example, therapists can ask clients to fill in the blank as they imagine themselves in situations using overpracticed strategies such as avoidance or demands for special treatment:

"When you are [*doing your strategy*], how do you see yourself? I am. ..."
"How do you see others? People are. ..."
"How do you experience the world? The world is. ..."

Theoretically, core beliefs and underlying assumptions are closely linked. Therefore therapists can also inquire:

"If [relevant underlying assumption] is true, what does that say about you? I am. ..."
"About others? People are. ..."
"About the kind of world you live in? The world is. ..."

By definition, core beliefs are likely to be strongly held and emotionally evocative. For this reason, therapists identify core beliefs in the context of a positive therapeutic alliance after other conceptualizations have been collaboratively constructed. During work with core beliefs, the therapist should be alert to client distress and expect activation of strategies and underlying assumptions central to presenting issues. Clients often develop a range of underlying assumptions and strategies that mask the distress associated with core beliefs (J. S. Beck, 1995). Underlying assumptions such as, "If I let down my guard, I will be abused," and strategies such as, "Keep a shield between me and others," can be identified and tested in the context of a positive working alliance. Of course, if a therapist determines that a client does not have the resources to manage intense emotion, core belief work may be deferred until client coping and resilience is further developed.

Using Imagery, Metaphors, and Diagrams

Any of the elements described in the previous sections can be expressed in imagery, metaphors, and diagrams. We have drawn our conceptualization model as a crucible (see Figure 1.1). The central ideas expressed in this book are captured in that image. We hope it will remind readers of the key ideas and how they link to one another. Similarly, clients some-times draw or describe an image that captures important aspects of their struggles and strengths. The power of images is that they sometimes lead to creative ideas for intervention. One client who had been strug-gling with a problem for many months without progress conceptualized her dilemma as just like pushing against a large boulder day after day with no success in budging it. A few days later, as she reflected on this metaphorical conceptualization, it occurred to her that she could move the boulder if she dug out the earth beneath the far side. This imaginal solution led her to a creative new approach to successfully resolving her dilemma.

Thus therapists should be alert to client images and metaphors. Whenever possible, these should be integrated into conceptualizations. Even when clients do not volunteer images, it can help to ask, "Do any images or memories come to mind that capture how you think this hap-pens?" Furthermore, we recommend that conceptualizations be written or drawn with the client, often as diagrams such as those shown in the various conceptualization figures in this chapter. Written conceptualiza-tions are easier to remember, can be empirically tested and edited over time, and offer an opportunity for the therapist and client to check their collaborative understanding of client issues and strengths.

Metaphors, images, and memories offer rich sources of information about beliefs, personal meanings, and strategies (Blenkiron, 2005; Teas-dale, 1993). Metaphors often capture both complexities and nuances in how people conceptualize themselves, other people, and the world. Images are equally phenomenologically rich and usually strongly and directly linked to emotional responses (Hackmann, Bennett-Levy, & Holmes, in press). Client metaphors and images make valuable contri-butions to case conceptualizations because they are easy to remember, packed with information, and often offer sources of creative ideas to facilitate change. Clients may also relate particular stories, songs, or memories that incorporate rich symbolic meaning to the client. Any symbolic elements incorporated into a case conceptualization are likely to improve understanding at a deep resonant level for the client.

Figure 3.1 shows the initial conceptualization drawn by Rose and her therapist to capture her presenting issues. Although it is a clear description of what Rose described, this conceptualization is a bit com-plex for her to easily remember. Over time, Rose and her therapist sim-plified her conceptualization, favoring use of imagery and metaphors that were easy for her to remember. The image of her mother walking across the street, head held high, while men heckled her was already very familiar to Rose. Based on observations of other women at work and behavioral experiments she conducted, Rose created a vivid image

of her "manager self," who was comfortable and confident making asser-
tive responses to sexist remarks. She also found it helpful to create a
comical image of her favorite comedian, Ellen DeGeneres, who made
deadpan, silly comments in response to criticism. Rose was able to call
on each of these three images to guide her responses to sexism in the
workplace depending on which was most appropriate to the circumstances. Simple case conceptualizations often have greater utility than
complex ones. Figure 3.4 shows the much simpler conceptualization
Rose was using by the eighth week of therapy that incorporated the
images that were most helpful to her.

Notice that her simpler conceptualization includes new ideas gained
in therapy that guide her responses to disrespectful remarks. Rather
than detailing each thought, feeling, and behavior, useful metaphors
and images are used to capture "packages" of responses that Rose can
easily tap when she remembers the image. This simpler conceptualization helped Rose develop and practice a repertoire of adaptive responses
to perceived disrespect from others. Depending on the situation, Rose
could adopt her mother's quiet nonconfrontive manner, her new asser-
tive response style she labeled her "Manager Self," or a humorous set of
replies derived from Ellen DeGeneres. Each of these response sets was
rehearsed in session until Rose could practice them confidently. Rose
carried Figure 3.4 on an index card as a quick reminder.

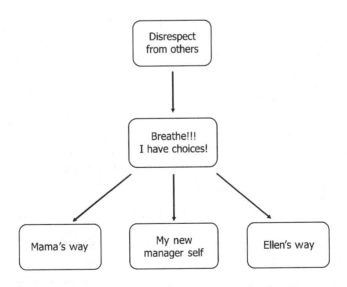

Figure 3.4. Rose's simple case conceptualization.

A Framework of Checks and Balances

In this chapter we have showcased the second of our three principles of case conceptualization—collaborative empiricism. By providing a framework of checks and balances, collaborative empiricism increases the odds that case conceptualization will be a creative crucible for understanding and change. A positive therapy alliance and therapy structure foster collaboration during case conceptualization, especially when alliance and structure operate in tandem. An empirical approach relies on a therapist's knowledge of relevant theory and research insofar as this provides a good fit with client experience. To ensure that a conceptualization maps well onto client experience, therapists stay curious and employ scientific methods such as observation, Socratic dialogue, and behavioral experiments to construct and evaluate case conceptualizations.

The next chapter details the third principle of our model, incorporation of client strengths. Although client strengths were alluded to in several case examples in this chapter, many therapists have greater experience assessing and conceptualizing problems than strengths. Chapter 4 elaborates the processes involved in a strengths focus and expands on the benefits of incorporating strengths throughout the case conceptualization process.

| Chapter 3 Summary |

- Collaboration is attained and maintained via explicit discussion, a positive therapy alliance, therapy structure, and optimal balancing of alliance and structure throughout the course of therapy, including conceptualization.
- An empirical framework for case conceptualization entails (1) integration of client data with empirical literature, and (2) use of observation, Socratic dialogue, and behavioral experiments to actively test conceptual models to see whether they fit and predict client experiences.
- Collaborative empiricism is used to identify links among cognitions, behaviors, emotions, and physical states occurring within the client's broader life context; client strengths and relevant cultural factors are included.
- Conceptualizations are written down with the client, often in a diagram that shows links among the elements. In addition, they incorporate client images and metaphors whenever possible.

Chapter 4

Incorporating Client Strengths and Building Resilience

A consulting psychiatrist who is also a CBT therapist is asked to meet with Zainab, a 31-year-old married woman who is hospitalized on a medical floor of the community hospital following a serious suicide attempt.

ZAINAB: Go away. I'm not broken, I don't need fixing. (*The voice from beneath the bed covers speaks in clear English, with a strong accent.*)

THERAPIST: I've been asked by the staff to meet with you to see whether there are any ways I can help.

ZAINAB: I don't want your help; go away, I said. (*silence*)

THERAPIST: OK, I understand. I will let the nurse know and speak with your husband.

Zainab is mother to four young children and employed as a classroom assistant. Her family emigrated from a North African country 5 years ago. Zainab has so far refused to discuss her problems with any of the hospital staff. Thus the details of her suicide attempt have been pieced together from information provided from her husband, Muhammad. He reports symptoms that suggest Zainab experienced a psychotic break several weeks ago. Prior to her suicide attempt, she became increasingly isolated and afraid. When her husband and children were out at the beach one Sunday Zainab intentionally swallowed an overdose of pills. A neighbor discovered her in a coma and called emergency services.

While Zainab has been desperate to leave the hospital as soon as possible, nurses comment that she will not speak in detail about her life, and her husband Muhammad seems "lost." The psychiatrist has been asked to assess whether Zainab poses an ongoing risk to herself and also to try to engage her in treatment if appropriate. Given Zainab's clear message that she does not want help, the psychiatrist decides to speak with her husband:

THERAPIST: Muhammad, I have been asked to speak with Zainab to try and see whether there is anything I can do to help her. She seems to be suffering a lot but says she does not want my help.

MUHAMMAD: I know, I know. She is a very good person, and she is very ashamed to be in this position; she is frightened and worried about what will happen to her. She wants to be with our children very much.

Muhammad explains that Zainab recently started to hear voices saying her two children were special. These voices denigrated Zainab, asserting she was not good enough to be their mother. In the days leading up to Zainab's suicide attempt, the voices began to insist that she should be cast out so the family could return to their home country and live with one of their uncles and aunts, who were members of a revered religious family. Muhammad explains that 5 years ago the family had been forced to leave their country because Zainab's father is a writer who has published articles critical of government authorities. Her father also lives in exile. Muhammad's parents are devout Muslims and disapprove of Zainab's father's political stance.

THERAPIST: The voices sound really frightening. Did Zainab turn to anyone for help?

MUHAMMAD: She spoke with me, but I did not know what to do. Zainab is so proud and strong; she thought that to ask for help outside our family was impossible. (Smiles.)

THERAPIST: (with curiosity) Why are you smiling?

MUHAMMAD: When we moved here 5 years ago, none of us spoke English. Zainab learned quickly so that she could find work. She also taught me English so I could find work. Then she taught our children because her English was better than mine. You know she is a pillar in our family; (smiling broadly) we nicknamed her "the pillar." We know a few other families from our home country here and we are a community; Zainab has made us a community that helps each other. Also, where she works, they have phoned me and they really want her to come back. (*As he speaks, he looks increasingly proud of her achievements.*) But, she could not ask for help. (*His expression changes and he begins to look lost and scared again.*)

THERAPIST: When you use this term, *pillar*, what do you mean?

MUHAMMAD: That she is strong … steady … she stays strong. (*Although there is a sense he could say more, the therapist decides not to inquire further at this time.*)

INSIDE THE THERAPIST'S HEAD

This psychiatrist faces some important choice points about how to best help Zainab. He uses an emerging preliminary conceptualization to inform these choice points. He hypothesizes that Zainab has a core belief about herself as "strong" that is founded in considerable evidence of her self-efficacy. Zainab herself does not want to be treated as if she is "broken." The psychiatrist wonders whether help focused on Zainab's strengths and rebuilding her resilience would interest her and be sufficient to restore her to positive functioning.

Our book is about both relieving distress and building resilience. Zainab's voices and the fear and shame she feels in relation to these voices cause her a lot of distress. Zainab's resourcefulness and others' view of her as a pillar are encouraging strengths. Client strengths provide the building blocks for resilience so incorporation of strengths into case conceptualization is a first step toward restoring or building client resilience.

This chapter explains how to assess and conceptualize using a strengths focus. Strengths-based conceptualizations that foster resilience can be a useful part of CBT. We first outline how to identify client strengths and incorporate these into case conceptualizations. Next we define resilience and show how it can become the focus of a case conceptualization. Finally, we present a rationale for incorporating resilience goals into CBT.

IDENTIFYING STRENGTHS

Unlike Zainab, most clients want and expect to talk about their problems at the beginning of therapy. Even so, it is important for the therapist to ask about and express genuine interest in client strengths. In times of intense distress, clients often forget they have internal and external resources. Therapist inquiries about strengths, skills, and support can remind the client of resources that may prove immediately helpful. Also, therapists who search for strengths obtain a more holistic view of their clients. Clients who are invited to reveal positive qualities as well as struggles are likely to leave an initial therapy session with more confidence that their therapist "knows" them. The balance of gathering information about difficulties and strengths varies from client to client. Some clients are eager to disclose positive aspects of their lives; others may be put off if the therapist does not solely address presenting issues. Therapists can routinely inquire about strengths and use clients' responses to judge what detail to gather regarding these in initial sessions.

Imagine what Zainab's psychiatrist would see if he had used an exclusively problem-focused lens. He would see a withdrawn, frightened, incommunicative woman with psychosis, living in an alien culture with a husband who appears depleted of coping resources. A strengths-focused lens enables the psychiatrist to see a person generally high in self-efficacy, who has negotiated a difficult move to a new country, has a supportive family, and is regarded by others as a "pillar," yet for some reason is struggling with psychosis and suicidal intent. Incorporating strengths into the initial conceptualization provides a more balanced view of Zainab.

Although a therapist can directly ask the client to identify strengths, it is often more helpful to explore areas of the client's life that are going relatively well. For example, a client who complains of work stress can be interviewed about life at home, relationships with friends, hobbies, and other interests. By expressing curiosity about areas of the client's life that are going well, the therapist communicates to the client that he or she is interested in all of the client's life, not just problem areas. Relatively successful areas of the client's life can then be linked to therapy goals, as in the following dialogue between David and his therapist:

THERAPIST: I imagine your whole life has not been wrapped up in [these problems]. Are there any areas of your life that generally make you happy, perhaps even now?

DAVID: Right now, not really.

THERAPIST: Well, how about before these problems began?

DAVID: I used to volunteer at the pet shelter. I did like that.

THERAPIST: That sounds interesting. What did you do there?

DAVID: I groomed the animals. My specialty was the dogs. I really liked working with them.

THERAPIST: What do you like about working with dogs?

DAVID: Well, a lot of them are pretty scared at the shelter. Some show this by being quite aggressive and others act very submissive. I had a knack for settling down the aggressive ones and calming the frightened ones.

THERAPIST: That sounds tough.

DAVID: Not so much for me. I took pride in my ability to work with all types of dogs.

THERAPIST: It sounds like you have some real talent when it comes to handling dogs.

DAVID: Yes, I suppose I do.

THERAPIST: We might want to tap into some of those talents when it comes time to handle some of these problems you are having at work and home.

DAVID: How do you mean?

THERAPIST: Well, I'm not sure. But maybe if you think about it, we'll be able to find some similarities between those dogs and some of your family members and coworkers.

DAVID: (*laughing*) Oh, I can think of a few people who act worse than the dogs!

THERAPIST: (*laughing*) See? You just might need those dog-handling skills in the rest of your life, too!

Identification of strengths often helps clients creatively imagine more effective behaviors in areas of difficulty. Clients often operate with more resilient belief systems in areas of strength and competency (Mooney & Padesky, 2002). These resilient belief systems can help clients persist in the face of obstacles when pursuing therapy goals. For example, David may have beliefs that help him stay calm with aggressive dogs (e.g., "He is just frightened and trying to protect himself," "She will settle down if I don't act aggressively in return"). Once identified, these beliefs also might help during conflicts with family members and coworkers.

When clients arrive at therapy sessions in states of extreme distress it may appear difficult to find evidence of strengths. Clients may deny that any area of life is going well. For example, severely depressed clients often see themselves as devoid of worth and ability; they frequently deny possessing any positive qualities or areas of success. The following dialogue illustrates one way therapists can identify strengths when clients see only struggles and problems:

THERAPIST: I think I have a pretty good idea now of some of the struggles you have been going through. Before we end our session today, I'd like to find out a bit about what has carried you through these past few months.

KATRINA: I don't know what you mean.

THERAPIST: Well, times have been very tough for you. You must be doing something to keep yourself on your feet in the face of all these pressures and losses you've experienced.

KATRINA: I'm not on my feet at all. I'm a wreck. I've just fallen apart and can't get anything done in my life. I've ruined my friendships and destroyed my family's confidence in me.

THERAPIST: I do understand how things look very bleak to you. Yet I remember when we set an appointment time you said it had to be before 4 o'clock because you wanted to be there when your children came home from school.

KATRINA: I have to be at home after 4. There is no one else to do that.

THERAPIST: Yes. And it seems to me it must be very difficult to be a parent when you are feeling so low.

KATRINA: I'm not a good parent right now.

THERAPIST: Perhaps not. But, from what you said earlier, it sounds like you manage to talk to the children, make their dinner, and put them to bed even though you feel very poorly all the while you are doing it.

KATRINA: Yes. Any parent has to do that.

THERAPIST: And those things can be hard to do after a long day, even under the best of circumstances. (*pause*) Yet you are managing to do it under the worst of circumstances. How do you do that?

KATRINA: Well, I just don't see a choice. My children are too young to care for themselves. I'm not doing anything special.

THERAPIST: So you do it out of a sense of duty? Or love?

KATRINA: Both duty and love. It is a parent's duty to raise children. And I do love my children, even though I don't show it very much to them when I am this upset.

THERAPIST: So, it the midst of these terrible circumstances, your sense of duty and love for your children help you keep going ... even when you'd rather just give up.

KATRINA: Yes, I suppose so.

THERAPIST: Even though this may seem like just a small thing to you, I really admire your ability to keep up your duties and express your love for your children when you feel so badly. I've known many parents who do not do that even when they are happy.

KATRINA: Really?

THERAPIST: Yes. I think those small things you do for your children, even if you don't always do them very well when you are feeling so poorly, speak positively about who you are inside as a person.

In this interchange the therapist introduces an area of strength Katrina has not identified. When clients are highly self-critical and despondent, the therapist can be alert to identify small positive behaviors the client performs on a daily basis. Katrina manages small daily positive behaviors as a parent. Other common daily behaviors that clients might perform consistently even when distressed include good grooming (clothing choices, shaving, fixing hair), going to work, caring for a pet, keeping up a garden, or showing up for sports activities. Any common daily activity maintained during distress is symbolic of some value the client holds that can be viewed as a strength. These values and strengths may only be implicit, and clients may minimize them through the cognitive biases that are typical of emotional disorders (Beck, 1976).

Personal Values

Personal values often function as sources of strength for people because they inform people's choices and behaviors. Thus it helps for therapists to show interest in client values so these can be incorporated into conceptualizations. For instance, when the therapist in the above example expresses open appreciation and admiration for how difficult it can be to carry out daily duties when depressed, Katrina begins to see herself as possessing some positive qualities. She acknowledges that she chooses to care for her children even though she no longer feels able to do many other activities of daily living. Although a depressed client will undoubtedly focus on how poorly she is parenting, the therapist's recognition of the strength despite her distress can be quite meaningful to the client.

Notice that the therapist does not overplay the depressed client's display of strength. An empirical understanding of depressive thought processes helps this therapist realize that an overly positive statement such as, "Even when depressed you show great love toward your children," is likely to be knocked down by depressive thoughts such as, "It's not great love when you criticize and yell at them all the time." Instead, the therapist anticipates and incorporates Katrina's potential for self-criticism by summarizing, "Those small things you do for your children, *even if you don't always do them very well when you are feeling so poorly*, speak positively about who you are inside as a person."

Client values can be understood as beliefs about what is most important in life. These beliefs typically are relatively enduring across situations and shape clients' choices and behaviors. Incorporating values into conceptualizations as part of a client's belief system enables us to better understand clients' reactions across different situations. Katrina's therapist can hypothesize a value such as, "It is important to show love toward my children." Because this is an enduring value, it continues to drive Katrina's behavior even when she becomes so unmotivated that she stops other behaviors that are not rooted in her values.

In the case of Zainab the therapist can hypothesize the value, "It is important to be strong for my family." This value proved a source of resourcefulness when Zainab navigated the challenges of immigration to a new country and culture. However, it is noteworthy that this value also helps us understand why the denigrating voices Zainab heard as part of the psychosis (e.g., "you are not good enough to be a mother to your children") were so devastating; she thought she had violated her own values. In this way Zainab's presentation illustrates how values and beliefs can simultaneously serve both protective and predisposing functions. Her view of herself as a pillar gave her strength, yet because it was so important for Zainab to be a pillar for others, she was more vulnerable when she began to hear voices because she believed she was weak and could not help others if she needed help herself. In this way, positive beliefs can be just as debilitating as negative beliefs when they are rigidly held and prove a mismatch to situational requirements.

Cultural Strengths

As demonstrated in Chapters 2 and 3, personal and cultural values can be important strengths for clients. Recall the case example in Chapter 3 of Rose, a Hispanic woman experiencing problems at work. Rose's personal and cultural values were incorporated into a conceptualization of how she reacted to coworkers' taunts ("Women in my culture are quiet in public when men criticize them"). Rose and her therapist reconceptualized these values as a source of power, "In this work culture, coworkers' taunts are a form of posturing: I can *choose* to act out of my cultural values or act within the work culture, whichever seems most effective." Rose's ability to choose between these options helps her be more resilient. She can either quietly accept taunts or respond to them within the parameters of work culture norms.

Sometimes aspects of a client's life or culture represent both strengths and dangers. In the case of Ahmed (see Chapter 2), his faith was a source of strength to him, yet he also recognized that some people were prejudiced against his faith and these people could represent a danger to him and his family. When cultural discrimination is a focus of therapy, it is especially important for the therapist to ask about and validate positive strengths within the client's culture. Without explicit validation of positive aspects of culture, the client often assumes the therapist agrees with cultural biases against him or her (American Psychological Association, 2000, 2003). In Chapter 8 we consider the issue of therapist values and how these intersect with clients' personal and cultural values.

INCORPORATING STRENGTHS INTO CASE CONCEPTUALIZATIONS

Strengths can be incorporated at each stage of therapy. Goals can be stated as increasing strengths or positive values (e.g., be more considerate) as well as reducing distress (e.g., feel less anxious). As we demonstrate in Chapter 5, therapists can routinely ask about positive goals and aspirations in early sessions and add these to the client's list of presenting issues. Discussions of positive areas of a client's life often reveal alternative coping strategies to those used in problem areas. These often more adaptive coping strategies can be identified as part of the same process that identifies triggers and maintenance factors for problems (see Chapter 6). When it is time for behavioral experiments to alter maintenance cycles, the client can practice alternative coping responses drawn from more successful areas of life. Later in therapy, positive assumptions and core beliefs prove just as important as negative ones when forming longitudinal case conceptualizations (see Chapter 7).

Although identified strengths can be incorporated at each stage of case conceptualization, this has not typically been demonstrated in the CBT literature. There has been a much greater emphasis on identifying precipitating, predisposing, and perpetuating factors for problems. In this text we advocate the inclusion of strengths whenever possible during case conceptualization. To illustrate, see Figure 4.1. It shows Rose's conceptualization as seen in Figure 3.1, but with her strengths now listed on the left side of the diagram.

Rose identified her strengths after the conceptualization in Figure 3.1 was drawn. Her therapist collaboratively derived the strengths overlay shown in Figure 4.1 with a few additional questions:

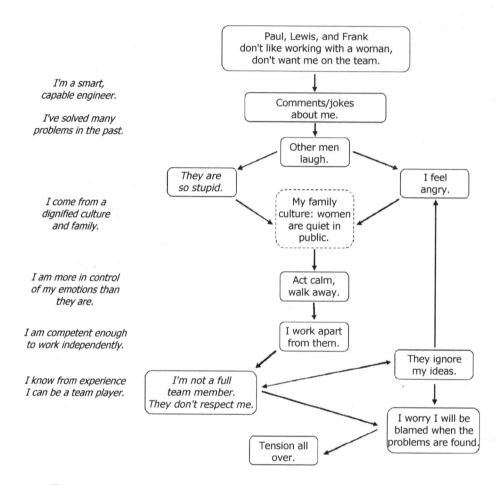

Figure 4.1. Rose's conceptualization with her strengths listed (on the left).

THERAPIST: There is at least one thing missing from this diagram of your work difficulties, Rose.

ROSE: What?

THERAPIST: This picture shows what is happening, but it doesn't include the strengths you have that can help you resolve this problem.

ROSE: What strengths do you mean?

THERAPIST: Look at the diagram. See if you can find some hidden strengths. For example, why were you added to this work team in the first place?

ROSE: Because they needed help.

THERAPIST: And why do you think management chose you to help?

ROSE: I'm a smart and capable engineer. I solved many problems for my other team.

By helping Rose highlight her strengths as an engineer as well as her familial and cultural strengths of dignity and self-control, the therapist adds important dimensions to the written case conceptualization. Inclusion of strengths boosts client awareness of resources that can help. Rose realized that she might be able to use her engineering problem-solving skills to help resolve the problem she was having with her coworkers. Recognition of strengths can buoy client confidence, strengthen collaboration, and point to interventions that build on client capabilities. Adding strengths to the case conceptualization diagram helps both client and therapist remember these resources whenever the conceptualization is consulted.

Early in therapy, conceptualizations identify strengths that have helped clients cope to date. Sometimes strengths are identified in one area of the client's life that are relatively absent in areas of concern. In this case, these proven strengths are added to conceptualizations to inform the best choice of CBT intervention. Interventions that involve strengths practiced in other areas of a client's life may be more effective because they may help the client bypass long-standing factors involved in maintaining problems. As therapy progresses, strengths are added to explanatory conceptualizations. Sometimes these conceptualizations reveal overused strengths that contribute to distress. A common example of this phenomenon occurs in couples' conflicts when one partner has well-developed management and problem-solving skills at work, yet finds these same skills applied with a partner at home are a handicap to the couple's communication.

In addition to preexisting strengths, CBT helps clients develop new emotional, cognitive, behavioral, and interpersonal skills. Newly developed strengths are also highlighted throughout therapy so the client is aware of available skill sets when facing difficulties. To this end, clients are encouraged to keep a therapy notebook. In addition to records of observations and homework assignments, this notebook can include summaries of new beliefs, skills, and tools gained during therapy. Toward the end of therapy, clients are invited to imagine with the therapist how various strengths and skills can assist the client in managing future challenges as well as promoting continued positive development. In fact, client strengths become a central focus of conceptualizations that promote continued client growth and development. This process is highlighted in Chapter 7.

FROM STRENGTHS TO RESILIENCE

As defined in Chapter 2, resilience is a broad concept that refers to how people negotiate adversity to maintain their well-being. The term describes the psychological processes through which people draw on their strengths to adapt to challenges. Ann Masten (2001), a clinical researcher who has investigated resilience in a number of studies, coined the phrase "ordinary magic" to describe resilience. She writes: "The great surprise of resilience research is the ordinariness of the phenomena. Resilience appears to be a common phenomenon that results in most cases from the operation of basic human adaptation processes" (p. 227). Later in the same article she continues: "Studies of resilience converge on a short list of attributes. ... These include connections to competent and caring adults in the family and community, cognitive and self-regulation skills, positive views of the self, and motivation to be effective in the environment" (p. 234). Others have added dimensions such as physical health and having meaning in one's life (Davis, 1999).

Resilience has multiple dimensions; there are many pathways to it, and people do not need strengths in all areas to be resilient. Thus resilience is perhaps "ordinary" because there are many different combinations of strengths that, joined together, help someone be resilient. Masten draws an important distinction between strengths and resilience. *Strengths* refer to attributes about a person such as good problem-solving abilities or protective circumstances such as a supportive partner. *Resilience* refers to the processes whereby these strengths enable adaptation during times of challenge. Thus, once therapists help clients identify strengths, these strengths can be incorporated into conceptualizations to help understand client resilience.

For example, throughout her life Zainab demonstrated particular strengths such as a gift for learning languages, good physical health, and high energy. These strengths enabled her to be quite resourceful during challenging times. She responded to her family's move to a new culture by learning English and finding work. In Zainab's case, resilience refers to how her strengths interacted with her life circumstances to enable her to adapt to a new culture. At the same time, Zainab's experiences illustrate that resilience is not an absolute or fixed quality. Resilience is a dynamic process across situations and time (Luthar, Cicchetti, & Becker, 2000; Masten, 2001, 2007; Rutter, 1987). When challenged with psychosis, Zainab's resources were overwhelmed. Although she turned to her husband for help, his support was not enough to erase her despair and prevent her suicide attempt.

CONCEPTUALIZING CASES IN TERMS OF RESILIENCE

Once strengths are identified, how can therapists incorporate these into a conceptual model of client resilience? All the forms of conceptualization taught in this book can be used and adapted to conceptualize resilience. Each of the existing CBT models such as the generic CBT model of emotion (Beck, 1976, 2005), functional analysis (e.g., Hayes & Follette, 1992), the five-part model (Padesky & Mooney, 1990), explanatory conceptualizations of triggers and maintenance factors, as well as longitudinal conceptualizations can be *translated to focus on resilience.* Resilience can be conceptualized using the same three levels of case conceptualization described in Chapter 2: (1) descriptive accounts in cognitive and behavioral terms that articulate a person's strengths, (2) explanatory cross-sectional (triggers and maintenance) conceptualizations of how strengths protect the person from adverse effects of negative events, and (3) explanatory (longitudinal) conceptualizations of how strengths have interacted with circumstances across the person's lifetime to foster resilience and maintain well-being.

Relevant theory and research can be integrated with the details of an individual case using the heat of collaborative empiricism. Because resilience is a broad multidimensional concept, therapists can either adapt existing theories of psychological disorders (see Box 1.3) or draw from a large array of theoretical ideas related to resilience found in the positive psychology literature (see, e.g., Snyder & Lopez, 2005).

Zainab's psychiatrist decided to conceptualize her case in terms of resilience. He thought Zainab would respond more positively to that than to a problem-focused one ("I'm not broken"). First, the therapist identified several of Zainab's strengths through interviews with Muhammad. At his next interview with Zainab, he emphasized these as well as the metaphor of the "pillar" that had particular meaning to Zainab because it was her nickname in her family:

THERAPIST: Muhammad has told me how you are the pillar of your family, Zainab. (*Zainab glances at the therapist and then looks down again.*) I understand you were the first to learn English and that you taught the rest of the family. Everyone wants you to come home. (*Zainab nods slightly.*) If you are willing, I would like to talk with you about what might help you go home more quickly. Would that be all right with you?

ZAINAB: (*Quietly*) Yes.

This dialogue shows how a positive therapeutic alliance is advanced when therapists are attuned to and interested in a person's strengths, values, and positive goals. Zainab engaged with the therapist only when he communicated that (1) he wished to work with her strength (metaphor = "pillar") and (2) he was interested in helping her work toward her primary goal (i.e., returning home). As emphasized throughout this text, collaborative conceptualization is recommended as a check and balance. Zainab's involvement in her case conceptualization is necessary to correct erroneous therapist inferences and also to fuel her commitment to the treatment plan. Her therapist uses the strengths view of Zainab he obtained from Muhammad to engage Zainab in her goal of returning home. Zainab is more willing to collaborate with her therapist on a strengths-based conceptualization because in her mind she is "not broken and does not need fixing."

Figure 4.2 shows a five-part model drawn by Zainab and her therapist to develop a better understanding of how her strengths operated when she emigrated to her new country. This conceptualization makes explicit how positive thoughts, emotions, and body reactions are mutu-

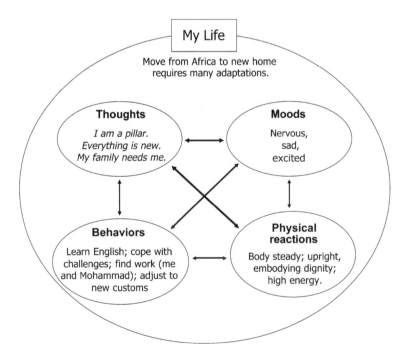

Figure 4.2. Descriptive conceptualization of Zainab's strengths.

ally reinforcing and lead to adaptive behavior. This conceptualization became a springboard to discussion of how she might use these strengths to deal with the critical voices she heard and the other pressures that led to her suicide attempt. A person like Zainab who has a recent and acute onset of difficulties, yet has demonstrated active and successful functioning in most areas over many years, is ideally suited for CBT focused on restoration of preexisting resilience. A client with a chronic history of mental health difficulties who has displayed little resilience might be better suited to CBT oriented toward building new strengths as a basis for resilience.

Identifying Resilient Strategies and Beliefs

Noticing the strategies a person employs to manage adversity is often an easy first step toward conceptualizing resilience. Strategies usually can be observed and may be behavioral (e.g., persisting in efforts), cognitive (e.g., problem solving, acceptance), emotional (e.g., humor, reassurance), social (e.g., seeking help), spiritual (e.g., finding meaning in suffering), or even physical (e.g., sleeping and eating well). People are often not aware of the strategies they use to be more resilient. Highlighting these in a case conceptualization increases the likelihood the person will consider their use during future challenges.

People who cope resiliently tend to construe events positively, including objectively challenging events. These interpretations involve positive expectancies (e.g., "I have faith this will work out"), self-efficacy (e.g., "This is tough, but I have coped with worse times"), and optimism (e.g., "We will be able to manage this"). Sometimes clients are not aware of these thoughts. Conceptualizations of resilience bring these interpretative biases into awareness so clients can choose how to respond during challenging times. Consider the following exchange in which Zainab describes filling out a job application with her husband one evening.

ZAINAB: Some of the questions, we just laughed you know. At home people would never ask such questions. The form was very long, and it took us all evening.

THERAPIST: How did you manage to keep your sense of humor during this one evening, presumably after you had been working all day?

ZAINAB: Yes, I had been at work, and then we read to the children and put them to bed. I was tired. I don't know how I found it funny. Maybe *because* I was tired.

THERAPIST: Thinking back to that evening, what sorts of thoughts were running through your mind as you were laughing?

ZAINAB: We were just being silly, you know, saying, "These questions are so stupid!" (*Looks thoughtful.*) I was happy for Muhammad, it is so important to him to be earning money for the family. I was happy to see him laughing; you know this has been so difficult for him. (*Looks uncertain; makes eye contact with the therapist as she speaks*) It is important to me to help Muhammad, to be strong for him.

THERAPIST: To be like a pillar.

ZAINAB: Yes, to support him like a pillar.

A growing body of evidence suggests that people who are resilient positively interpret events and employ adaptive strategies in both challenging and neutral situations (Lyubomirsky, 2001; Lyubomirsky, Sheldon, & Schkade, 2005). This is evident in Zainab's report of the evening they filled out the job application. Her thoughts are about Muhammad and his well-being. She wants to support him and finds that humor makes a difficult situation easier. When conceptualizing resilience it is important that the therapist is alert to notice times like this, when clients operate resiliently, and capture the thoughts related to these situations.

Resilience core beliefs and underlying assumptions often reflect core human concerns of autonomy (e.g., "I enjoy a challenge and can face it on my own when I need to"), competence (e.g., "I am persistent"), affiliation (e.g., "My partner will support me through this"), and connection to a larger humanity (e.g., "Many people struggle with these issues; I'm not alone"). Resilience core beliefs and underlying assumptions are elicited in relation to difficulties faced because resilience is only required in the face of challenges. For example, resilient underlying assumptions can be identified by asking the client to complete this sentence, "If I face serious challenges in my life, then. ..." The following questions can be asked to identify client beliefs and personal qualities related to resilience:

- "What rules or beliefs can help you be resilient in this situation?"
- "Ideally, what qualities would you like to show in the face of these obstacles?"
- "What beliefs [about you/others/the world] help you show these qualities?"
- "If you coped in the best way you can imagine, what would you be thinking [about yourself/others/the world]?"
- "What rules would you follow? If ... then. ...."
- "What qualities would someone you see as a role model show?"
- "What rules or beliefs do you think guide them to respond in these ways?"

Metaphors, Stories, and Images

Metaphors, stories, and images provide a shorthand conceptualization that communicates the rich interplay of beliefs, emotions, physical states, and strategies that define resilience. Metaphors, stories, and images need to come from the individual to have personal meaning and resonance. For example, many people might think of a pillar as too rigid to be resilient. However, for Zainab the pillar symbolized ancient wisdom, faith, and strength that lasted through centuries.

Some of the metaphors, stories, and images developed with our clients are listed here. Each of these was unpacked in therapy discussions to understand the resilient core beliefs, underlying assumptions, emotional responses, and behavioral strategies that they encompass:

- "I am a pillar, not broken; I don't need fixing." Zainab's underlying sense of strength was tied to the image of a specific pillar near her home where she grew up that is thousands of years old and has lasted through many generations. This metaphor had its foundations in her Muslim faith.
- "The compost and the flower." For this client, distress (the compost) and resilience (the flower) became one and the same. The flower needs compost and itself becomes compost. This client's values were strongly influenced by Buddhism and this metaphor had its roots in Buddhist teachings (Thich Nhat Hahn, 1975).
- "I am learning to live in the light." This client's long history of mental health problems led to her becoming "very familiar with the dark." For her, recovery involved learning to live in the light, a worthwhile and sometimes frightening experience.
- "The orchid and the dandelion." This was a metaphor from a research paper (Boyce & Ellis, 2005) suggested to a client who was highly sensitive. The metaphor described how some people need very little to thrive (dandelions can flower in a concrete driveway) and some people need just the right conditions to thrive (orchids). This metaphor led the client to pay more attention to creating healthy conditions in her life so she could thrive.
- "My mental heath problems are like a chronic physical health problem such as diabetes." This is a common analogy and communicates the need to use simple yet effective coping resources to manage daily life. This person managed self-care (diet, sleep, routine) and medication (lithium) in the same way that someone with diabetes manages their diet and uses insulin.
- "My mental health problem is my 'teacher.'" This is how Gwyneth Lewis, a renowned Welsh poet, describes her experience with

recurrent depression. Rather than allow her negative beliefs to escalate, when she becomes depressed she asks, "What do I need to learn? What part of my life is out of balance?" (Lewis, 2002).

- "Hiking on an unknown trail." One man struggled with pressures in his daily life, yet he handled extreme challenges quite adeptly when he was in the wilderness. By accessing his "hiker" self, he responded more resiliently to daily challenges by following his personal hiking principles: slow down, read the signs, review options, make choices, and follow these choices with steady effort until it is time to reevaluate progress.

The following dialogue is an example of how a therapist can unpack the meaning in a metaphor, story or image. In this session, the therapist met with both Zainab and Muhammad:

ZAINAB: My father was always secular and I myself am also secular. But Muhammad is a devout Muslim and sometimes we argue about the children. To me, it is important for the children to make up their own minds about this.

INSIDE THE THERAPIST'S HEAD

The therapist has a hypothesis. Zainab's voices contain strong religious content, condemning her for her inability to provide her children with an appropriate religious upbringing. He is also aware of some tension between Zainab and Muhammad's families of origin around Zainab's religious values. The therapist is wary of discussing religious values, especially given his limited knowledge of the Muslim faith, and so he is uncertain about how best to proceed. He decides to use his limited knowledge to explore this issue with Zainab and Muhammad using guided discovery. Note how guided discovery supports an open questioning style, which is especially helpful because the therapist knows little about Islam or about the couple's religious beliefs and behaviors.

THERAPIST: This sounds like an important difference between you. I do not know much about Islam; perhaps you can explain to me what it means to you to be secular.

MUHAMMAD: You must understand, I do not agree that Zainab is not a good Muslim. This is something she thinks. She holds many of the values of Islam; there is an idea that Islam has five pillars ...

THERAPIST: (*looking at Zainab*) Is this related to why people say you are a pillar?

MUHAMMAD: (*stepping in again, seemingly wanting to protect Zainab*) Yes, because they feel that Zainab is an example of one of the pillars of Islam. There is the pillar of Zakah, which you might understand as giving money to others. Always she has done this, not just with money but with her time and heart as well, this is why we call her a pillar.

THERAPIST: So in this respect, in this sense you agree. In what areas do you disagree?

MUHAMMAD: It is true that I pray five times every day, where Zainab does not. But in other ways Zainab is a better Muslim than me. Because of what happened with our families she is afraid we will disagree and I will want to return home. (*The therapist is mindful that Muhammad is doing all the talking, but Muhammad is regularly referring to Zainab.*)

ZAINAB: That is true. I feel that I have let you down. I feel guilty about what has happened.

MUHAMMAD: Instead I feel grateful to you. (*Zainab smiles at Muhammad; he reciprocates.*)

ZAINAB: (*looking at Muhammad*) I think that unless I am a good Muslim in every respect you and others in our community will look down on me.

MUHAMMAD: (*looking at Zainab*) People look up to you as a good Muslim.

The therapist was able to work with Zainab and Muhammad to address some of Zainab's underlying assumptions (e.g., "If I am not a good Muslim in every respect, then Muhammad and others in my community will look down on me"). Zainab and Muhammad were able to discuss this important issue and agreed they jointly could teach their children about Islam and spiritual values. In the past, her conditional assumption and guilt prevented her from talking more fully with Muhammad. Without her input, Muhammad needed to "mind read." Clearly, religion had played a pivotal role in the messages Zainab heard from the voices. This dialogue illustrates how religious beliefs can both fuel distress and play a pivotal role in resilience. As Ann Masten notes, religious systems "engage fundamental human adaptive systems in multiple ways, from teaching self-regulation through prayer or meditation, prescribing rules for living and rituals for major life passages, to fostering emotional security through attachment relationships" (Masten, 2007, p. 926). For Zainab, religious faith was both a predisposing and a protective factor.

The image of the pillar provided a helpful metaphor for Zainab to access resilient beliefs and strategies connected to her faith. Resilient metaphors, stories, and images are most likely to be useful when they are tied to a client's important values, goals, or aspirations. As her therapist learned more about the role of the pillars in Islam, he was able to make clearer links between Zainab's resilient strategies and her values of providing for and protecting her family; these values reinforced her commitment to be resilient (see Figure 4.3). Her therapist asked Zainab questions about the physical pillar in her hometown mosque that resided in her mind as the image she held of herself. These inquiries led Zainab to reflect on the importance of reinforcing a pillar's strength so it could withstand pressures and earth movements. Thus Zainab's own metaphor yielded another perspective on allowing herself to receive help: she was not broken; she was shoring up the foundations (pillar) that supported her family and community. Receiving help was thus transformed for Zainab into a principle for maintaining her resilience and strength.

The enduring strength of a pillar and Zainab's beliefs about the pillar at the mosque in her hometown provided a model for what she needed to do to stay well and free from the distressing voices. To shore up her strength as a pillar, Zainab accepted her psychiatrist's help to

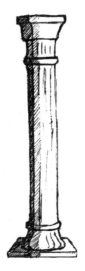

Core Beliefs

Self-as-a-pillar
(strong, steady, and enduring)

Underlying Assumptions

*When I protect and provide for my family,
I am like a pillar.*

*When I am a pillar, I look at the troubles of
the world and know these are only temporary.*

Strategies

Protect and provide for my family.
Resourceful coping at work and at home.

Figure 4.3. Zainab's conceptualization.

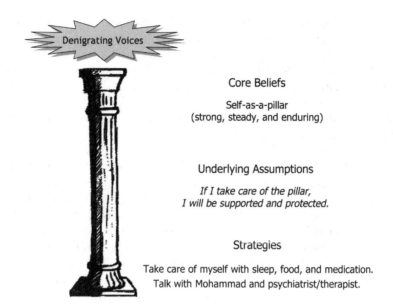

Core Beliefs

Self-as-a-pillar
(strong, steady, and enduring)

Underlying Assumptions

*If I take care of the pillar,
I will be supported and protected.*

Strategies

Take care of myself with sleep, food, and medication.
Talk with Mohammad and psychiatrist/therapist.

Figure 4.4. Zainab's conceptualization using the metaphor of a pillar to connote how her beliefs and coping behavior could keep her free from the denigrating voices.

test out whether the voices were real or within her own mind. Guided by empirical research on psychosis, her psychiatrist spent time helping Zainab learn the voices were not as powerful as they seemed, which significantly reduced their frequency and her distress (Morrison, 2002). Zainab learned new ways to understand the voices, her psychosis, and her reactions to these voices.

Zainab sketched how accepting support could protect her from the voices, which she could still vividly remember even though she was now stabilized on medication (see Figure 4.4). The picture she drew prompted Zainab to remind herself that she was like a pillar, "strong and steady," and that as long as she took care of herself she would be able to stay strong for others and also to manage the voices if they reappeared. At least in the short term this meant continuing on antipsychotic medication, testing out her thoughts and beliefs about the voices, speaking with Muhammad regularly about how she was doing, and attending outpatient appointments with the psychiatrist. In this way, her original metaphor and core belief of herself as a pillar that blocked access to help when she became overwhelmed was modified to become more resilient. Zainab was able to tap into her former resilience and broaden its applications through the addition of new underlying assumptions and strategies, which helped her manage this new challenge to her mental health.

Once Zainab returned home she came back regularly for follow-up sessions, including joint sessions with Muhammad. This work focused on building and maintaining her resilience as she gradually resumed her roles at home and work. It also strengthened Zainab's relationship with her psychiatrist, who helped monitor her reactions to various life stressors and remained available to help Zainab and Muhammad if her functioning deteriorated.

Just as all conceptualizations do, conceptualizations of resilience provide guidelines for intervention. Diagrams and models drawn to capture resilience are likely to provide rich ideas for how clients can address presenting issues and move toward therapy goals. Client values and strengths identified in these conceptualizations can inform the types of interventions in which a client is willing and able to engage. For example, a client who enjoys sports may be more likely to use sports-related physical activity during behavioral-activation treatment of depression.

In summary, conceptualizations of resilience:

- Provide a sense of the whole person, not just problematic issues.
- Broaden potential therapy outcomes from alleviation of distress to include resumption of normal functioning and improved quality of life.
  —Early phases of therapy can use clients' strengths to ameliorate distress.
  —Middle phases of therapy can use clients' strengths to work toward positive therapy goals.
  —Later phases of therapy can help clients consider how resilient applications of their strengths can help them work toward longer-term goals.
- Can help develop a positive therapeutic alliance.
- Provide guides to change.

RESILIENCE AS A THERAPY GOAL

Therapists often consider amelioration of client distress the most important therapy outcome. It is an outcome that CBT therapists generally view as primary; they assume that their clients share this view. However, a recent large survey of people receiving mental health services revealed the most important outcomes for clients are: attaining positive mental health qualities such as optimism and self-confidence; a return to one's usual, normal self; a return to usual level of functioning; and relief from symptoms (Zimmerman et al., 2006). While relief from symptoms is an important outcome for clients, positive mental health and normal functioning are also very important. Mental health problems, especially long-standing difficulties, tend to erode proactive behaviors toward positive goals. Thus it is helpful to evaluate therapy outcome on three dimensions:

1. Amelioration of distress.
2. Building resilience.
3. Proactive movement toward positive personal goals.

As shown in Box 4.1, Seligman conceptualizes three domains of happiness: the pleasant life, the engaged life, and the meaningful life (Seligman, 2002). While Seligman's goal is to conceptualize happiness, his framework also provides a helpful way to think about client strengths and resilience, different stages of CBT, and how to assess therapy outcomes. The first domain, the pleasant life, refers to people's natural desire to maximize pleasant and minimize unpleasant experiences. It encompasses the experience of positive emotions associated with intrinsically pleasurable activities and personal orientations of optimism and hope. In the early phases of therapy clients typically express considerable distress. The amelioration of symptoms is a pressing concern. Positive therapy outcome for distress is typically assessed using symptom measures such as the Beck scales (Beck, Brown, Epstein, & Steer, 1988; Beck, Steer, & Brown, 1996). Symptom relief and maintenance of these gains is usually a prerequisite for a return to normal levels of functioning. In this way, CBT helps clients to redress the balance toward a more pleasant life.

Box 4.1. Domains of Happiness

Pleasant life	Maximizes sensual pleasure and minimizes unpleasant experiences. Includes reminiscence about the past, engagement in hedonistic pleasures in the present, and anticipation of future events.
Engaged life	Use personal strengths (e.g., integrity, wisdom) to participate fully in life, through work, family, or recreation.
Meaningful life	The experience of contributing to institutions larger than the self; service to others.

Note. After Seligman (2002).

The engaged life, Seligman's second domain of happiness, describes people who use their strengths to fulfill personally meaningful goals. Seligman describes strengths as personal qualities such as kindness, integrity, wisdom, the capacity to love and be loved, and leadership. As CBT progresses, therapy goals can shift to helping clients identify and deploy their strengths to work toward an engaged life in which they experience psychological, physical, and social fulfillment. Improvements at this level can be assessed by instruments that measure broader quality of life like the World Health Organization Quality of Life (WHOQOL) tests (Ryff & Singer, 1996). Clearly Zainab's flexibility, linguistic abilities, and concern for her family are important strengths. Zainab's wish to return to her family and new home reflects her commitment to living an engaged life.

The third domain is the meaningful life, that is, belonging to and serving positive institutions including families, communities, work settings, educational settings, political groups, or even nations. Helping others is often cited as one pathway toward positive mental health and resilience (Davis, 1999). In later phases of CBT, therapists may help clients identify values and goals that can enable them to lead more meaningful lives. In Zainab's case, service to her family and community provided the meaning in her life. She did not need the psychiatrist's help to resume a meaningful life once her functioning improved. As was true for Zainab (see Figure 4.4), conceptualizations of resilience often incorporate core beliefs and underlying assumptions that link personal experiences to broader human experience and also highlight how one can contribute to others' lives. In this way CBT can help people function more fully and enjoy a meaningful life.

In general, therapists can consider a number of questions to determine when it might be helpful to ask a client if he or she would like to include a goal of building or restoring resilience:

- Is resilience connected to important client concerns?
- Is it related to the presenting therapy issues?
- Would greater resilience help clients work toward therapy goals (e.g., because the client has a history of recurrent problems in these areas)?
- Does the client see advantages and seem committed to becoming more resilient?

Building resilience can be incorporated into every stage of CBT. Client goals and conceptualizations can guide a therapist to the most appropriate approaches. However, throughout therapy therapists can be alert to opportunities to help clients build resilience through new learning, positive reinforcement of strengths, encouragement of positive client values, and formation of healthy social relationships. Barbara Fredrickson (2001) developed a theoretical framework to conceptualize how clients can broaden and build resilience. She theorizes that when a person experiences positive emotional states their repertoire of beliefs and strategies broadens. Emotional states of joy, pride, happiness, contentment, interest, and love momentarily make a wider array of resilience core beliefs, underlying assumptions, and strategies accessible. Recall the example of Zainab helping Muhammad complete a job application. Bringing humor to the task enabled Zainab to access beliefs and strategies that might not have been available if she was feeling fear or guilt. These beliefs and strategies that are uncovered in the exploration of positive experiences can be applied, in turn, to build personal resources of resilience and broaden their use across physical, social, spiritual, and psychological life domains.

Building and restoring resilience can be the main goal of therapy or it can be adjunctive to other therapy approaches. In the case of Zainab, restoring and broadening her former resilience was a central treatment goal.

VIEWING DISTRESS THROUGH A STRENGTHS LENS

In Zainab's case, the therapist identified strengths that were distinct from her presenting issues. However, therapists can also view client distress through a strengths lens. Nearly every client difficulty encompasses strength when therapists use a strengths-focused lens to view it. For example, overly dependent clients are highly skilled in the art of getting help. Awareness of risk and danger is a strength with evolutionary benefit even though it is troublesome for an anxious client who possesses it in such high degree (Sloman, Gilbert, & Hasey, 2003).

When we conceptualize presenting issues with clients, it is important to use language that communicates the positive functional value of their beliefs and strategies. The following capsule summary provides an example:

THERAPIST: You are skilled at getting help from people, something you learned growing up when you chose to stick close to your sister at school to avoid the bullies on the playground.

KEISHA: Yeah, it was weird to hang out with kids 3 years older, but it meant that the girl-gang in my year couldn't touch me.

THERAPIST: Now, you still have this ability to make friendships. But is it a bit difficult for you to know when to stick close to friends and when to give people a bit of space?

KEISHA: Yes. I guess what I want is to learn to choose when to stick close to people and when to give someone space.

This constructive reframe of an area of client difficulty recognizes strength embodied within a problem. Strengths-based language enables clients to reconceptualize a difficulty in a way that is normalizing and opens up new behavioral possibilities. In the dialogue above, the therapist introduces the idea of choice, an idea that Keisha picks up in the final part of the exchange: choosing to stick close or give people space. Many of the therapist–client dialogues involving Zainab in this chapter make use of language that helps her move toward her goals. If her therapist had used problem-focused language this may have reinforced her sense of herself as "an inadequate mother and Muslim."

A variant on this perspective is asking the client about strengths borne out of the adversity they have experienced. Below are a few ways therapists can introduce this theme:

- "You have suffered from depression for a long time. In my experience, people who have been depressed so long develop some skills or tools they use to cope with it. What helpful things have you learned?"
- "I'm sorry you endured such abuse as a child. How did you manage to get from that childhood to this adulthood? What strengths pulled you through?"
- "You've been battling cancer on and off these past 10 years. How have you managed it? ... You know, I sometimes hear people say that serious illness has positive effects as well as negative. Has the cancer had any positive effects on your life?"

For clarity, we have made a distinction between conceptualizations of problems and conceptualizations of resilience. However, as the examples in this text illustrate, either type of conceptualization will include client core beliefs, conditional assumptions, strategies, and sometimes emotional and physical components. Whether these elements enhance risk or resilience will depend on the context. Zainab's core belief she was a pillar for her family and community was functional in helping her make the transition to a new country. However, this same core belief was not functional when she needed to respond to her denigrating voices. Her therapist worked with Zainab to introduce greater flexibility by stressing the importance of self-care including the option of asking for help from her family as well as her psychiatrist (Figure 4.4).

The goal of CBT is to introduce flexibility so that beliefs and strategies can be used in different ways at different times, depending on the demands of a situation and client goals in that situation. For example, Zainab learned to evaluate the strength of her pillar's foundation on a regular basis. When she felt positive and strong, she devoted considerable time and energy toward caring for her family and community organizations. When her mood worsened or her voices returned, Zainab put more energy into strengthening her own foundations through delegation of tasks, allocating more time to her own sleep and self-care needs, and requesting help from others. The primary foci of her therapy sessions were to help her develop self-observational skills, underlying assumptions, and strategies that enabled her to make these assessments of her well-being and respond effectively.

STRENGTHS, RESILIENCE, AND LEVELS OF CONCEPTUALIZATION

Conceptualization is an evolving process. At the beginning of therapy, clients describe an array of presenting issues and symptoms. Therapists can identify and incorporate strengths into initial conceptualizations of these presenting issues. Over time, explanatory conceptualizations are developed to capture the clients' and therapists' understanding of presenting issues, triggers, and maintenance factors. This is a good time to also begin conceptualizing clients' resilience—to learn how their strengths protect them during challenging circumstances. In later stages of therapy, longitudinal conceptualizations of resilience can explain how strengths have interacted with circumstances across the person's lifetime. This is a time for therapists and clients to form proactive plans for how to use historic and newly acquired strengths to foster future resilience and improve well-being.

In the next three chapters we offer a detailed case example to demonstrate this evolutionary development of case conceptualization throughout the course of therapy with a single client, Mark. These chapters integrate the three principles of case conceptualization outlined in these opening chapters: levels of conceptualization (Chapter 2), collaborative empiricism (Chapter 3), and incorporation of strengths and resilience (Chapter 4). As we follow the case of Mark, we show how these principles of case conceptualization guide him and his therapist in charting a path to meet the twin therapy goals of relieving distress and building resilience.

Chapter 4 Summary

- Client strengths are included in case conceptualization to boost awareness of current client resources and to form a foundation to build resilience.
- Resilience describes how people use their strengths to negotiate adversity.
- Resilience can be conceptualized using the same three levels of case conceptualization described in Chapter 2:
  - Descriptive accounts in cognitive and behavioral terms that articulate a person's strengths.
  - Explanatory (triggers and maintenance) conceptualizations of how strengths protect the person from adverse effects of negative events.
  - Explanatory (longitudinal) conceptualizations of how strengths have interacted with circumstances across the person's life to foster resilience and maintain well-being.
- When building resilience is an explicit therapy goal, client and therapist are more likely to make proactive plans to use identified strengths to foster future resilience and improve well-being—important goals to many clients.

Chapter 5

"Can You Help Me?"
Descriptive Case Conceptualization

THERAPIST: Mark, perhaps you could tell me what led you to call the clinic.

MARK: I don't know where to begin; my life is just a mess.

THERAPIST: I am sorry to hear that, it sounds like things are tough right now. In what ways does your life feel like a mess?

MARK: Well, I worry about my health, I worry about my work, I worry that I will let my family down, I worry about stupid things like whether the gas stove is off even though I have checked it lots of times.

THERAPIST: It sounds like a number of things are distressing you. Are there other ways your life feels like it is a mess?

MARK: Well, I get angry a lot with people at work, and I am feeling down. I am feeling so fed up, and so low, I just don't feel I can cope. (*Begins to look very dejected.*) Like I said, my life is a mess.

This opening dialogue between Mark and his therapist demonstrates that presenting issues can be diverse and overwhelming for the client and, sometimes, even for the therapist. Clear descriptions help organize presenting information and, in the process, often reduce overwhelming feelings and hopelessness. In this chapter we show how the therapist achieves the first level of case conceptualization: describing the presenting issues in CBT terms. Generally, therapists begin with descriptive case conceptualizations because it is necessary to sketch out the territory and characteristics of presenting issues before it is possible to explain how problems are maintained or developed. Thus a clear description of client concerns is a prerequisite to forming a treatment plan that is likely to help.

To construct an initial case conceptualization, the therapist first needs to understand Mark's personal experiences and then integrate these details of his life with CBT theory and research. This chapter demonstrates how the therapist gathers and begins to blend the three key elements within the case conceptualization crucible: particularities of the case, CBT theory, and research. We then show how an initial descriptive case conceptualization helps Mark and his therapist determine treatment goals. Throughout this chapter we illustrate the principles of collaborative empiricism and incorporation of client strengths.

ELEMENTS IN THE CRUCIBLE: PARTICULARITIES OF THE CASE

The first stage of understanding an individual client involves generating a list of presenting issues. We deliberately use the term "presenting issues" rather than presenting *problems* to keep the language neutral and thereby enable an even-handed and constructive description of the issues brought to therapy. Often clients will suggest a broader list of topics for therapy when these are described as "presenting issues" rather than "presenting problems." For example, some clients want to discuss positive life changes, and more neutral language allows these topics to be added to the list.

The process of generating the presenting issues list involves identifying the basic issues, describing and rating their impact, and then prioritizing them for the therapy. These steps are summarized in Box 5.1, together with some important functions each step serves. The following sections show how this process unfolds with Mark and his therapist.

Helping the Client Identify Presenting Issues

Making a presenting issues list requires collaboration. To elicit Mark's collaboration, his therapist offers a rationale for why it is important to specify which areas need to be addressed:

THERAPIST: Mark, there are clearly a number of important areas we need to address if we are going to help you stop feeling like your life is a mess. In order to make sure you get as much benefit as possible

---

Box 5.1. Process and Perceived Value of Listing, Rating, and Prioritizing Presenting Issues

Process	Value
Listing of presenting issues	Reach collaborative agreement for therapy focus. Helps maintain therapy emphasis on central issues that led person to seek help rather than responding to "issues of the week." Helps provide details necessary for an initial descriptive conceptualization by providing information about each issue and how the person is coping. Specific details sometimes illustrate potential relationships between issues and may therefore allow a better targeted treatment of a common feature. For example, a woman may be worried her partner will leave her, that she will lose her job, and that she spends too little time playing with her children. All of these problems may be consequences of excessive Internet usage. Her overuse of the Internet will be prioritized.
Impact ratings	Impact ratings help ensure the list is very specific and salient to this particular person. They help the therapist see the world from the client's perspective and demonstrate the therapist's interest in the client's experience, which strengthens the therapy alliance.
Prioritization	Reduces overwhelmed feelings by framing the list as an opportunity to deal with one issue at a time, effectively, and in small stages. Helps build structure across therapy sessions because several sessions are often required for each issue or set of issues.

---

from therapy, let's make a list that can remind us of everything that we want to achieve in our time working together. Does that sound OK?

MARK: Yeah, I suppose so, I just don't know where to start; there seems to be so much.

THERAPIST: Perhaps we could start with the issues affecting you the most in the last few days and weeks. How is that? (*Mark nods.*) What is bothering you most right now?

MARK: Well, I think the main difficulty is just feeling so low.

THERAPIST: We should write that down on our list. Could you write it down on this sheet for me? (*Mark writes down "Feeling very low."*) We will find out more about this issue for you, but before we do, what other issues would you like to put on this list?

The therapist actively encourages Mark to participate in developing the presenting issues list with verbal prompts and by asking him to write out the list in his own words. The primary focus is on the "here and now." Current concerns are most accessible to recall and they also include obstacles that will need to be overcome to help achieve meaningful change. Over time an understanding of the origins of presenting issues may develop, but it is not necessary for this initial descriptive level of conceptualization.

The presenting issues list is written in simple and concrete terms, using the client's own words. For the therapist, the list is the first stage of seeing the world through the client's eyes and thus discovering what case particularities belong in the conceptualization crucible. During Mark's initial assessment interview he generated the following presenting issues list: feeling very low, health worries, excessive worry about work, anger with work colleagues, and frequent checking of the gas stove and lights.

Identifying Avoidance

Clients sometimes don't report important presenting issues that are masked by avoidance, especially when their avoidance minimizes distress. In the following dialogue, Mark's therapist searches for and begins to examine areas Mark is avoiding.

THERAPIST: Mark, are you not doing any tasks that you feel you should be doing?

MARK: Definitely. I am avoiding meetings, and I think it is becoming a real problem.

THERAPIST: In what way?

MARK: Well, I know that people are commenting about me not being there, but I should present my work at these meetings, and I haven't done the work, so I don't go.

THERAPIST: What would happen if you did go?

MARK: I would feel like a total failure, like I am useless because I am so far behind. If anyone asked me about my work I think I would just fall to pieces. So I cannot go to these meetings, it would be unbearable.

THERAPIST: How long has it been like this?

MARK: About 3 months now.

THERAPIST: Mark, can you remember the last time you attended a meeting and presented some of your work and it seemed to go OK?

\ | /   **INSIDE THE THERAPIST'S HEAD**

Having outlined the problematic side of Mark's avoiding tasks at work, the therapist sees an opportunity to explore Mark's strengths related to this issue. Because Mark is so despondent, the therapist also sees this as an opportunity to help him begin to explore alternatives and build hope.

MARK: Yeah, 6 weeks ago I presented a paper relevant to next year's budget.

THERAPIST: How did you feel during and after the meeting?

MARK: Well, beforehand I was really worried. You know, thinking about it a lot . . .

THERAPIST: I understand, but during the presentation how did it go? You seemed to think it might have gone OK.

MARK: Well, I had to be really focused on what I was presenting, so it seemed fine. I didn't have time to worry during the presentation, you know, and afterward people seemed to appreciate having the information.

The therapist's questions reveal that Mark has begun to avoid tasks at work he used to be able to do. Following this dialogue, Mark is invited to add "not attending meetings" to his presenting issues list. Mark readily identified avoiding tasks at work. For some people avoidance is so long-standing that it is taken for granted and not identified as an issue. In these cases the therapist needs to listen carefully for what is missing from the description of the person's life, drawing on cultural knowledge and what is typical for a person in similar life circumstances. Hence, to develop a presenting issues list the therapist needs to ask both about what the person is doing and what he or she is not doing.

Incorporation of Strengths

As is typical, in the opening session Mark did not spontaneously mention any strengths or aspirational issues to put on his presenting issues list. However, his therapist observed Mark was able to engage in a collaborative relationship easily. Also, Mark described his experiences in terms of thoughts and emotions, which were signs that CBT is an amenable treatment match for him (Safran, Segal, Vallis, Shaw, & Sanstag, 1993). Comments Mark had made earlier suggested that his wife and family are generally supportive. Mark offered side comments that indicated he used to have a number of hobbies. Each of these resources and strengths can help Mark during treatment. In addition to making these covert observations, it is important that Mark's therapist asks directly about strengths.

Identification of strengths should not emerge simply as a by-product of general assessment. There are two main reasons for this: (1) Mark may not be aware of his strengths at this point in time, and (2) explicit questions may reveal strengths not immediately apparent to the therapist. Observe how Mark's therapist explicitly inquires about strengths:

THERAPIST: Mark, we spent a lot of time today discussing issues in your life with which you want help. I also want to find out what is going right in your life. Would that be OK?

MARK: I don't see why, it feels like nothing is going right.

THERAPIST: It can certainly feel that way sometimes. Perhaps I can explain this a bit more. If we can find out what is going right for you, we can help you build in more of the good things and less of the bad. People sometimes have strengths in an area of life that is going well; these can help us figure out a better way of coping in the areas that are harder to manage.

MARK: OK.

THERAPIST: So what things would you regard as your strengths?

MARK: It feels odd even thinking about it this way, I am not sure.

THERAPIST: Most of us find it hard to identify our strengths. What would your wife say are your strengths and good qualities?

MARK: She would say I am a good father and husband, even though I do not see it that way.

THERAPIST: How about your colleagues, what would they say are your strengths and good qualities?

MARK: They would say I am hard working, conscientious, and reliable.

THERAPIST: That's a good start. Why does your wife think you are a good father and husband?

MARK: Well, I really love my kids, I love being around them. I like to play games with them, and I make them laugh. I try to be consider-ate to Clare, like bring her breakfast in bed on Sunday so she can have a break from the kids.

THERAPIST: I can see you are smiling while you say this. That is nice to see.

MARK: But I have been so low of late that I am not sure that they know how much they mean to me.

THERAPIST: So it sounds important that we help you with this. What other strengths do you have?

MARK: I am very organized and thorough. I do my job to a high standard ... well, I used to! I care about people, my friends and my mother and brother. I am quite good at music, but I have not played for ages. (*Seems to brighten further.*)

Following this dialogue, the therapist encouraged Mark to write these strengths on his presenting issues list page in a separate section labeled "Strengths" (see Box 5.2 on p. 132). Mark wrote: "Organized; care about family and friends; good musician, love music; enjoy being a father and husband." Discussion of his strengths shifted the emotional tone of the session, and Mark seemed to feel a bit better about himself. As explained in Chapter 4, positive emotional states broaden clients' thinking (Fredrickson, 2001), potentially opening up discussion of strengths and resilience that would not be reported if the focus of a session was entirely on problems and negative emotional states. Moreover, inclusions of strengths can help build the therapy alliance and also may offer potential routes for creating change. Purposefully eliciting strengths during this early descriptive level of conceptualization begins to lay the groundwork to help Mark build a positive and resilient view of himself as someone who can cope with difficulties.

The client keeps a written copy of the presenting issues list in his or her therapy notebook. The therapist also keeps a copy in his or her notes for easy reference when considering the agenda for each therapy session. The presenting issues list sets out the areas therapy will address. As such, it is likely to change over time. Progress on the issues on the list will be considered at scheduled review sessions. Additional issues may emerge or be added to the list once greater trust has been established within the therapeutic relationship. Experiences such as having been a victim of sexual assault or problems such as erectile dysfunction may only be discussed later in treatment, especially if the client experiences shame regarding these types of issues.

Describing the Impact of Presenting Issues

CBT therapists often use problem checklists as part of intake procedures. While these can be a useful starting point, it is important that presenting issues be understood in terms of the impact on the individual; that is, how much each issue leads to distress and disruption in the person's life. Consider Mark's initial presenting issues list: feeling very low, health worries, worrying excessively about work, indecision, difficulty with checking the gas stove and lights, anger with work colleagues, and not attending meetings. Although this list helps us know some of Mark's concerns, we still need to explore their unique meaning to Mark. The next step typically is to explore the meaning and impact of these issues. Once this is done, Mark and his therapist can prioritize the order in which the issues will be addressed in therapy.

Exploration of the impact of a client's presenting issues reveals important details about the client's life, what he or she values and how current difficulties and strengths affect quality of life. To begin, therapists can ask open-ended questions such as:

> "In what ways does [relevant issue] affect you?"
> "In what ways does this [relevant issue] affect those around you?"
> "What would you be able to do if you did not have to face this issue?"
> "What would key people in your life [partner, children, colleagues, friends] say about how this [relevant issue] affects you and your life?"
> "When this was not a [relevant issue], how was your life different?
> "What were you thinking and doing differently when the [relevant issue] was not a part of your life?"

These questions demonstrate curiosity about how the person's life has been affected and how the person's resilience has been protective (e.g., "What were you thinking and doing differently when the [relevant issue] was not a part of your life?"). Following these general questions, the therapist pursues a fuller understanding with genuine curiosity. It is important to encourage the client to fully disclose details that might otherwise be overlooked. In the following exchange, notice how the therapist pursues greater detail to complete the picture of how low mood affects Mark:

THERAPIST: We have a list of the main issues we want to work on. Next, it would be really helpful if you can tell me a little about how each of these affects your life. For instance, what impact does low mood have on your life?

MARK: I am just so depressed all of the time.

THERAPIST: It sounds like quite a problem for you, feeling depressed all the time. To help me really understand what it is like for you, can you tell me *how* depression affects you?

MARK: I feel tired all the time.

THERAPIST: That is helpful to know. So what impact does feeling tired have on you?

MARK: I don't exercise anymore, or see my friend John, and I cannot be bothered to play piano, which I used to enjoy.

THERAPIST: It sounds like this low mood stops you from doing a lot of things you used to do. Are there other ways feeling low shows itself in your life?

MARK: I find I cannot be bothered at work.

THERAPIST: What do you mean by that?

MARK: Some days I just sit staring at the pile of work I am supposed to do and I just can't get things done properly, to the right standard or on time. So I just don't bother.

THERAPIST: Next to where it says "Feeling very low," we need to write some of the ways that this shows up in your life. Can you write these down? (*Mark writes down "Not seeing John, not exercising, not bothering at work, and not getting my work done on time." Both look at Mark's summary.*) So, Mark, can you summarize the ways in which feeling low is affecting on your life?

MARK: It affects my friendships, my motivation, and my ability to get my work done.

INSIDE THE THERAPIST'S HEAD

The therapist also looks for variation in Mark's experiences to identify exceptions to the general experience of feeling low. These exceptions are used to help identify potential areas of strength and resilience.

THERAPIST: Now, tell me about the last specific time when you had a day when you were feeling OK, not down.

MARK: (*after a pause*) Actually, last Thursday was a pretty good day. I remember I woke up, looked out of the window, it was a beautiful blue sky, and I thought, "Today is going to be OK." I remember listening to music in the car on the way to work and enjoying it. I even sang along a bit. I enjoyed a joke with some colleagues over lunch and didn't really procrastinate on any of my work. I e-mailed a good friend at work suggesting we get together, and he wrote right back and said OK—I was kind of surprised. But you know, it didn't last because that evening I got to thinking about all the things I should have done differently at work. Pretty soon I started to feel low again.

THERAPIST: Thanks, Mark. It's good to hear about a day when you had some good experiences. If I understood correctly, when you felt things were a little better you took the initiative in connecting with your friend and managed to work without procrastinating. How did you think about yourself last Thursday?

MARK: I don't remember. But I did feel better that day ... not such a mess.

As they explore the impact of presenting issues, Mark and his therapist develop a shared understanding of Mark's life and the specific ways in which his current difficulties disrupt his life. At the same time, Mark's therapist asks about times when Mark's difficulties are not present; these are likely to be circumstances associated with Mark's coping constructively. The balance between careful description of struggles and strengths helps reveal potential sources of resilience and instill hope. At the beginning of therapy, however, Mark is more likely to be focused on difficulties than strengths. To put his difficulties in perspective, it helps to ask Mark to rate the perceived impact of his presenting issues.

Rating the Impact of Presenting Issues

Ratings help identify which areas of a person's life are subjectively the most distressing. Only the client knows the relative impact of each issue. In the following dialogue Mark's therapist introduces the rating concept.

THERAPIST: Mark, you are telling me you have been feeling low and sad for a few months now and that this has affected your life in a number of ways. In particular, you don't enjoy your family like you used to, you don't exercise anymore or see your friend John, and you cannot be bothered to play piano, which you used to enjoy. You also think you are not managing at work as well as you used to. Have I got that right?

MARK: Yeah, that is me, a real mess.

INSIDE THE THERAPIST'S HEAD

Here the therapist notes Mark's use of overgeneralization (Kernis, Brockner, & Frankel, 1989), but elects to stay with the primary task of rating the impact of low mood. While the therapist could socialize Mark to the cognitive model and show how his "good Thursday" does not fit with being "a real mess," the choice is made to complete impact ratings so therapy tasks can be prioritized. The therapist believes this forward progress will help Mark more than testing a negative thought, especially since Mark does not yet have the skills to continue thought testing after this session.

THERAPIST: I need to understand how much of a problem this is for you if we are going to be able to figure out which issues we need to start to address first. On a scale from 1 to 10, with 1 being no problem at all, 5 being a moderate problem, and 10 being a really major problem, where would you put this problem of feeling low and sad?

MARK: It is pretty bad, about an 8.

THERAPIST: It sounds like this is an important issue that we will need to help you manage.

MARK: I would like that. I want to get this sorted out.

There is no set threshold for deciding when an issue needs to be a therapy priority. However, when a score is low, perhaps 3 or 4 out of 10, the therapist and client can discuss whether it represents such an area of difficulty that it is necessary to address in therapy, especially if there are a number of other issues with greater impact ratings.

Prioritization of Presenting Issues

After Mark has rated each of his presenting issues, he and his therapist consider the order in which to address them. Presenting issues can be prioritized in a number of ways, such as by their importance, by what causes the most distress, by how easy they may be to change, or by their urgency. Distress, ease of change, and urgency often interact. For example, a presenting issue may be very distressing, very long-standing, and unlikely to easily change. Such an issue may be given a lower immediate priority than an issue producing less distress but perceived as more likely to change.

Prioritization criteria such as distress, ease of change, and urgency are determined by asking questions such as "What is bothering you most?"

or "Which of these issues do you think is the best place to begin?" or "When you look at your impact ratings, which issues do you think are the most important to work with first?" Sometimes one presenting issue is contingent upon another. For example, someone with severe depression needs to be able to get out of bed in the morning before resuming a regular job. Evidence-based therapy protocols also inform prioritization. The CBT protocol for moderate to severe depression suggests behavioral activation as the first step of treatment, especially to target low motivation (Beck et al., 1979); this recommendation is supported by research (Dimidjian et al., 2006; Jacobson, Martell, & Dimidjian, 2001).

When Mark prioritized his presenting issues, he gave highest importance to his low mood and the effect this had on his work. Low mood was

---

Box 5.2. Mark's Presenting Issues List, Prioritized

1. **Feeling low:** I feel like a failure a lot of the time, feel sad, and do not enjoy myself with my family or do pleasurable things like play piano. Other signs are not seeing John, not exercising, not bothering at work, and not getting my work done on time. (8)

2. **Worries about my health:** This stops me from eating and drinking in public places and stops me from going swimming with my children. (8)

3. **Worrying about work:** Every evening my mind is full of worries about work. This leads me to spend over an hour each night thinking through the day, and so I am tense in the evening and do not talk to my wife, which makes her angry. (6)

4. Difficulty making **decisions:** I put off making decisions. When I have to make a decision I spend hours on the Internet or reading magazines to find out which is the best decision, but then I end up confused and unable to act. (6)

5. Problems with **checking:** I spend time each night checking the gas stove, doors, electric sockets, and water faucets. If I do not do this I get very agitated. (5)

6. Getting very **angry** with people at work: When I think over the day I get resentful that others can say off-hand comments, act unhelpfully, and get away with it, and yet I have to be really careful how I act. (5)

7. **Not attending meetings:** When I haven't done the work, I avoid meetings. (4)

STRENGTHS

1. **Organized**
2. **Care about family and friends**
3. **Good musician, love music**
4. **Enjoy being a father and husband**

his most frequent and distressing issue. He and his therapist also agreed that low mood could be readily addressed because there were so many examples of it during each week. Mark's worries about his health were a serious issue that had affected him almost daily for nearly 20 years. Given the long-standing nature of his health concerns, Mark chose these as second priority. The order in which Mark prioritized all his presenting issues is shown in Box 5.2, which Mark wrote in his own language, clearly describing the impact of each issue in specific and concrete terms along with his subjective severity ratings.

The Presenting Issues in Context

While our focus has been on presenting issues that are experienced in the here and now, client concerns are understood within the larger context of the person's current life and history. There are many good reasons for conducting a relatively comprehensive biopsychosocial assessment (cf. Barlow, 2001; Lambert, 2004). As shown in the case of Rose in Chapter 3, the genuine bullying of her work colleagues contributed to her difficulties, and her cultural background affected how she felt able to manage this experience. Similarly for Ahmed (see Chapter 2), cultural context was an important element in understanding his presenting issues. So far, our understanding of Mark has not yet considered this broader context.

What areas should Mark's therapist explore? Box 5.3 highlights assessment areas that may be important to an emerging case conceptualization. This listing is broad and detailed and can be adapted according to the needs of different clients and circumstances. For example, in forensic settings, forensic history and risk assessments are essential and would normally be gathered in detail for every client. In private practice settings, the degree of necessary forensic detail might be determined according to the client's response to a broad opening question such as, "Have you ever had any legal difficulties that relate to [these presenting issues]?" As this question highlights, therapists only need to be concerned with history that has relevance for the presenting issues. An arrest for underage drinking may not be relevant 30 years later if the client does not have a current substance misuse problem.

Collaboration during Assessment

In early phases of assessment and conceptualization it is important that therapists balance the need to build a strong therapeutic relationship with the need to gather contextual information. There is a potential tension between a therapist's need for a comprehensive assessment and the client's desire to get help with the presenting issues. Therapists manage

Box 5.3. Areas to Consider in a Biopsychosocial Assessment

MULTIAXIAL DIAGNOSTIC WORK-UP
- Note especially any Axis I, II, and III comorbidity as well as severity and chronicity of problems.

CURRENT LIFE SITUATION
- Relationship with partner (satisfaction/dissatisfaction)
- Home (satisfaction/dissatisfaction)
- Work (aspirations, satisfaction/dissatisfaction)
- Leisure/relaxation
- Relationships with friends and family/social support
- Current stressors/concerns
- Financial resources/difficulties
- Health problem(s)/input from health professionals
- Spiritual or religious issues (satisfaction/dissatisfaction)
- Goals and aspirations

HISTORY
- Family history (mother, father, siblings, extended family, other significant figures)
- Cultural backgrounds: racial, ethnic, gender, sexual orientation, spiritual, generational
  Often overlooked: assessing the impact of match or mismatch with the community one is in
- Childhood sexual and/or physical abuse/neglect/emotional and practical support
- School and education
- Employment history
- Relationships (sexual partners, friends, and family)
  Often overlooked: domestic violence and sexual behavior
- Past psychological difficulties
  Often overlooked: substance abuse
- Coping with past difficulties: include assessment of personal and social strengths
- Major life events or trauma (e.g., unwanted sexual experiences in adolescence and adulthood)

PSYCHIATRIC HISTORY
- Treatment for previous psychological difficulties
  Often overlooked: past therapy failures
- Previous suicide attempts/self-destructive behavior/hospitalizations

---

Box 5.3 (cont.)

MEDICAL HISTORY

- Significant comorbid medical conditions like chronic pain
- Medications history
  Often overlooked: prescription medication misuse and abuse

FORENSIC HISTORY (OFTEN OVERLOOKED)

SAFETY AND RISK

- Risk of self-harm or suicide
- Violence at home
  Often overlooked: risk to others

OBSERVATION

- Person's presentation (physical, emotional, ease with expressing problem[s])
- Significant personality traits (e.g., wanting to please, hostility, externalizing, dependency)
- Cognitive functioning: cognitive distortion in memory or perception
- Intellectual level
- Ease of attaining rapport
- How the therapist reacted to client overall, and at key points in the meeting
- Person's response to questions, comments, and early therapeutic interventions
  Often overlooked: client skills and motivation to change

---

this tension in many different ways. Some therapists conduct a broad assessment before therapy begins. Such assessment may include pretherapy screening interviews, a battery of preappointment measures, informant interviews, and structured history questionnaires. Other therapists gather just enough assessment information to begin treatment and then gather additional relevant assessment information as therapy proceeds. Often, a balance between these two approaches is struck whereby clients complete a detailed written history to give to the therapist at the beginning of therapy. For this purpose, two of the authors use an Aid to History Taking Form (see the Appendix at the end of the book) as an efficient way of collecting important information prior to the first assessment session. This form provides relevant contextual information that can be reviewed by the therapist at the beginning of therapy and explored in greater detail with the client as needed throughout therapy.

Mark completed an Aid to History Taking Form (see Appendix 5.1), which provided his therapist with demographic information, Mark's initial perceptions of presenting issues, and contextual background information. His therapist was able to draw heavily on this information in the initial CBT sessions. Mark's therapist noted the following areas as important issues to keep in mind during therapy:

- Mark had a history of depression that he could date to early adulthood. However, the most recent onset was 2 years ago when his father died, he accepted a promotion at work, and his second child was born.
- He reports asthma and eczema and no other medical conditions.
- Mark grew up in a family with moderate income and was in the cultural majority in his community in terms of race, religious affiliation, and ethnicity. He learned gender roles common to his community (e.g., men and boys were expected to care for women and girls).
- Mark's excessive health worries began at age 18 years.
- Mark has been with his partner Clare for 14 years, and the marriage appears to be happy.
- Mark's father suffered from bipolar disorder and attempted to kill himself when Mark was 8.
- Mark's father's condition led to periods of family distress with parental arguments and financial pressures.
- Mark's mother could be quite critical, and she sometimes was rather preoccupied with Mark's father's mental health when Mark was growing up.
- Sometimes Mark's mother asked him to assume more of a parental than a sibling relationship toward his brother David, who was quite a few years younger.
- Mark had an important relationship with his grandfather, who was a role model and supported Mark at difficult times, including his father's suicide attempt.
- Music was an important and enjoyable activity for Mark since late childhood.

His therapist also looks to rule out important areas that potentially might affect therapy:

- Mark did not report suffering any physical, sexual, or emotional abuse as a child.
- He did not report a history of self-harm.
- He does not currently abuse alcohol or other substances.

Each section of the Aid to History Taking Form may provide vital information for understanding the development and maintenance of Mark's presenting issues. Throughout the initial stages of CBT the therapist is alert to information that may bear on the presenting issues and uses clinical judgment about what to consider and when to consider it. Although Mark's therapist noted the issues above, she chose to focus initially on Mark's presenting issues and goals. At the same time, she kept in mind that any of these other issues might grow in significance as she and Mark began to work toward his goals.

Empiricism in Standardized Assessment Tools

CBT therapists typically use standardized assessment tools to assess depression, anxiety, and other presenting issues. The advantages of using relevant standardized measures of mood and behavior is that the therapist can compare an individual client's responses with previous clients' as well as responses of large groups of people from research studies. In addition, when standardized questionnaires are given multiple times throughout treatment, they can be used to evaluate the effectiveness of therapy. Client and therapist can discuss changes in scores and compare these with the client's subjective perceptions of improvement or a decline in functioning. The therapist can compare changes on standardized measures with those obtained in outcome research to see whether he or she is obtaining the expected results with a particular treatment approach. If not, this can be a signal to reexamine the conceptualization or treatment plan. For these important reasons, Mark's therapist introduced two standard mood measures in the initial session, and Mark agreed to complete these weekly to track therapy progress.

At intake, Mark scored 20 on the Beck Depression Inventory–II (BDI-II; Beck et al., 1996) which placed him in the mild/moderate level of depression range. On the Beck Anxiety Inventory (BAI; Beck et al., 1988) his score was 26, indicating moderate anxiety levels. This information was discussed with Mark: "I notice on this measure of depression you completed this week that you scored in the mild/moderate range for depression and moderate range for anxiety. Do these levels fit with your experience of your low mood and how anxious you feel?" If Mark had not reported low mood or anxiety in the interview, his therapist might have prompted, "Do you think we should add depression and anxiety to our list?"

Although the BDI-II and BAI are not diagnostic instruments they provide useful baseline measures of depression and anxiety symptoms that contribute to diagnostic criteria. Also, individual item scores sometimes prove useful in identifying additional presenting issues. For instance, item 9 on the BDI-II inquires about suicidal ideation. If Mark had rated this item more highly (or if he reported a history of self-harm), then a more comprehensive assessment of suicide risk would have been undertaken. On the BAI, Mark endorsed the following items as most distressing: unable to relax, a fear of the worst happening, and a fear of dying. His ratings could prompt questions that might lead quickly to identification of Mark's health worries.

Consistent with the principle of focusing on strengths, we advocate that therapists also use outcome measures that assess strengths and well-being. Psychotherapy and psychotherapy research tend to focus on dissatisfaction and dysfunction, not on satisfaction and function (Fava, Ruini, & Belaise, 2007; Ryff & Singer, 1996, 1998). A handbook by Lopez and Snyder (2003) is a resource for therapists seeking appropriate measures of well-being. In addition to the Beck instruments, Mark's therapist used a measure that assesses quality of life in a number of domains (Gladis, Gosch, Dishuk, & Crits-Christoph, 1999), the World Health Organization Quality of Life Brief scale (WHOQOL; Harper & Power, 1998). The WHOQOL surveys physical, psychological, social, and environmental quality of life to highlight positive factors in a client's life as well as areas for concern. Mark's profile indicated that he experiences quite impaired quality of life particularly in the physical, psychological, and social domains.

The assessment information and presenting issues list help specify and organize client details as well as place these in context. This process helped organize experiences that had become amalgamated in an unhelpful way in Mark's mind. Clarity on these presenting issues sets the stage to help Mark develop descriptive conceptualizations for his struggles.

Mark's therapist now needs to add relevant CBT theory and research to the crucible. The following section illustrates how the therapist unpacked Mark's presenting issues and linked them to relevant cognitive-behavioral models.

ELEMENTS IN THE CRUCIBLE: THEORY AND RESEARCH

Mark's therapist used two common descriptive case conceptualization methods to link Mark's presenting issues with CBT theory: functional analysis (Kohlenberg & Tsai, 1991) and the five-part model (Padesky & Mooney, 1990). While we emphasize these two conceptualization approaches in this chapter, therapists can use any framework that links a client's presenting issues to evidence-based theories. Factors therapists can use to choose an appropriate conceptualization approach are described in Box 5.4.

Box 5.4. Deciding Which Conceptualization Schematic to Use	
Question	**Issues to consider**
Is an evidence-based theoretical model directly relevant to the case? (see Box 1.3)	Can this model be used to describe the presenting issues in cognitive-behavioral terms?
Which conceptual model or descriptive approach is most likely to build collaboration, draw out client strengths, and elicit hope in this key early stage of therapy?	Use clinical judgment and be attentive to client feedback.
What is the simplest possible framework that provides a good-enough level of description?	The best conceptualizations are as simple as possible without losing essential meaning.

Functional analysis is a method that maps behavioral theory onto presenting issues by examining behavioral contingencies (Kohlenberg & Tsai, 1991). The five-part model, described in Chapter 2, is a widely used method to describe presenting issues in biopsychosocial terms (Greenberger & Padesky, 1995; Padesky & Greenberger, 1995). Both functional analysis and the five-part model can be used collaboratively to meet many of the initial functions of case conceptualization: linking theory, research, and practice; normalizing presenting issues; increasing empathy; and organizing large amounts of complex information (see Chapter 1, Box 1.1).

Functional Analysis: ABC Model

Behavioral research demonstrates that behaviors can be learned and extinguished on the basis of patterns of association, reward, and punishment. The following simple acronym distills functional analysis into a format that is readily accessible to clients and therapists in the early stages of conceptualizing presenting issues:

A (antecedent)—B (behavior)—C (consequence)

Antecedents refer to the contexts associated with the onset of behaviors. These can be associations, conditions, or triggers for the behavior. Antecedents can be external to the person (e.g., meetings at work) or internal (e.g., particular thoughts). For the purposes of case conceptualization the behaviors highlighted in this model are typically "molar" or higher-order behaviors such as behavioral avoidance (Martell, Addis, & Jacobson, 2001). It is important to note that in functional analysis, behavior can include cognitive processes such as worry. Consequences are typically direct rewards (e.g., praise) or secondary rewards that come from avoiding aversive experience (e.g., reduction in anxiety after avoiding a meeting).

During the descriptive stage of case conceptualization functional analysis can be used to map how, when, and where behaviors occur, noting the consequences (behavioral contingencies) across different contexts (Martell et al., 2001). Thus functional analysis helps articulate the presenting issues in functional terms. Therapist and client can identify molar behaviors within the presenting issue and use the ABC model to determine how these behaviors link to contingencies. The following transcript shows how Mark and his therapist described Mark's avoidance at work in functional terms:

THERAPIST: Mark, you told me when you feel low you withdraw into yourself and this creates problems at work because you start putting off work tasks. People at work notice this. (*Mark nods, indicating that this is an accurate capsule summary.*) Can you say more about what sorts of tasks you have been putting off?

MARK: (*Thinks for a few seconds.*) I can just about do trivial tasks like keeping up with routine e-mail. But anything that requires a lot of concentration, is more complex, or involves other people, I put off. Sometimes I can't put things off because other people are in charge of the project and I *have to* turn up, but I'll do the minimum because I just can't face doing more. So I guess anything that requires effort or other people.

THERAPIST: Tell me a bit about what happens in the hours before you put a task off. Can you remember a specific time you did this recently?

MARK: Last week I had to put together some figures for a budget. Mary asked me to do it, but set a vague deadline. I didn't do it. I guess I couldn't face it because I felt plain low; I didn't think I had the energy to do the research. I worried I would get it wrong and when others noticed it was wrong I would get the blame. I just got really wound up and uneasy, like I wanted to run. (*Starts to cry.*)

THERAPIST: It's OK, Mark. I can see this is upsetting for you, which is why we are looking at it together. Take your time.

MARK: (*trying to pull himself together*) I just try not to think about it.

THERAPIST: I can understand that. What we are doing here is not easy.

Let's see if we can work together to figure out how putting off tasks at work makes sense for you.

> **INSIDE THE THERAPIST'S HEAD**
>
> Mark's tearfulness emphasizes how distressing the antecedents are (feeling low, lack of energy, and worry). The therapist chooses to use this moment to empathically build hope, using functional analysis as a method to understand Mark's distress. She notes that Mark has also communicated the use of avoidance ("I try not to think about it") as a way of relieving distress.

THERAPIST: You have told me about a number of important things that were going on beforehand, and I'm going to write them down. Let's call those "Antecedents," which means "things that happened before." (*Writes "Low mood," "Lack of energy," "Worry about failure," "Anxious," "Try not to think about it."*) Now, I'm going to write down what you then did in the situation when you were feeling upset. I'll put this under "Behaviors." (*Writes "Avoid complex tasks," "Avoid tasks involving other people," "Put things off."*) Is anything missing?

MARK: No, that is what it is like.

THERAPIST: Can you tell me what happens to the worry and anxiety afterward?

MARK: I feel really relieved that I won't have to do it. (*Smiles sheepishly, but this quickly turns into a look of worry as he seems to get carried away by another thought.*) But then I begin worry about losing my job. (*Looks distressed again.*)

THERAPIST: I can see that would be upsetting. Let's write both of those things under "Consequences." (*Writes "Reduced anxiety," "Worry about losing my job"* [see Figure 5.1].) Looking at the board, Mark, can you summarize what you think we have found out about this problem of putting off tasks at work?

MARK: Well, I do it because I feel low and tired and I am sure I'll screw it up, and afterward I feel relieved that I don't have to do it. But the relief doesn't last long!

THERAPIST: That's a good summary. Let's look at this situation we have mapped out. This is the "ABC" model for understanding behaviors. "B" is for behavior. The "A," or antecedents, help us figure out *when* you avoid tasks at work, and the "C," or consequences, can tell us a

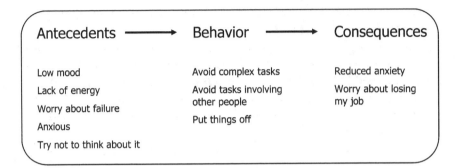

Figure 5.1. Mark's work avoidance: functional analysis.

lot about *why* you avoid tasks. We can see you avoid things because of the relief you feel. Unfortunately, avoidance is not working as well as you'd like, because pretty soon you start worrying again. We'll talk more about that later, but for now you've done a great job of mapping how, when, and why you avoid things at work in ABC terms. Is there anything you want to add, ask, or say about this?

MARK: People are starting to notice I am not doing things. The next day I e-mailed Mary and said I was too busy and suggested she ask someone else to do it. I am doing that a lot.

THERAPIST: Do you want to add that to our agenda for today?

MARK: Yes, should I write this down in my therapy notebook?

THERAPIST: That's a good idea. Near the end of our time today, when we talk about tasks for next week, I'll make a note to make sure we come back to this.

In this example, Mark's avoidance has positive consequences (short-term relief from distress) that reward his behavior and also negative consequences (increased worry about losing his job and incomplete work projects that weigh on Mark). When there are dissonant consequences (costs as well as benefits), therapists can constructively use functional analysis to identify preferred behaviors that might have greater benefit with fewer costs, as illustrated in this subsequent dialogue between Mark and his therapist:

THERAPIST: So when you avoid or put things off, you tend to feel a little better, but at a cost. You don't make progress in your work and you worry about losing your job.

MARK: Yeah.

THERAPIST: Ideally, how would you like things to turn out when you approach a task?

MARK: (*thinking*) I don't know. I have been avoiding things for so long. I almost can't imagine doing it differently.

THERAPIST: It's hard changing habits. You mentioned that last Thursday went well, and you did not put things off. Can we learn anything from that experience?

MARK: I would like to think I could have more days like that, but it felt like a one-time event.

THERAPIST: OK, can you think of someone whom you respect for how they handle work projects? Someone who seems to prioritize their work effectively?

MARK: Well, there is this fellow at work named Peter. He is really good at dealing with things without getting in a mess. He doesn't worry about things, and when he makes a mistake he just sort of admits it and then does the next thing right. He doesn't get all caught up in it, in worrying. I want to bottle what he has. (*Laughs.*)

THERAPIST: (*laughing too*) If we could bottle not worrying too much that would be easier for sure. So, ideally you would like to approach tasks not worrying about them going wrong. You would acknowledge everything you did well, and if there were any mistakes admit them but not get caught up in worrying about them. Instead, get on with the next task. How different is this from how things normally turn out for you?

MARK: Lots different!

THERAPIST: Does Peter's way seem like something you could do?

MARK: Not really ... I don't know, I guess ... You know last Thursday after I had had a good day ... the worry wasn't so bad, really. I was able to not get caught up in it so much.

THERAPIST: OK. So when you have a good day you are less likely to get caught up in the worry and more likely to get on with your work. (*Mark nods.*) Let's come back to that later, then, when we start thinking about goals for our work together. But for now we can see that worrying about work leads you to avoid tasks, put them off, and this makes you feel more tense and creates difficulties in completing tasks. The only benefit of avoidance is that you feel better in the short term. There may be alternative ways of dealing with tasks that are closer to how you would like things to be, closer to how Peter seems to do things, and closer to how you do things on a good day too.

As shown in this extended example, contemporary behavioral approaches that use the ABC model of functional analysis (cf. Martell et al., 2001) are entirely consistent with the principles of a collaborative, constructive, and empirical approach to case conceptualization. They have the advantage of generally being readily acceptable to clients and are relatively easy to apply therapeutically with many of the issues clients bring to therapy.

The Five-Part Model

While functional analysis provides a simple model based on behavioral contingencies, cognitive-behavioral therapists often want to include client interpretations and appraisals of experience as distinct and important conceptualization factors. Therapists can expand their descriptive framework by articulating key presenting issues in terms of the five-part model (Padesky & Mooney, 1990) introduced in Chapter 2. While still simple enough for clients to readily understand, this biopsychosocial model differentiates overt behaviors from thoughts, emotions, and physical reactions. As demonstrated in the case of Ahmed, the five-part model can also incorporate the impact of cultural and other environmental influences that may affect client's responses, even though these are not physically present as observable antecedents.

Environment and Emotion Factors

The following dialogue illustrates how Mark's health concerns were elicited using the five-part model. As before, his therapist focuses on a recent and specific example to develop a comprehensive description. She diagrams the information as the discussion proceeds. The completed diagram can be seen in Figure 5.2.

THERAPIST: On your presenting issues list you wrote, "Worries about my health." I would like to find out a little bit more about this issue. Is that OK? (*Mark nods.*) Perhaps you could tell me about a recent time these worries affected you.

MARK: Yes. I was out shopping with my wife and family last weekend, and we went to a café to have a drink and something to eat. I thought I saw some lipstick on the coffee cup and then I just felt awful, so worried.

THERAPIST: This sounds like a good example. Does this happen often?

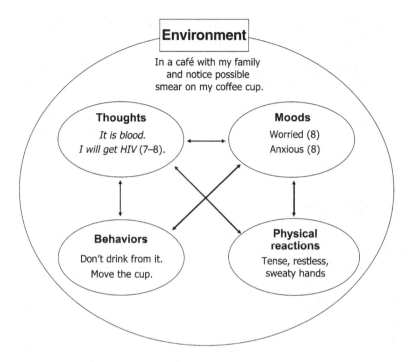

Figure 5.2. Completed five-part model for Mark's health worries.

MARK: It varies, but most weeks there will be two or three examples of this sort of thing.

THERAPIST: OK. I am just going to summarize what we are saying here by drawing this out. So you were in the café and you noticed lipstick on your coffee cup. (*Writes this down.*) I call this the "environment" you were in. (*Writes this.*) And you say you felt awful, very worried, and anxious? (*Mark nods.*) If you remember how we used the scale before of 1 to 10, how bad was this experience?

\\ | / INSIDE THE THERAPIST'S HEAD

Mark's therapist notes that this example could signal either obsessional worry or health anxiety. Mark's thoughts will help differentiate between these two issues. The five-part model is introduced to gather the information necessary to make this clinical decision. The decision will inform the treatment plan because it will guide the therapist to the most relevant evidence-based therapy approach.

MARK: It was bad, about an 8.

THERAPIST: It sounds like a tough situation. I have written down "Anxious," with your rating, "8," under "Moods." Let's look at this so far, to check that I have gotten it right.

Mark readily identified that he felt awful in this situation. Since this is the first component of the five-part model spontaneously described by Mark, the therapist writes it just below the situational factor, environment. The next step is to further inquire about this experience, collaborating with Mark as the five-part model helps to organize the details he provides.

Physiological Factors

THERAPIST: So you were feeling really worried. When you felt this bad, what else did you notice?

MARK: I felt very restless, and quite wound up and tense.

THERAPIST: So you noticed lots physical sensations and body experiences. Did you notice anything else?

MARK: My hands were sweaty.

THERAPIST: I am going to add those to the picture. Can we call these physical reactions?

MARK: That's fine.

THERAPIST: So when you felt worried you noticed yourself feeling restless and your hands were sweaty. What do you think caused these reactions?

MARK: Well, it was the anxiety I was feeling.

THERAPIST: OK. So I am going to draw a line between "Moods" and "Physical reactions."

Behavioral Factors

THERAPIST: OK, Mark, so you were in the café feeling anxious, noticing that you felt tense, restless, and sweaty. How did you cope? What did you do?

MARK: Well, I knew I could not drink the coffee, but I thought my wife would see and get angry with me for not even being able to drink without it being an issue. In the end, I pretended to drink from the cup. Then when she went to the toilet, I moved my cup to an empty table.

THERAPIST: You would not drink from the cup because you had noticed a lipstick mark and you ended up moving it to another table. Is that right? (*Mark nods.*) Let's put that down under "Behaviors." Behaviors will include all the actions you take. How did you feel when you moved your cup?

MARK: Less anxious, less tense.

THERAPIST: OK, so can I draw a line indicating that your feelings were influenced by your behavior?

MARK: Definitely, as soon as I got rid of the cup I felt better.

An emerging understanding of Mark's health concerns is clarified with the addition of each element in the five-part model. Just like his work avoidance, Mark's avoidance of drinking from the cup provides relief from his anxiety.

Cognitive Factors

The fifth element of the five-part model emphasizes the importance of understanding the appraisal or interpretation of a situation. Not everyone feels anxious when they notice a possible lipstick mark on a coffee cup. Mark's therapist wondered what this meant to him. Mark's interpretation or appraisal of this experience should explain his emotional reaction and behavioral avoidance. It will also help his therapist determine whether Mark's distress is caused by obsessional thinking, which emphasizes control and responsibility, or health worries, which emphasize the uncertainty of health risks (Salkovskis & Warwick, 2001).

THERAPIST: You could not drink from the cup because you noticed a lipstick mark and you ended up moving it to another table. OK, so you are really struggling with these worries that you will. ... Sorry, I am not sure I understand what would be so bad about drinking from the cup? What would have happened if you had drunk from it?

INSIDE THE THERAPIST'S HEAD

If Mark has difficulty describing his thoughts, his therapist is ready to help Mark articulate his thoughts. For example, the therapist might use imagery to evoke the café situation or even set up a behavioral experiment in session in which Mark is invited to drink from a used coffee cup with a red mark on it in order to elicit associated thoughts.

MARK: I was really worried that it could have been blood, or saliva on the cup and that I would get HIV.

THERAPIST: So you worried that you would contract HIV?

MARK: Yes.

THERAPIST: No wonder this is a concern for you. Anyone who thought they would get HIV would feel worried. So perhaps to understand this situation fully we need another box I'll call "Thoughts." What should we write in there?

MARK: The smear is blood and I will get HIV.

THERAPIST: Mark, rate how strongly you believed in the café that you could have gotten HIV from that cup. Rate your belief when you felt most anxious. Use "1" for "I don't believe it all," and 10 for "I believe it completely."

MARK: It felt pretty realistic. If I drank from the cup my belief that I would get HIV was about a 7 or 8. Sometimes my concern about it reaches a 9 or 10.

THERAPIST: So to understand why you felt so anxious it helps to appreciate that you were pretty concerned you might get HIV. So we can see the connection between "notice a possible smear" and your thoughts and draw an arrow between "Thoughts" and "Moods." (*Completes the five-part model as shown in Figure 5.2.*) What do you make of this diagram? Does it capture what it is like for you?

MARK: Definitely, it is just what it is like for me.

This initial descriptive conceptualization of Mark's health worries demonstrates links between his cognitive, emotional, physiological, and behavioral responses to particular environmental cues, in this case a smear on a cup. The specific details captured in Figure 5.2 highlight his distress and the disruption to his life. Mark's therapist was able to write down the information as it was gathered so that Mark could begin to see the links between each of the elements of his experience. At this stage the therapist has not yet inquired about the relationships among all five parts. Therefore, bidirectional arrows only reflect the relationships reported thus far.

The five-part model can be used flexibly. The order in which elements are identified can vary according to what parts of the experience are most salient to a client. Generally, therapists are encouraged to write down observations in the order the client presents them. Thus when Mark noted feelings and body sensations first, these were written first, even though his thoughts were highly relevant to the therapist in terms of distinguishing between OCD thoughts and health worries. Mark was also asked to rate the strength of his beliefs and distress. These ratings add depth to the descriptive conceptualization because they establish the extent of his health concerns. If Mark did not believe strongly that he could get HIV from the cup then it would be hard to understand the extent of his distress. In that case, his therapist would need to ask additional questions until Mark's level of distress was explained by the conceptual model.

Descriptive Conceptualizations as an Opportunity for Normalization

Further discussions with Mark revealed that his HIV worries led to avoidance of eating or drinking in nearly all public places. He believed food, dirty cutlery, or dishware could increase his risk of acquiring HIV. Mark closely studied dishware, glasses, and cutlery in order to determine how clean and hence "virus free" they were. Similarly, Mark did not go swimming with his children because he believed he was at increased risk of HIV infection from pools. While all these circumstances were highly distressing to Mark, he revealed these details with some reluctance to his therapist. People often worry that their behaviors or thought processes signal that they are odd or crazy. This concern can be reinforced by family and friends who identify particular beliefs as illogical or even ridiculous.

Descriptive conceptualizations can be used as vehicles to normalize clients' experiences. This is one of the functions of conceptualization (see Box 1.1). Imagining life events from the client's perspective is one of the first steps a therapist can take toward normalization. Even though drinking from a cup will not transmit HIV, the therapist can imagine what it would feel like to hold that thought. In light of this appraisal, the resulting anxiety makes sense. The therapist can then honestly say to Mark, "I understand why you were so distressed. If I thought drinking from a cup would give me HIV, then I would be anxious too." Therapy will help Mark investigate his erroneous appraisals. In the meantime, descriptive conceptualizations help him see that his reactions make good sense in the context of his interpretations of the situation.

Five-Part Model Descriptions of Low Mood and Other Presenting Issues

Mark and his therapist also used the five-part model to conceptualize his low mood. They focused on his evening routine because Mark reported he nearly always felt low during that time of day. Mark's habit was to spend an hour or more each evening scrutinizing his recollections of each encounter during the day. He tried to remember anything he said that was incorrect or possibly contentious. His nightly review convinced Mark he did nothing right and, as a result, he would lose his job. His thoughts raced ahead, imagining that when he was without a job he would lose his house and his wife and children would see him as a failure.

Mark's therapist organized these observations into the five-part model as shown in Figure 5.3. While many of these same issues emerged in the functional analysis of Mark's work avoidance (Figure 5.1), the five-part model also specifies Mark's interpretation of the situation associated with his distress. Mark's low mood seems characterized by a view of himself as inept and a failure. Notice connections are drawn between all the circles in Figure 5.3. This drawing is consistent with the theoretical idea that depressive feelings, thoughts, physiological states, and behaviors are *reactivated* during a recurrent depression (Lau, Segal, & Williams, 2004).

Descriptive conceptualizations using schematics like the five-part model can be developed for each of Mark's presenting issues. However, it is more likely only one or two prioritized presenting issues will be

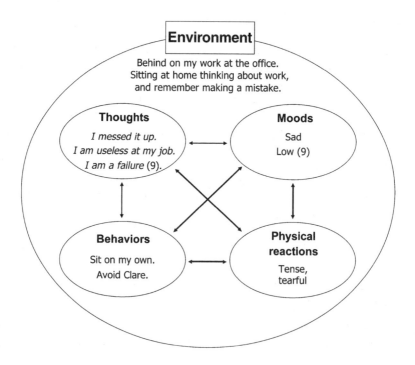

Figure 5.3. A five-part model conceptualization of Mark's low mood.

described in this manner. These serve as useful frameworks to begin to understand Mark's experiences. In addition, they introduce the central idea of CBT theories to Mark. That is, he begins to observe how his thoughts, moods, behaviors, and physical reactions interact within the environmental context of his life. Thus descriptive conceptualization frameworks add cognitive theory to the crucible in terms the client can understand. At this point, the conceptualization crucible contains general cognitive theory interwoven with the particularities of the case, understood through a detailed description of Mark's presenting issues. We have begun to turn up the heat via active collaboration and empiricism, gathering observational data and organizing it within conceptual frameworks.

Clinical Summary

When Mark's therapist combines these additional sources of information with the clinical interview data, the following picture emerges of Mark:

Mark is in his mid-30s, married with two children, successful in his work but currently experiencing work difficulties due to mild to moderate depression and moderate anxiety. He has long-standing fears of being infected with HIV. His social life is constricted, partly due to family commitments and yet also hampered by a pattern of social withdrawal when his mood deteriorates. More broadly, he is from a white, working-class environment and describes his upbringing as generally happy although his father suffered bipolar disorder. His presenting issues are severely affecting his quality of life. He has experienced depression for 2 years following a particularly difficult time in his life during which three life events intersected: the death of his father, a work promotion involving additional duties, and the birth of his second child. He describes a particularly close relationship with his maternal grandfather, which grew especially strong during a period in his childhood when Mark's father was in the hospital following a suicide attempt.

Diagnostic Impressions

From the various sources of information use in Mark's assessment, his therapist derived the following provisional diagnostic impressions for Mark within the DSM-IV-TR (American Psychiatric Association, 2000) multiaxial system:

Diagnostic Summary

Axis I: Major depressive disorder, recurrent, in partial remission
           Rule out obsessive–compulsive disorder
           Rule out hypochondriasis
Axis II: Avoidant personality traits
Axis III: Asthma, eczema
Axis IV: Occupational problems (possibility of losing his job)
Axis V: 55

CBT theories of particular diagnostic profiles provide fertile bases from which to hypothesize likely client beliefs, appraisal processes, and behaviors. Thus diagnoses guide a CBT therapist to promising fields of literature and research.

CASE CONCEPTUALIZATION AND GOAL SETTING

By the end of this assessment phase of therapy, Mark and his therapist have identified his presenting issues, rated their impact, and prioritized their importance. In addition, Mark's therapist has completed initial diagnostic impressions, collected baseline measures of depression and anxiety symptoms and, using functional analysis and the five-part model, helped Mark form initial descriptive conceptualizations of his highest-priority issues: low mood and HIV worries. Important contextual information from Mark's developmental history and current life situation has been noted. Like Mark's therapist, readers of this chapter are probably already formulating hypotheses about potentially helpful treatment plans. However, before treatment begins it is important for Mark to set treatment goals so therapy is focused toward the goals he wants to achieve. As is done with case conceptualization, goals are defined collaboratively:

THERAPIST: Before we begin working on these presenting issues, it will help to know what your goals are. We know how things are for you now. How would you like them to be? How will we know whether we are making progress? For example, with your top-priority issue, low mood. ... What do you hope we accomplish in therapy?

MARK: I want to feel less sad, not feel that I am a failure so much of the time.

THERAPIST: OK, how would we define feeling less sad? On that 1 to 10 scale, where your mood is 8 right now, how would you like to feel?

MARK: A 1 would be good.

THERAPIST: That would be great. Just as a check, were you at a 1 most of the time before you felt depressed?

MARK: Not really. My mood goes up and down. Maybe normally, when I'm not so low, my mood goes between 1 and 5, depending on what's happening in my life.

THERAPIST: So what mood level would seem like good progress to you, if you are at an 8 now?

MARK: I suppose if I was at 5 or lower most of the time—maybe below 5 most of the time. Yeah, that would be pretty normal. What do you think?

THERAPIST: That sounds good to me. If you felt this way, below 5 most of the time, what would you be doing that you do not do at the moment?

MARK: I'd play piano regularly and see my friend John at least once a week.

THERAPIST: And would there be any changes with Clare or the children?

MARK: Yes. I would like to get this mood out of my head so I experience happiness with them every day.

THERAPIST: OK, have you got that presenting issue list? Let's write down your goals on the other side. So the first is to feel less sad, 5 or less, and second to play piano again. A third is to see John once a week, and a fourth to experience happiness every day with Clare and the children. How do you feel about these as goals?

MARK: Good. I would like to be able to do this.

With his therapist's help, Mark identifies goals that represent personally defined improvement in mood. Goals can be further specified as short term, medium term, and longer range. A short-term goal is achievable within a month or two, a medium-term goal toward the end of a period of treatment (approximately 10 to 20 sessions, or 6 months), and a longer-term goal may be targeted posttreatment, during the next year or more. A short-term goal for Mark in relation to his low mood may be to "start playing piano again." Medium-term goals may include "feeling much less sad (less than 5), to see my friend John every week, and to experience happiness every day with Clare and the children." A longer-range goal might be "to keep myself well and cope better with future periods of depression." Longer-term goals are particularly addressed in relation to personal development as illustrated in Chapter 7.

Ideally, goal setting is linked to conceptualization. It is possible to articulate a goal in terms of changes in thoughts, feelings, and behaviors. When a descriptive conceptualization has been reached using functional analysis, goals can be set by comparing current actual behaviors and desired behaviors. McCullough (2000) suggests that therapists ask clients to contrast actual outcomes of behaviors with ideal outcomes. Mark's therapist used this approach in reference to the functional analysis in which Mark described how he put off work tasks (behavior) that worried him (antecedent). His ideal outcome was to not worry so much, accept mistakes, and get his work tasks done:

THERAPIST: Mark, you said earlier that ideally you would like to be more like Peter at work. You'd like to acknowledge what you did well and admit any mistakes, but not get caught up in worrying about them. You thought this would help you overcome avoidance of tasks. I think you wrote this down in your therapy notebook?

MARK: (*looking at his therapy notebook*) Yes, here it is.

THERAPIST: I said we'd come back to this. Are these responses you'd like to have as goals at work?

INSIDE THE THERAPIST'S HEAD

There is compelling evidence that avoidance and rumination maintain and worsen low mood (Nolen-Hoeksema, 1991). Thus Mark's therapist highlights this process to alleviate distress and protect Mark from future difficulties.

MARK: Yes, it feels tough because I have such ingrained habits, but I'm sure it would really help me to be more like Peter.

THERAPIST: What words can we use to describe an ideal yet realistic goal you could have for how you manage your work tasks each day?

MARK: Mmm. How about, "Manage my tasks more like I imagine Peter does it, taking credit for good things that happened and admitting mistakes without getting too caught up with them and putting off my work for fear of making a mistake?"

THERAPIST: Sounds good to me. Why don't you write that down?

Goals for Mark's HIV worries were facilitated by reference to the five-part model developed to conceptualize Mark's HIV worries (Figure 5.2):

THERAPIST: How will we know that we have made a difference with your HIV worries?

MARK: I wish I knew. Sometimes it just feels better and I think to myself, "I'm better." Then it seems to get so bad, I worry it will never go away.

THERAPIST: You raise a really important point. How can we tell the difference between whether you are really over your worries or are just temporarily free of the concern?

MARK: (*Thinks for a moment.*) Maybe if I could go places and be able to cope if I see a mark on a cup, maybe convince myself I was going to be OK?

THERAPIST: That might be one sign. (*pause*) Let's look together at the diagram we drew together about this issue. (*Shows Mark Figure 5.2.*) Looking at this, what would need to be different for you to know you had improved?

MARK: Well, I suppose if I felt less worried, and less tense and restless when I was out eating.

THERAPIST: What sort of rating would show your worry was less of a problem?

MARK: About a 2, I suppose.

THERAPIST: OK, is there anything else that would need to change when you are out at cafés?

MARK: I need to be more relaxed and not so worried about things having HIV. I know it is really unlikely, and that other people are not bothered, but it really gets me.

THERAPIST: OK, so one goal is to feel less worried, less restless. A second may be to no longer believe that you are going to contract HIV. How little would you need to believe you were in danger for us to know we had helped?

MARK: About a 2 or 3 again.

THERAPIST: OK, we will write that down as another goal. Is there any other change that will show us we have tackled this issue effectively?

MARK: I should be able to eat in public places without examining the utensils and dishware. I would be able to go swimming with my children.

These last two dialogues show how descriptive case conceptualizations are used to help organize goal setting. As is often the case, Mark's therapist conducted descriptive conceptualizations only for Mark's highest-priority issues. Later in therapy, lower-priority issues can be conceptualized as needed once progress has been made on the highest-priority concerns. While not all of Mark's issues were conceptualized in the opening sessions, broad goals were identified for the top five priorities on Mark's presenting issues list as shown in Box 5.5. These goals appeared to be realistic, achievable, and relevant to Mark. For the most part, they are specific in terms of providing observable outcomes. His goals also seem to be within Mark's control; achieving these goals does not depend on changing someone else.

The therapist will keep all of Mark's presenting issues and goals in mind as therapy proceeds. Even though the focus is on one or two issues at a time, explanatory levels of case conceptualization may end up explaining more than one presenting issue. For example, Mark's checking

---

Box 5.5. Mark's Goals

MY THERAPY GOALS

1. **Feeling low:**
   - Feel better and not such a failure—feel 5 out of 10 or less for sadness most days.
   - See my friend John at least once a week.
   - Play piano several times a week.
   - At work, manage more like I imagine Peter does—take credit for good things that happen and admit mistakes without getting too caught up with them. Do my work without fear of making a mistake; attend all work meetings.

2. **Worries about my health:**
   - Feel less worry, a 2 or 3 out of 10 instead of 8.
   - Believe I am at less risk of getting HIV, perhaps believe it's only a 2.
   - Be able to eat and drink in public places.
   - Go swimming with my children at the public pool.

3. **Worrying about work:**
   - Not spend so much time each night thinking about the day (less than 10 minutes).

4. **Difficulty making decisions:**
   - Be more relaxed making decisions. Actually make a decision instead of searching endlessly on the Internet for advice; anxiety ratings less than 5.

5. **Problems with checking:**
   - Spend little (5 minutes at most) or no time each night checking house appliances.
   - Do this without becoming agitated; anxiety ratings of 4 or less.

Box 5.6. Guidelines for Setting Goals

- Ensure goals relate closely to the presenting issues.
- Specify short-, medium-, and longer-term goals (not necessarily all at the start of therapy).
- Draw on descriptive conceptualizations to help specify what constitutes change.
- Are goals within the person's control? Do they seem realistic?
- People need success to generate hope: emphasize achievable goals early in therapy.
- Is one goal contingent or dependent upon another? If so, which has to be tackled first?
- Are the goals measurable (e.g., reduced score on a symptom measure, reduced time spent in an unhelpful activity, increased rate or time spent in positive activities)?
- Do the goals reflect more than the reduction of distress? Do they represent positive, meaningful growth for the person?
- Building resilience is a valuable goal for most clients.

---

behavior might be conceptually similar to his health worries. Or explanatory conceptualizations that address his low mood may simultaneously address Mark's goal to enjoy his role as father and husband more.

Box 5.6 presents guidelines for goal setting, emphasizing links to case conceptualization. For more information about setting goals in CBT, see Padesky and Greenberger (1995, pp. 58–68) or Westbrook, Kennerley, and Kirk (2007, pp. 154–156).

FROM "COMPLETE MESS" TO DESCRIPTIVE CONCEPTUALIZATION

In the opening dialogue of this chapter Mark described his life as "a complete mess." This chapter shows how Mark and his therapist unraveled that "mess" to reach a mutual understanding of the range, impact, and priority of Mark's presenting issues. In addition, his therapist used two descriptive case conceptualization methods, functional analysis and the five-part model, to link Mark's presenting issues with CBT theory and research. These descriptive conceptual models helped Mark identify key cognitive and behavioral treatment targets and also define relevant treatment goals. The chapter summary box below highlights key elements of these processes for the reader.

Collaborative empiricism characterizes the relationship between

Mark and his therapist as they construct these initial descriptive conceptualizations and specify treatment goals. Descriptions of Mark's presenting issues are derived using observations of his experience informed by cognitive theory and research. Mark's therapist consistently asks whether the emerging account "rings true" to help prevent a reliance on unhelpful heuristics (see Chapter 2). Active inquiries regarding Mark's strengths and what is right in his life encourage him to set therapy goals that include positive growth and development of resilience. In all these ways, collaborative empiricism begins to build heat in the crucible that can lead to lasting positive change.

Although the purpose of conceptualizations at this early point in therapy is a clear description of presenting issues, therapists also scan for common themes across presenting issues that provide clues to deeper levels of conceptualization. After these initial therapy sessions, the therapist hypothesized that Mark's issues might be knitted together by a theme of high standards and expectations. Mark worries about mistakes and expects terrible consequences from his errors, which are maintained by rumination and avoidance. This theme might connect his work anxiety, HIV worries, checking behavior, indecision, and perhaps even precipitate his low mood. This emergent hypothesis will be examined in Chapter 6 as Mark and his therapist consider what triggers and maintenance factors account for his vulnerability to these presenting issues.

Chapter 5 Summary

- A presenting issues list organizes the *particularities of the case* in the crucible.
- To develop a presenting issues list a therapist:
  —Provides a rationale to enlist the client's help.
  —Identifies issues in the "here and now" using client language.
  —Searches for areas of avoidance that may mask important presenting issues.
  —Actively inquires about strengths and their relevance to the presenting issues list.
  —Draws on additional contextual information to help provide a full and detailed list, including: referral letter(s), standardized assessments, clinical interviews, and observation.
  —Gathers specific details to promote understanding and facilitate client ratings of how strongly presenting issues affect functioning and quality of life.
- The therapist links presenting issues to *CBT theory* in the crucible by

using descriptive case conceptualization methods such as functional analysis or the five-part model to formulate presenting issues in CBT terms. Knowledge of disorder-specific CBT models informs therapist inquiries regarding client experience.

- *Research* is the third element in the crucible. Knowledge of relevant research guides the therapist to potentially useful theoretical models, key processes associated with emotional, behavioral, cognitive, and social difficulties, as well as comparative outcome evidence for potential treatment approaches.
- Goals for treatment are personally and specifically defined using the prioritized presenting issues list and the descriptive CBT conceptualizations of these issues.

Mark's Completed
Aid to History Taking Form

AID TO HISTORY TAKING

The purpose of this questionnaire is to obtain some information about your background, which may help us to understand your situation. We will have the opportunity to discuss your difficulties with you in detail, but we may not have the time to discuss all aspects of your history and situation. This form gives you the chance to provide us with a fuller picture and to do this at your pace. Some questions are quite factual, whereas others are of a more subjective nature. If you find any parts of the form difficult, please leave these blank and we can discuss these at your appointment. In the meantime, if you have any trouble completing any of the sections please do not hesitate to contact us. **All of the information you provide on this form is confidential.**

YOUR PERSONAL DETAILS

Name	*Mark*	Marital status	*Married*
Date of birth	*04-08-1971*	Religion	*Christian*
Sex	*Male*	Date	*06-07-2007*
Occupation	*Retail Manager*	Telephone	

YOUR DIFFICULTIES AND GOALS

Please briefly list the three main issues that have led you to seek help.

1. Feeling low and depressed.
2. Worries about my health.
3. Finding it hard to relax and switch off, I always end up checking things.

Please state what you want to achieve by attending our center.

1. I want to feel better and have more control over my worries.

YOU AND YOUR FAMILY

1. Where was your place of birth? _Boston, MA_

2. Could you please give some detail about your **FATHER** (if known)
   - What is his age now? _____
   - If he is no longer alive, at what age did he die? _64_
   - How old were you when he died? _34_
   - What is, or was, his occupation? _Heating engineer_

Please tell something about your father, his character or personality, and your relationship with him.

Dad was a kind, hard-working man. He cared about people but sometimes let his cares get the better of him, and he became depressed. He was diagnosed with manic depression when he was hospitalized one time, and after that his medication mostly kept him well. He used to do well for periods of time, but would then seem to collapse for a while. Gradually he would pull himself together. I used to worry about him as a boy. He tried to kill himself when I was 8, but seemed to feel better afterward: I think he must have had some help (don't know for sure). My mother looked after him a lot. There were times when I was growing up that he would get out of control and spend lots of money, have arguments with my mother, and it made things tough at times. He was not in great physical shape for the last couple of years, and suffered quite a lot with all his health problems. We got along, but he found it hard because of his physical and mental health to give much back. I miss him.

3. Could you please give some details about your **MOTHER** (if known)
   - What is her age now? ___67___
   - If she is no longer alive, at what age did she die? _____
   - How old were you when she died? _____
   - What is, or was, her occupation? ___Housewife_____

Please tell something about your mother, her character or personality, and your relationship with her.

She is caring and kind, she wants the best for me and my brother. When we were growing up she took care of Dad, helping him manage his ups and downs. She can be a bit critical, and she always makes comments about how I am raising my kids; she seems to think I am doing it all wrong. We get along OK but because of her comments she upsets my wife a lot, and it is difficult for me because I feel stuck in the middle.

4. If there were/are any problems in your relationship with your parents, please describe the most important one(s).

My mother sometimes does not give me and my wife, Clare, enough space. She can be a bit too quick to comment on our parenting, and even though she means well it comes across as criticism and it upsets Clare. I feel that I have to try and help my mother since Dad died, and Clare gets annoyed that I am going around to help my mother when I should be back helping her and the kids.

How much does this bother you now? (please circle)

Not at all   A little   (Moderately)   Very much   Couldn't be worse

Your brothers and sisters (if known)

5. How many children, including yourself, are there in your family? ___2___

Please give us their names and other details listed below. Include yourself and please start with the **eldest**. Please also include any step- or half-siblings or any other children adopted by your parents and indicate who they are.

Name	Occupation	Age	Sex	Comments
David	Painter/Decorator	29	(M)/F	David lives 400 miles away, so we do not see much of him.

6. Please describe any important relationships with your siblings, whether helpful or problematic for you.

David and I get on reasonably well; I am older, so we did not have much in common for a long time, but it is nice when we see each other. We only catch up occasionally because he lives a long way away. When we were younger I was more like a father or uncle than a brother to him. I had to look after him quite a lot.

7. What was the general atmosphere like at home?

Loving, caring, but our mother could be a bit critical toward us, and I always seemed to be expected to look after David, which was tough given he was 7 years younger than me. Dad's ups and downs cast quite a long shadow over the family. He would do OK but then could get out of control. He spent a lot of the family money and acted pretty badly toward my mother at times. We knew he was not well, but it was still pretty hard at times.

8. Were there any important changes, for example, moves or any other significant events, during your childhood or adolescence? Include any separations from the family. Please give approximate ages and details.

Dad was hospitalized once when I was about 8, and things were pretty rocky for a few months. I lived with my grandfather for awhile because of Dad. It was all pretty stable except when Dad would get really down, or become manic.

9. Was there someone else who was important to you during your childhood (e.g., grandparents, aunts/uncles, family friend, etc.)? If so, could you tell us something about them?

I was close to my grandfather on my mother's side. He took David and me fishing, swimming, camping a lot; you know, we would go away for weekends and in the summer sometimes longer. When my dad was hospitalized my brother and I lived with him for a few months. He is a great guy, he has a lot to offer, generous with himself, a real "can-do" attitude.

10. Has anyone in your family ever received psychiatric treatment? (Yes) No Not sure

11. Does anyone in your family have a history of mental illness, alcohol, or drug abuse? (Yes) No Not sure

If yes, please complete:

Family member	List specific psychiatric, alcohol, or drug problem
1 Father	*Manic depression*
2	
3	
4	

12. Has any member of your family ever made a suicide attempt?   (Y)/N

If yes, how is this person related to you?

_____ *Father* _____

13. Has any member of your family died from suicide?   Y/(N)

If yes, how is this person related to you?

_____

YOUR EDUCATION

1. (a) Please tell us something about your schooling and education.

I attended a local high school and got pretty good grades. I went to college in retail management, and then I went to work for a retailer, where I have done some short courses.

    (b) How did you enjoy school? Were there any particular achievements or difficulties? Which were the most important ones?

School was OK. I did all right. I enjoyed it on the whole, but I had asthma and eczema, and the other kids teased me. I hung out with friends who liked to listen to music and we had a band for a while.

How much does this bother you now? (please circle)

(Not at all)   A little   Moderately   Very much   Couldn't be worse

YOUR WORK HISTORY

1. What job or main role do you currently do?

Retail Manager—35 staff report to me.

2. Please tell us something about your past working life, including the jobs and trainings you have done.

I have worked in retail for a long time—5 years in my current job. I have had various training courses—human resources, disciplinary procedures, communication skills, etc.

3. Have there been any particular difficulties? Which were the most important ones?

No major problems, although 2 years ago a colleague left and I had to do his work as well as my own. At the same time we had some disciplinary procedures under way with a difficult-to-manage employee. It was a really tough time because my second child was born then, and it was hard coping with little sleep and the extra responsibility.

EXPERIENCES OF UPSETTING EVENTS

1. Sometimes things happen to people that are extremely upsetting—things like being in a life-threatening situation like a major disaster, very serious accident, or fire; being physically assaulted or raped; or seeing another person killed, badly hurt, or hearing about something horrible that has happened to someone you are close to. At any time during your life, have any of these kinds of things happened to you?

(a) If "no," please check here. _____

(b) If "yes," please list the traumatic events.

Brief description	Date (month/year)	Age
1. Dad's overdose	June 1978	8
2.		
3.		

If *any* events listed: Sometimes these things keep coming back in night-   Yes   (No)
mares, flashbacks, or thoughts that you can't get rid of. Has this ever
happened to you?

If "no": What about being very upset when you were in a situation that   (Yes)   No
reminded you of one of these terrible things?

2. Did you ever experience physical abuse as a child?   Yes   (No)   Not sure

3. Have you ever experienced physical abuse as an adult?   Yes   (No)   Not sure

4. Did you ever experience sexual abuse as a child?   Yes   (No)   Not sure

5. Have you ever experienced rape, including date or marital   Yes   (No)   Not sure
   rape?

6. Did you ever experience emotional or verbal abuse as a   Yes   (No)   Not sure
   child?

7. Have you ever experienced emotional or verbal abuse as   Yes   (No)   Not sure
   an adult?

YOUR PARTNER AND YOUR PRESENT FAMILY

1. About your **partner(s)** (if applicable)

   (a) Please briefly describe any previous important relationship(s), in chronological
       order. Please include how long they lasted and why you think the relationship(s)
       ended.

   I had a few casual relationships in my teens and early 20s. I met
   Clare when I was 22, and we have been together since.

   (b) Do you have a partner now? If yes,

      How old is s/he?   *34*

   What is her/his occupation?   *Part-time biology teacher*

   How long have you been together?   *14 years*

   (c) Please tell us something about your partner, her/his character or personality, and
       your relationship with her/him. What do you like about the relationship?

   Clare is very caring, a great mother and wife. She is very orga-

nized and matter of fact. She gets things done and does not worry about money or things like that.

(d) If there are any problems in your relationship with your partner, please describe the most important one(s).

We do pretty well. We have the usual arguments, mainly about my mother. This happens particularly when we have not slept well.

How much does this bother you now? (please circle)

Not at all   A little   (Moderately)   Very much   Couldn't be worse

2. How is your sex life? Do you have any difficulties in your sexual life? If so, please try to describe these.

No.

How much does this bother you now? (please circle)

(Not at all)   A little   Moderately   Very much   Couldn't be worse

3. About your **children** (if known)

(a) If you have children, please list them in order of age. Please indicate any children from previous marriage(s) and adopted children; indicate who they are.

Name	Occupation	Age	Sex	Comments
Jessica		9	M/(F)	
James		2	(M)/F	

(b) Please describe your relationship with your children. If there are any difficulties with your children, please describe the most important one(s).

They are both doing well.

How much does this bother you now? (please circle)

(Not at all)   A little   Moderately   Very much   Couldn't be worse

YOUR PSYCHIATRIC HISTORY

1. Have you ever been hospitalized for any emotional or psychiatric reason?   Y/(N)

If yes, how many times have you been hospitalized? _____

Date	Name of hospital	Reason for hospitalization	Was it helpful?

2. Have you ever received outpatient psychiatric or psychological treatment?   (Y)/N

If yes, please complete the following:

Date	Name of professional	Reason for treatment	Was it helpful?
June '04	Dr. A	Medication for mood	Y/(N)
August '06	Dr. B	Medication for mood	(Y)/N

3. Are you taking any medication for psychiatric reasons?   (Y)/N

If yes, please complete the following:

Medication	Dosage	Frequency	Name of prescribing doctor
Prozac	20mg	daily	Dr. Cristoph

4. Have you ever made a suicide attempt?   Y/(N)

If yes, how many times have you attempted suicide? __

Approx. date	What exactly did you do to hurt yourself?	Were you hospitalized?
		Y/N

YOUR MEDICAL HISTORY

1. Who is your general practitioner?

Name	Dr. Cristoph
Practice address	Cristoph and Partners 4 Oak Street

2. When was the last time you had a physical checkup? ___3 months ago___

3. Have you been treated by your GP or been hospitalized in the past year? (Y)/N

If yes, please specify. ___I have gotten mood medication___

4. Has there been any change in your general health in the past year? Y/(N)

If yes, please specify. ___physically I am pretty much OK___

5. Are you taking any nonpsychiatric medications or over-the-counter drugs at the moment? (Y)/N

Medications	Dosage	Frequency	Reason
1. Asthma inhaler		As needed	Asthma attacks
2.			

6. Have you ever had or have a history of (check all that apply)

☐ Stroke   ☐ Rheumatic fever   ☐ Heart surgery

☑ Asthma   ☐ Heart murmur   ☐ Heart attack

☐ Tuberculosis   ☐ Anemia   ☐ Angina

☐ Ulcers   ☐ High or low blood pressure   ☐ Thyroid problems

☐ Diabetes

7. Are you pregnant or do you think you may be pregnant?   Yes   (No)

8. Have you ever had fits, seizures, convulsions, or epilepsy?   Yes   (No)

9. Do you have prosthetic heart valve?   Yes   (No)

10. Do you have any current medical conditions?   (Yes)   No

If yes, please specify:

___Asthma, eczema___

11. Do you have any medication or food allergies?   Yes   (No)

If yes, please specify:

ALCOHOL AND DRUG USE HISTORY

1. Has your alcohol use ever caused any problems for you?   Y/**N**

2. Has anyone ever told you that alcohol has caused a problem for you or complained about your drinking?   Y/**N**

3. Has your drug use ever caused any problems for you?   Y/**N**

4. Has anyone ever told you that drugs have caused a problem for you or complained about your drug use?   Y/**N**

5. Have you ever been "hooked" on a prescribed medication or taken a lot more of it than you were supposed to?   **Y**/N   *If yes, please list those medications:*

_____

6. Have you ever been hospitalized, entered a detox program, or been in a rehabilitation program because of a drug or alcohol problem?   **Y**/N   *If yes, when and where were you hospitalized?*

_____

YOUR FUTURE

1. Please mention any particular satisfaction that you draw from your family life, your work life, or any other areas that are important to you.

I am proud of my family, and I enjoy being with my wife and children.

I play piano; I love music really.

I think I do a good job at work, but I am not coping as well as I would like.

2. Could you tell us something about your plans, hopes, and expectations for the future?

I would like to be more relaxed about life and not be so on edge about things. Then I would be able to enjoy more things with my children and wife, rather than be a burden on them.

3. Please could you let us know how you felt completing this questionnaire?

It was OK, a bit long.

Thank You

Chapter 6

"Why Does This Keep Happening to Me?"
Cross-Sectional Explanatory Conceptualizations

THERAPIST: It is good to see you again, Mark. As part of our agenda for today, can you give me a quick overview of how this past week has been for you?

MARK: Well, I had a bad time last Saturday. I was out with my family and then it just hit me like a wave. I just felt so down, so useless, like such a failure. It was all I could do to stop myself from crying. I kept it together until we got home and then I went to bed. That's not normal. Why does this keep happening to me? I am such a mess.

THERAPIST: I am sorry to hear it was so bad for you on Saturday. It sounds like a really difficult day. Would you like to spend some time today figuring out why that happened on Saturday and what we can do to help?

MARK: I've been here before. It gets better for a while, I think I am doing OK, and then bang! It's back to square one. It's not normal to be feeling this way for no reason.

THERAPIST: Perhaps if we can figure out what led to you to become so upset on Saturday this will help us understand why your mood dropped so quickly. Shall we put this on our agenda for today?

MARK: Yes, because I don't know why my moods keep crashing.

Like most clients, Mark wants to know why he keeps having difficulties, especially when his drop in mood seems to come out of the blue. To answer his question, we need to move from a descriptive to an explanatory level of case conceptualization. In clinical terms, Mark is searching to understand the precipitants or *triggers* of his mood shifts. In addition, Mark and his therapist can look for what *maintains* or perpetuates his presenting issues. Maintenance factors can explain why Mark's issues have not remitted over time as many transient worries and mood problems do. These cross-sectional explanatory conceptualizations link CBT theory and client experience at a higher level by identifying the key cognitive and behavioral mechanisms underpinning clients' presenting issues. We call them cross-sectional because Mark and his therapist will look across numerous situations in which presenting issues are activated to identify the common triggers and maintenance factors.

This chapter shows how explanatory conceptualizations of triggers and maintenance factors guide the therapist's choice of treatment interventions. Because explanatory conceptualizations are expected to predict intervention outcomes, the outcomes of interventions are used to evaluate the "fit" of the conceptualizations. Interventions chosen to respond to triggers and maintenance factors ideally will lead to reduced distress, one of the desired outputs of the crucible. Interventions can also draw on and expand Mark's strengths so he simultaneously builds greater resilience. If Mark can build resilience he reduces the risk he will be "back to square one" after a period of improvement. Throughout this chapter the key processes of collaboration, empiricism, and incorporation of client strengths are highlighted.

DEVELOPING CROSS-SECTIONAL CONCEPTUALIZATIONS

While the search for explanatory factors can occur in a number of ways, in this chapter we suggest a four-step process as summarized in Figure 6.1. First, the client and therapist gather and describe several recent examples of the highest-priority presenting issue—in Mark's case, low mood. Second, the therapist explores whether specific client experiences fit with evidence-based CBT models. This is done as the client and therapist collaboratively look for themes and commonalities among recent examples as a way to identify triggers and maintenance factors. Third, the therapist uses the explanatory conceptualization derived in the second step to select and implement therapy interventions. Finally, in the fourth step, the effects of the interventions are used to evaluate

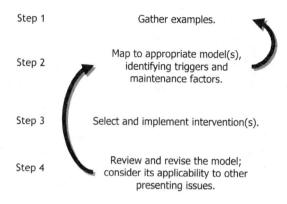

Step 1   Gather examples.

Step 2   Map to appropriate model(s), identifying triggers and maintenance factors.

Step 3   Select and implement intervention(s).

Step 4   Review and revise the model; consider its applicability to other presenting issues.

Figure 6.1. Cross-sectional case conceptualization: A four-step process.

the conceptualization's "fit." Appropriate revisions to the conceptualization are made. The process is circular, with each step offering feedback to support or alter previous steps.

The process of developing cross-sectional explanatory conceptualizations builds on the information used in the descriptive conceptualizations. In Mark's case, these are the ABC and five-part descriptive models illustrated in Chapter 5. As conceptualization moves from description to explanation, the therapist shares relevant knowledge of theory and research with the client, especially as these pertain to trigger and maintenance factors. Client observations are compared with theoretical models to see where these converge and diverge. Socratic dialogues are employed to help the client observe personal processes that create and maintain distress even when these closely match a theoretically or empirically derived model. Socratic dialogue is also employed to evaluate whether results of therapy interventions support or refute the explanatory conceptualizations derived.

Although Chapter 5 emphasized detailed descriptions of presenting issues, people usually experience some variation in their presenting issues according to time and place. The explanatory phase of CBT conceptualization articulates the external (e.g., situations, interpersonal context, external reinforcements) and internal (e.g., cognitions, emotions, physical sensations, internal reinforcements) factors linked to variations in experience and connects these to cognitive and behavioral theories. These levels of understanding help explain the personal meaning of triggers and the functional aims of strategies even when they serve to maintain difficulties (see Chapters 2 and 3).

CROSS-SECTIONAL EXPLANATORY CONCEPTUALIZATION OF LOW MOOD

Step 1: Gather Examples Related to Mark's Mood

Mark prioritized low mood/depression as the first issue to address. His therapist decided to use a functional analysis approach to gather examples in which Mark's low mood was triggered. The ABC approach was selected for its simplicity, Mark's familiarity with it, and its emphasis on antecedents. Using the situation described in the opening dialogue of this chapter, the therapist employs Socratic dialogue to uncover triggers for Mark's abrupt mood change on Saturday. The intense affect shift reported by Mark suggests this situation is highly relevant to understanding his low mood.

THERAPIST: If we look at Saturday in a bit more detail, maybe we can figure out what leads you to feel so bad, apparently out of the blue. Let's try to find what triggered this experience on Saturday.

MARK: I'm not sure what happened.

THERAPIST: Maybe the ABC model we used last session will help. Remember, "A" stands for antecedent, which is another word for trigger. Can you tell me what you were doing just before you noticed a change in how you felt?

MARK: As I said, we were out shopping. I thought I was doing well, and then it hit me.

THERAPIST: Can you remember where you were when it hit you?

MARK: I was in the line waiting to pay for some lamps that Clare wanted.

THERAPIST: Can you picture yourself in your mind, now as we talk about it?

MARK: Yes. I was standing there feeling OK. My daughter Jessica was with me and we were joking about Clare's choice of lamps. Then I just hit rock bottom.

THERAPIST: When you say "rock bottom," do you remember what set that feeling off?

MARK: I am really not sure. (*His brow is furrowed as he remembers the moment.*) It was so intense. It seems so odd now that it should have happened that way. (*Pauses for a few moments.*) I know—all of sudden I remembered a work meeting coming up on Monday that I was not ready for. I got a tight feeling in my stomach. A few minutes later I realized I was not paying any attention to my daughter, and I just felt awful, like such a failure.

THERAPIST: You look upset now when you remember.

MARK: Yeah, I feel awful.

THERAPIST: Even so, stay with those feelings a bit so we can figure this out. What do you think triggered your crash in mood?

MARK: It was thinking about work again.

THERAPIST: OK, let's think about this in terms of the ABC model. For the trigger, the "A," what should we write?

MARK: (*leaning in to look at the paper on which the therapist is writing*) I started thinking about the work meeting.

THERAPIST: OK, so that sounds like the trigger or antecedent, so we will put that under "A." Thinking about the effect it had on you, what should we put in the Consequences section? This is the impact on you in terms of how you felt.

MARK: I felt really bad.

THERAPIST: OK, so we will put "I felt really bad" under "C." And when you remembered the meeting what was the behavior? What did you do when you thought about the work meeting?

MARK: I just thought about how I was not ready for the meeting, how it was important and once again I would be useless, not up to the job. I felt so bad I asked Clare if we could leave and I went home to bed.

THERAPIST: So you thought about how you were not ready for the meeting and then you went home to bed. Is that right?

MARK: Yeah.

THERAPIST: OK. So let's look at the ABC model we have drawn [Figure 6.2]. At the beginning of our session you asked what makes your mood change so rapidly. Looking at this model, what do you think triggered your mood crash on Saturday?

MARK: I was thinking about work, what a bad job I am doing, and how useless I am.

THERAPIST: And I remember another piece you mentioned. You said you felt worse when you realized you weren't paying attention to your daughter.

MARK: Yes, I'm useless as a dad, too.

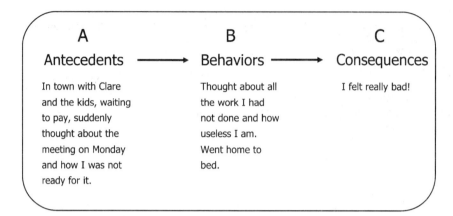

A
Antecedents ⟶ **B** Behaviors ⟶ **C** Consequences

A Antecedents	B Behaviors	C Consequences
In town with Clare and the kids, waiting to pay, suddenly thought about the meeting on Monday and how I was not ready for it.	Thought about all the work I had not done and how useless I am. Went home to bed.	I felt really bad!

Figure 6.2. An ABC functional analysis for the "collapse" in Mark's mood.

Mark and his therapist begin to address Mark's first question regarding what causes his moods to seemingly come out of the blue. Mark identifies a thought ("I'm useless") that occurs to him as a response to being unprepared for work on Monday and also his perceived neglect of his daughter. In this instance we can see how these reactions to his initial thoughts about work probably led to his "mood crash," and yet we do not know whether these reactions are typical and common. Therefore, Mark was encouraged to gather other examples of distressing experiences and add them to a worksheet using the ABC format. Such examples can be developed as a homework task or collaboratively completed in session on paper or a whiteboard. Figure 6.3 summarizes the examples Mark and his therapist gathered.

Step 2: Fit Mood Examples with an Appropriate Model of Triggers and Maintenance Factors

In step 2 the therapist considers whether Mark's experiences fit relevant CBT models and theories. This involves having enough data to infer themes that potentially fit a theory. The single event on Saturday was not sufficient to infer the typical causes of his low moods. However, once Mark identified a number of examples where his mood plummeted, he and his therapist could review these to identify common triggers and maintenance factors.

Triggers

Many things can trigger client reactions. As demonstrated via the five-part model, thoughts, emotions, behaviors, physical reactions, and events

Antecedents	Behaviors	Consequences
In town with Clare and the kids, waiting to pay. *Suddenly thought about the meeting on Monday and how I was not ready for it.*	*Thought about all the work I had not done and how useless I am.* *Went home to bed.*	*I felt really bad.* *Felt sad and tearful.*
Made a mistake at work on the monthly finance report.	*Stopped working, looked for other mistakes, did not finish the report on time.*	*Sad.* *Went home early.*
Received e-mail at work asking about the report that I had not completed.	*Left work early.*	*Sad, but also relieved to be away from work.*
At home thinking about my late report.	*Lost in my thoughts, ignored Clare.*	*Argued with Clare.* *Felt bad and low.*
Tried to work on report in the evening.	*Did not finish it because of poor concentration.*	*Canceled a night out with John again.* *Felt really sad.*

Figure 6.3. Examples of distressing situations for Mark using the ABC format.

in our life constantly interact and influence each other. Changes in any one or several of these might trigger Mark's low mood. Moods can be triggered either internally (as a reaction to certain thoughts, physical reactions, or behavior) or externally by particular types of events or situations. Mark and his therapist are interested to find whether there are any common triggers for his low mood across a number of situations:

THERAPIST: We have a few examples listed here (*pointing to Figure 6.3*) when your mood has gone down. Do you notice any patterns in what we've found?

MARK: I am a bit surprised. Even though I think I am down all the time, I realize there are times when it is much worse than others.

THERAPIST: What do you make of that?

MARK: Well, it is good, I suppose. At least I am not a total mess all the time.

THERAPIST: So if it is not all the time, what do you think triggers your low mood?

MARK: Looking at this, it is clear that I feel bad when I think about work and the bad job I am doing. And I know I do that a lot.

THERAPIST: Yes, it certainly does look like thinking about work is an important trigger that brings your mood down. How do you feel looking at this now?

MARK: Pretty useless, actually. I seem to make lots of mistakes.

THERAPIST: It can seem that way when we pay attention to these things. Let's stick with this, though, and keep asking, "Is there anything else that triggers low moods?"

MARK: Well, it seems clear it is thinking about all the mistakes I make at work.

THERAPIST: OK, so perhaps we need to write that down as an answer to your question today about what triggers your low mood. What can you write to summarize this?

MARK: Something like, "When I think about mistakes at work it triggers my low mood."

INSIDE THE THERAPIST'S HEAD

Mark's therapist notices that Mark's low mood is commonly triggered by perceived mistakes. Beginning at assessment, the therapist has been holding in mind that Mark is very conscientious. Although conscientiousness is a strength, this strength may be overdeveloped for Mark and lead him to greater vulnerability to feeling low when he makes mistakes. If so, Mark's therapist expects that he holds one or more underlying assumptions about making mistakes. She decides this is a good time to help Mark identify his underlying assumption(s) about making mistakes.

THERAPIST: Mark, what is it about making mistakes that is so upsetting to you?

MARK: I don't know, it just is upsetting.

THERAPIST: If you think about it, I bet you have a good reason. For example, "If I make a mistake, then … " (*Pauses so Mark can complete the sentence.*)

MARK: I could lose my job, lose my house, lose everything.

THERAPIST: I can see now why that would be so upsetting to you. And if we take it a bit further, what would it mean to you if you lost these things? What would it say about you as a person?

MARK: (*looking upset and shaky*) I would be useless, a waste of space.

THERAPIST: How do you feel when you say this to yourself?

MARK: Pretty low, actually. It is not good.

THERAPIST: I realize that talking about these things can be difficult, so thank you for telling me how you see it. It helps make sense of your current difficulties, because it seems that you believe something like "If I make a mistake, then it means I am useless, a waste of space," and this is connected to feeling low. Have I got that right?

MARK: That is it.

In this session, the therapist helps Mark identify underlying assumptions about making mistakes that link to his low mood. She also notes that Mark's depression seems linked to the negative core beliefs, "I'm useless" and "I'm a waste of space." It may already be obvious to Mark's therapist after several sessions that mistakes trigger his low mood. However, principles of guided discovery suggest that Mark's learning may be more meaningful and long-lasting if he identifies the trigger himself rather than if the therapist points out the pattern to him (Padesky, 1993). Once Mark identifies mistakes as a trigger, his therapist may take the opportunity to introduce Mark to theory and research on depression that suggest themes of achievement and failure in work are common triggers for many people's low mood (Bieling, Beck, & Brown, 2000). Knowing others react the same way might help normalize Mark's responses for him.

At the same time, Mark's individual experience is highlighted by identifying the personal meanings mistakes hold for him. Mark and his therapist have identified particular underlying assumptions about the dangerous consequences of mistakes. Due to his underlying assumptions and core beliefs, mistakes resonate with Mark more than with other people, or perhaps resonate more at this point in his life than they have previously. Making mistakes is a theme related to his low mood because it is associated with a powerful negative underlying assumption, "If I make a mistake then it means I am useless, a waste of space."

Of course, there are many times when Mark does not feel low, or he manages complex tasks without making, noticing, or becoming upset about mistakes. We advocate that therapists ask about these experiences as well, because more positive experiences reveal additional dimensions to the specific meanings of triggers. For example, Mark may not react to mistakes as negatively if he is working on a task on which other cowork-ers are also struggling. These are opportunities to understand what fac-tors might modulate or ameliorate low mood. The emergent understand-ing of key themes should help explain positive experiences as well as negative ones. Moreover, positive experiences are opportunities to con-ceptualize Mark's resilience. Understanding the cognitive and behav-ioral processes in operation when Mark manages difficulties successfully can inform an understanding of how he can stay well. Drawing out these processes is the same as with distress, but the focus is on understanding resilience.

For instance, the therapist can ask Mark about times he makes mis-takes at work and does not ruminate about them afterward, or times when he persists and accomplishes complex tasks at home. In Chapter 5 Mark described a day when his mood had been good. He described how he had not worried so much: "I didn't get caught up with negative thinking." His behavior resembled that of a colleague Peter, whom he regarded as effective at work. Mark's therapist used the ABC model to conceptualize this example of Mark's resilience in the face of thinking about mistakes at work (Figure 6.4).

Positive examples such as this one helpfully illustrate the specific-ity of triggers for low mood. In addition, they introduce a central tenet of the cognitive model that the same event can lead to different reac-tions depending on how the event is appraised and interpreted. Positive examples identify successes that Mark can link to a healthier view of himself. Understanding the positive consequences of resilient responses can encourage Mark to practice these more often in order to overcome

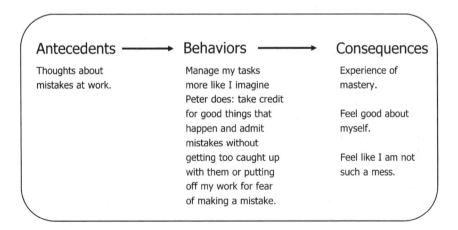

Antecedents ⟶ Behaviors ⟶ Consequences

Antecedents	Behaviors	Consequences
Thoughts about mistakes at work.	Manage my tasks more like I imagine Peter does: take credit for good things that happen and admit mistakes without getting too caught up with them or putting off my work for fear of making a mistake.	Experience of mastery. Feel good about myself. Feel like I am not such a mess.

Figure 6.4. An ABC functional analysis for Mark's resilience at work.

his low mood. The example in Figure 6.4 was a particularly powerful learning experience for Mark because he started to worry that evening and his mood dropped again. Within the same day, Mark was able to observe the behaviors that maintained a positive mood and triggered a low mood. Highlighting this contrast creates dissonance and can motivate clients to learn and rehearse more resilient behaviors (McCullough, 2000).

Understanding the Onset of Mark's Most Recent Depression

One way to evaluate an emerging explanatory conceptualization is to see whether it also accounts for the onset of a presenting issue. The onset of a person's presenting issues can refer to proximal onset (when the current issues began) or more distal onset (when the issues appeared for the first time). The current conceptualization of his low mood is that it is triggered by mistakes because Mark thinks making a mistake means he is useless. Did events during the recent and earliest onset of his depression tap into similar themes?

As noted on his Aid to History Taking Questionnaire (Appendix 5.1), Mark's current difficulties escalated over the previous 2 years following the birth of his second child and the death of his father. These two events in themselves were relatively uncomplicated. James was born when daughter Jessica was already 7. Clare's pregnancy and the delivery were without significant problems. Mark thought his father's death had positive aspects in that it released his father from long-standing health problems. The preparation for the funeral, the funeral itself, and a subsequent memorial service helped Mark grieve his loss. At the time, Mark said, "I feel at peace with his life and his death."

To understand the onset of Mark's low mood it is helpful to explore the consequences and meanings of what happened during the last 2 years and the coping strategies he used. After his father's death, he saw his mother more often. Mark reported that this exposed him and Clare to her frequent criticism, a characteristic of his relationship with his mother since childhood. In Mark's account, this evoked themes of being "useless." Around this time period Mark was promoted and took on more responsibility at work. Mark described being reluctant to take the promotion, but felt he had to provide for his expanding family. James was an infant during this period, so Mark and Clare experienced the reduced sleep and increased family demands common for couples with a new baby. As his increased workload, family duties, and caretaking of his mother continued, Mark described trying to manage by using strategies of working to a high standard and taking on more responsibility to make ends meet. As Mark reported in an early session:

"It was unsustainable. I was working harder and harder, constantly feeling like what I was doing was not good enough. All the while I was worried about Clare and the kids. You know, they were really young and that's tiring for Clare. Sometimes when my mother was staying with us I knew things would be tense with her continual criticism. I'd lie awake at night, replaying the day, trying to find a way through it all. I couldn't find a solution and I was getting more and more tired; eventually I wanted just to hide away and hibernate."

Making mistakes and feeling inadequate were at the heart of the onset of his most recent depressive episode. Hence, Mark and his therapist can be more confident that these are key themes to address. Although mistakes are a trigger of his low mood, his underlying assumptions help explain the meaning and impact of the triggers: "If I make a mistake, then I am useless." This certainly seems to explain why mistakes trigger his low mood. The therapist notes that this underlying assumption may have its origins in Mark's childhood, when this idea was congruent with his perception of his mother's constant criticism. Because the review of Mark's recent onset of depression supports the emerging conceptualization, he and his therapist returned to a focus on understanding and overcoming low mood in the present. The next step to accomplish this goal is to uncover what maintains his depression so they can intervene and interrupt the maintenance cycle.

Maintenance Factors

Just as many different factors can be triggers, there are many pathways to problem maintenance. When CBT therapists look for maintenance factors they usually first consider reinforcement factors. These include anything that increases a particular response. Reinforcement can be positive or negative. Positive reinforcement involves rewards and can be either internal (e.g., a positive feeling) or external (e.g., monetary rewards or praise). Negative reinforcement refers to the removal of an aversive circumstance and can also be internal (e.g., reduction in distress) or external (e.g., elimination of chores once mistakes are made).

Ironically, sometimes a person's chosen coping methods can maintain the problem. This is because people often prefer coping approaches that are immediately reinforcing; those that lead to immediate rewards or reductions in distress. Solving the root causes of distress can involve a temporary increase in discomfort. Therefore, CBT therapists identify the long-term costs of coping methods as well as the short-term benefits. Mark's therapist wonders whether Mark's preferred methods for dealing with his low mood may inadvertently maintain his difficulties. The following dialogue illustrates how Mark's therapist helps him link his avoidance with maintenance of low mood:

THERAPIST: We figured out that thinking about mistakes at work triggers your low moods because you equate making mistakes with being useless. We are building a picture of you as someone with high standards who tries really hard not to make mistakes. But you also had a question about why your low mood has not gone away and why you continue to feel so down. It seems to me if we can figure out the answer to that question, we might get some ideas about how to help you with your moods. Would it be OK with you if we talked about that now?

MARK: That is what I need help with, getting out of this mess.

THERAPIST: OK, let's see what we can figure out together. Looking at these examples (*pointing to Figure 6.3*), what do you think may keep the problem going?

MARK: (*Looks at Figure 6.3 for a minute silently.*) Well, it doesn't help when I just give up on things.

THERAPIST: What do you mean?

MARK: Well, when I was shopping and my mood crashed I just went home to bed. That didn't help, did it? It is not like I went and got ready for the meeting, or put time aside on Sunday to do it.

THERAPIST: That's a really good observation, Mark. (*Smiles encouragingly.*) What do you think led you to go home to bed like that?

MARK: Well, at the time it was just better to be away from the situation. I just wanted to be home and not think about it. It helped me a little at the time.

THERAPIST: So, at the time it helps a little to avoid your problems. Thinking about it now, how much do you think it helped in the long run?

MARK: In the end it made it worse, because the pressure just built up.

THERAPIST: So what if we draw an arrow between going home to bed and not being ready for the work meeting to remind us that avoidance might be something that keeps your problems going?

MARK: Yeah, I can see that.

Mark's therapist then suggests they review the other examples discussed previously to help establish whether this is a common pattern.

THERAPIST: Looking at this sheet (*showing Mark Figure 6.3*), are there other examples where you avoid your problems to temporarily feel better?

MARK: I did that with the example when I got the e-mail about the report. Instead of sorting out the report I just caved in and went home.

THERAPIST: How might doing that make your mood worse?

MARK: I didn't finish the report. The next time I went back to work the e-mail was still there. So then I felt even worse.

THERAPIST: Do you think you avoid a lot when you feel down?

MARK: Just look at the sheet (*pointing to Figure 6.3*). I avoid tasks at work, I avoid John, I avoid lots of things.

THERAPIST: So what can you write down to describe how this might keep you feeling down and stop you from feeling better?

MARK: When I avoid things, I make problems worse and this keeps my mood down.

Evaluating Conceptualization in Relation to Evidence-Based Models and "Fit"

Once Mark has had this opportunity to learn directly from his own experience, the therapist may contribute theory and research to the conceptualization crucible. Mark may be interested to learn that people with depression commonly withdraw from and avoid activities (Kuyken, Watkins, & Beck, 2005). Mark's behavior is consistent with research that shows avoidance acts as negative reinforcement by providing distance from a distressing situation (Martell et al., 2001). This simple hypothesis is derived from classic operant principles in behavior therapy (Ferster, 1973; Hayes & Follette, 1992). Thus Mark's observations are consistent with research, and this knowledge strengthens his therapist's confidence that CBT models for treating depression may help him.

Mark and his therapist drew the simple model shown in Figure 6.5 to summarize the trigger and maintenance model discussed in this session. To test the "fit" of this emerging explanatory conceptualization, Mark is encouraged over the next week to observe whether his low mood is triggered by thoughts of work and whether there are other triggers for low mood. In addition, he is advised to notice how often he uses avoidance and whether this seems to lead to a worsening of mood after a period of immediate relief. This direct observational test of the conceptualization is important as a check on the fit of the conceptualization.

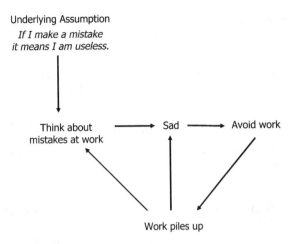

Figure 6.5. A simple conceptualization to illustrate triggers and maintenance of Mark's difficulties at work.

In the following session, discussion of Mark's observations reveals that avoidance does not sufficiently account for all of Mark's experiences.

THERAPIST: So on Wednesday, you noticed your mood worsened when you thought about your work a lot throughout the evening. That does not seem to fit with avoiding. Can you tell me a little more about that?

MARK: When I feel low at work I often leave or avoid tasks. But when I am at home I tend to sit and mull things over. I review all the mistakes I made that day and think about what a loser I am. I wonder, "Why can't I do anything right?"

THERAPIST: How does that make you feel?

MARK: Awful. I find so many things I have not done or have done badly that I feel worse and worse as the night goes on.

THERAPIST: So what does that tell you about the effects of thinking over your work like that?

MARK: Well, it doesn't seem to help. Although it sometimes seems like a good thing to do so I can know exactly what I have done wrong.

THERAPIST: Does reviewing your mistakes help you avoid making mistakes the next day or fix the ones you remember you made?

MARK: Not really. It makes me feel so bad I begin to think, "What is the point?" Then I end up staying up really late watching TV just to distract myself. When I go to bed I usually sleep badly and feel even less like working the next day.

THERAPIST: So at home you tend to ruminate or go over mistakes in your mind. Is that right?

MARK: That's me.

THERAPIST: And after you ruminate you feel worse and then stay up late watching TV and sleep poorly.

MARK: That's right.

THERAPIST: So perhaps we should add rumination to the model we drew last week (*points to Figure 6.5*). Where should we put rumination?

MARK: I think it should just go right above avoidance. I tend to either avoid or ruminate or do both at the same time. Both make me feel worse.

THERAPIST: Why don't you put it there? (*Waits while Mark adds rumination to the model.*)

MARK: I think I should draw an arrow from rumination right back to my low mood because even if work is not piling up, rumination makes me feel worse.

THERAPIST: That's a great idea. (*Waits while Mark adds the arrow as shown in Figure 6.6.*) Are there other ways in which rumination can affect you?

MARK: What do you mean?

THERAPIST: When you ruminate are you more or less aware of the mistakes you made that day?

MARK: Much more. I just start thinking about all the things I have done wrong, and then I remember even more things I have done badly or have not done at all.

THERAPIST: So when you ruminate you actually notice more mistakes, and that makes you feel bad. So we need to put that on the diagram too. (*Waits while Mark adds the arrow.*) So now we know both avoidance and rumination might be important reasons why your depression doesn't get better. How about the effect of rumination on what you do, your behavior?

MARK: It makes me feel like giving up; it makes it more likely I'll give up at work.

THERAPIST: So do we need to add another arrow in the diagram to

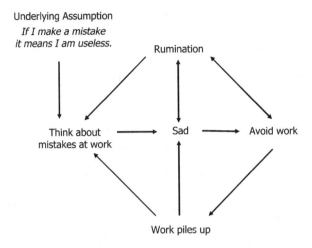

Figure 6.6. A conceptualization of Mark's difficulties at work that includes rumination as a maintenance factor.

describe the impact of rumination on what you do? (*Mark adds the arrow.*) You may not know this, Mark, but avoidance and rumination are common in people who are depressed. Fortunately, there are a number of things for you to try that can help you overcome both of these habits.

INSIDE THE THERAPIST'S HEAD

Mark's therapist recalls the conceptualization of Mark's resilience drawn in a previous session (Figure 6.4). She considers this a good time to remind Mark of that drawing and actively link these behaviors with overcoming rumination.

THERAPIST: Mark, last time we looked at a working day when your mood was pretty good (*points to Figure 6.4*). You said you "managed my tasks more like I imagine Peter does: taking credit for good things that happened and admitting mistakes without getting too caught up with them." What was the effect of behaving like this?

MARK: Well, I felt pretty good. (*Therapist sits silently and Mark thinks for a moment.*) You know, I just seemed to enjoy my day and thought to myself, "I enjoy my work and I'm OK at it."

THERAPIST: OK, so what effect does this have on what you do?

MARK: I can't say I stop to think about it very much.

THERAPIST: So you don't think about it, and it doesn't give space for worry or rumination? (*Mark nods.*) If you think about it, without ruminating (*both laugh*), what do you think is the effect of feeling pretty good at work, thinking that you enjoy your work, and are okay at your work?

MARK: Well, it makes it more likely I will carry on doing the right things; you know, acting kind of like Peter. So should I add all this to the diagram? (*Therapist nods* [see Figure 6.7].)

Just as Mark's therapist does in this session, therapists can help clients construct functional analyses of resilient coping experiences in parallel with those for triggers and maintenance cycles. Doing so brings adaptive patterns into focus for the client and suggests the possibility of alternative outcomes as described in Chapter 4. Therapists can ask the following questions to help clients conceptualize resilience:

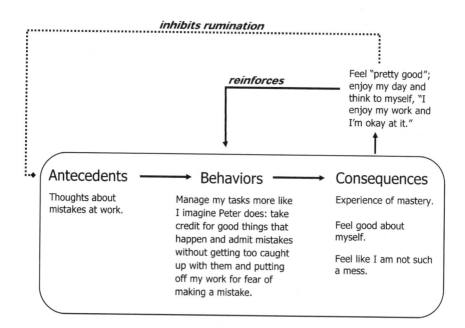

Figure 6.7. ABC for Mark illustrating resilience, with reinforcement built in.

- "How have you handled challenging situations in the past?"
- "What strengths, beliefs, or strategies helped?"
- "How might those experiences help you cope with this situation?"
- "What strengths, beliefs, or strategies can help you cope?"
- "What skills do you need to develop to cope with this situation?"
- "Can anyone else help you cope?"
- "What opportunities are there in this situation?"
- "What lessons can you learn?"
- "Who do you know who copes well with situations like this? How might he or she handle this situation?"
  —"What strategies would they use?"
  —"What beliefs would guide their actions?"

At this point, Mark and his therapist have constructed a working explanatory conceptualization that explains the triggers and maintenance of his low mood. They did this by gathering a number of typical examples of low mood and working collaboratively to discover the triggers and maintenance factors these situations had in common. The resulting conceptualization joins Mark's individual experiences with CBT models of depression and principles of reinforcement drawn from operant conditioning theory. They used the same ABC model to draw out the behaviors and operant principles maintaining his well-being and effectiveness at work on a day when Mark demonstrated resilience. His resilience conceptualization emphasizes reinforcing adaptive behaviors and Mark's success with inhibiting rumination. They are now ready for Mark's explanatory conceptualizations to fulfill their next function: informing CBT interventions.

Step 3: Select Interventions Based on Explanatory Conceptualization

Conceptualization in and of itself is not sufficient to improve a person's well-being (Chadwick et al., 2003). It is not usually helpful to solely promote insight, "I understand myself more now but I still do not feel any better." Instead, the purpose of conceptualization is to create an understanding of the presenting issues, which facilitates the selection of appropriate CBT interventions. Thus, one indicator of a good-enough case conceptualization is that it directs you to appropriate interventions.

Mark's therapist is aware of excellent source materials that guide therapists in the use of appropriate treatment principles and intervention methods for depression (Beck et al., 1979; J. S. Beck, 1995; Greenberger & Padesky, 1995; Martell et al., 2001; Padesky & Greenberger, 1995). Rather than applying these principles and therapy methods in a stereotypical fashion, Mark's explanatory conceptualization provides a rationale to select particular interventions from within this broad pool. Based on the conceptualizations shown in Figures 6.6 and 6.7, Mark and his therapist decide that interventions that target his maintenance processes of avoidance and rumination may be the most important for improving his mood.

Behavioral activation is proven to help improve mood and functioning in depressed individuals (Dimidjian et al., 2006; Jacobson et al., 1996). This behavioral treatment specifically targets avoidance and promotes an increase in pleasurable and rewarding activities. The examples Mark gathered of low mood (Figure 6.3) show he not only avoids work tasks but also has withdrawn from many rewarding and productive activities in his personal life. Thus the first intervention Mark's therapist chose was to help Mark schedule pleasurable and rewarding activities, including small steps to overcome avoidance.

For one week Mark recorded his current activities on an activity schedule (Beck et al., 1979; Greenberger & Padesky, 1995). A review of this record showed he spent a large amount of time at home ruminating about work-related mistakes. The consequence of his ruminative focus was that Mark did not engage in other potentially more rewarding activities. Mark's therapist actively searched for Mark's strengths and positive interests to find areas of activity that he might find pleasurable or otherwise rewarding. Careful investigation of Mark's strengths pays particular dividends because this exploration facilitates his behavioral activation:

THERAPIST: As you pointed out, your activity record shows how much time you spend ruminating about mistakes.

MARK: Yes, it fills my mind at night and ruins my life.

THERAPIST: I have an idea for what might help. It involves planning alternative activities, rewarding and pleasurable activities. What do you think of that?

MARK: That sounds OK.

THERAPIST: If you were not spending your time ruminating, what could you do instead that might be good for your mood?

MARK: Well, it would depend, I suppose. (*Mark reflects while his therapist remains quiet.*) I would like to play piano again. I have not done that for a long time.

THERAPIST: (*Leans forward, expressing interest and curiosity.*) How would that help?

MARK: I loved playing. At school I had a real talent for it. It was also something I really enjoyed.

THERAPIST: (*smiling*) That sounds great. How do you think you would feel if you could play regularly again?

MARK: Better, I guess.

THERAPIST: In what ways? For example, if you think about how that good day at work interrupted your rumination (*referring to Figure 6.7*), do you think playing the piano could help in the same way?

MARK: Well, I suppose if I am playing piano I am not kicking myself about work, so that would be good.

THERAPIST: Any positive aspects besides reducing rumination?

MARK: Well, I used to feel happy when I played. My children sometimes sit with me. And when I master a piece, sometimes I really get transported by the music.

Further detailed discussion of his musical interest and strengths led Mark to book a piano lesson so he would have structured support for rebuilding his skills. In addition to scheduling time to play the piano, he also made plans to contact his friend John to arrange some time together. These activities could boost Mark's mood as they reduced the time available for rumination about work and thus reduced the number of triggers, such as his thinking about mistakes.

Based on an understanding of Mark's triggers and maintenance factors, over the following weeks his therapist also helped him change his focus during rumination from self-criticism ("Why am I like this?") to an emphasis on problem solving ("What can I do about this tomorrow?"). This latter suggestion was derived from research that demonstrates this type of shift in ruminative focus has beneficial effects on both mood and problem solving (Nolen-Hoeksema, 2000; Watkins et al., 2007; Watkins & Moulds, 2005).

Avoidance was also addressed by encouraging Mark to draw on successes in other areas of his life where he demonstrated strengths and capacity to manage complex tasks. For instance, Mark recalled that he helped his mother sort out many financial and legal matters after his father died. Upon questioning, he remembered that he completed these complex tasks by breaking problems into small parts. Mark employed this principle in his current life to reduce his tendency to procrastinate on large tasks. Review of Mark's other successes at home led to a memory of how he helped his daughter, Jessica, overcome a fear of dogs. He described how he encouraged her not to run away when she saw a dog that frightened her. This memory inspired him decide to stay at work and finish his tasks even when he experienced sadness or anxiety, just as he had encouraged Jessica to confront her fear.

These interventions target key maintenance processes in the cross-sectional conceptualization. However, Mark and his therapist also need to address his underlying assumption, "If I make a mistake then it means I am useless." As long as this belief lies dormant, Mark is vulnerable to many triggers of low mood. Behavioral experiments are usually the intervention of choice to test underlying assumptions (Bennett-Levy et al., 2004; Padesky, 1997b, 2004). Therefore, his therapist helped Mark design a series of behavioral experiments to test his assumption that making mistakes means someone is useless.

In the first observational experiment, Mark actively looked for mistakes made by others at work. This experiment led Mark to recognize he did not judge others as useless when they made mistakes. Also, by noting other people's reactions to mistakes, Mark realized that others do not put the same importance on mistakes that he did. Discussions with his therapist uncovered an additional underlying assumption, "If I make a mistake then others will think less of me." While this assumption was consistent with many of his mother's comments regarding Mark's mistakes, Mark observed that his wife Clare and colleagues at work did not seem particularly critical or judgmental toward Mark when he made mistakes. Mark then bravely tested an alternative assumption that other people do not notice or care much about others' mistakes by deliberately making minor mistakes in presentations, documents, and meetings. Through this series of experiments Mark learned to accept that mistakes are a natural part of everyday experience and do not mean the person is useless, nor do they necessarily lead to bad outcomes.

Step 4: Review and Revise Conceptualization of Low Mood

Once interventions are chosen, their effects inform us whether the conceptualization has utility. If it does, it should adequately predict and explain intervention outcomes. Those interventions should also generally prove helpful in relieving client distress. If the interventions are not helpful or evolve in unexpected ways, the conceptualization needs to be revised to accommodate these experiences.

As described in the previous section, based on Mark's conceptualization of the triggers and maintenance factors for his low mood, he and his therapist initially chose behavioral interventions to interrupt rumination about mistakes at work, increase positive activities, and overcome avoidance. Simultaneously, he began the series of experiments described above designed to test his underlying assumptions regarding the meaning and consequences of mistakes. As expected, Mark's mood improved in the first weeks these interventions were implemented. Thus Mark and his therapist continued to review weekly events within the context of the conceptualization shown in Figures 6.6 and 6.7. During the third session after these interventions began, Mark raised a potential limitation to the conceptualization:

MARK: I know thinking about work is a big trigger for my low mood, but I noticed that when I get upset it is not always about getting things wrong at work. Like that time on Saturday—the more I think about it, it was not just the work that got me feeling sad.

THERAPIST: What else do you think made you feel so sad?

MARK: Well, I was in the line and thinking about work and the meeting and not being ready and being useless again, and those certainly made me feel anxious and down on myself. But the worst thing about it all was that I was holding my daughter's hand and I realized I was a million miles away in my mind. It made me think about what a failure I am as a dad.

THERAPIST: I remember you mentioning that before. How did that thought make you feel?

MARK: Completely miserable. (*Looks dejected; he looks downcast and his shoulders slump.*) You know, my dad was often not there for me and David when we were growing up. He was depressed for long periods, and sometimes we did not really see him. I really wanted my kids not to have to deal with that sort of thing.

THERAPIST: It sounds like it is important for you that your own low mood does not interfere with your time with your family.

MARK: It really is.

THERAPIST: So in addition to thinking about mistakes at work, thinking of yourself as a failure as a dad makes you feel bad. Do you feel this now? (*Mark nods.*) Do you think this is a separate type of thought, or do you think thoughts about mistakes and failures, whether at work or at home, is a theme that brings you down?

MARK: I think failure could be my theme song.

THERAPIST: So maybe we should spend some time today looking at this theme in a bit more detail.

INSIDE THE THERAPIST'S HEAD

The therapist recognizes that Mark's observation provides an ideal opportunity to introduce the concept of automatic thoughts and to teach Mark how to test these via Thought Records (Beck et al., 1979; Greenberger & Padesky, 1995). So far she and Mark have focused on maintenance behaviors (rumination and avoidance) and the underlying assumptions that make him vulnerable to having his low mood triggered by mistakes. However, the CBT theory of depression also highlights that negative automatic thoughts play a central role in maintaining depression (Beck, 1976). If Mark can develop skills in identifying and testing out his negative automatic thoughts, he may be able to prevent rapid mood drops like the one he just mentioned. In order to add this layer of understanding to their working conceptualization, Mark's therapist decides to gather additional examples of automatic thoughts.

THERAPIST: Perhaps we could collect some more examples of these distressing thoughts over the next week.

MARK: I have them all the time.

THERAPIST: It would be really helpful to write down some examples. Let me show you a Thought Record sheet that can help. For now, let's use this four-column worksheet. The first describes the situation you were in, who was there, and what you were doing. In the second column you write down your mood(s) and rate how you felt at your worst. For the third column I'll show you how to figure out what was going through your mind at the time so you can record that. Then in the fourth column we'll describe what you did to try to cope with or manage your feelings. I think this will become clear once we fill in this worksheet using the example you just gave. [The four-column Thought Record illustrated is a modified version of the seven-column Thought Record presented in Greenberger & Padesky, 1995.]

MARK: OK, so I was in the shop with Jessica buying lamps. My feeling was sadness. I thought to myself, "I am a useless dad. I'm a failure as a dad." The final column was I went home to bed.

THERAPIST: Wow, I can see that you understand the process involved.

MARK: Well, it is pretty similar to the ABC thing we have done before.

THERAPIST: That's true. Can you write down two or three more examples like this over the next week?

INSIDE THE THERAPIST'S HEAD

Mark's therapist notices the themes of being a failure and useless as a father are similar to those related to making mistakes at work. She begins to wonder whether these represent core beliefs that Mark holds about himself. If so, she does not know whether these core beliefs only emerge when Mark is depressed (in which case they may not require direct intervention) or whether they pervade his view of himself even when he feels better. If the latter is true, these negative core beliefs could make him particularly vulnerable to depression and may need to be addressed in therapy at a later point. She notes these themes, but she does not directly address core beliefs in this session; it would be premature given Mark's current knowledge and skills.

Before revising the conceptual model for Mark's low mood to incorporate his automatic thoughts, he and his therapist reviewed the examples Mark gathered during the preceding week (shown in Figure 6.8) in order to identify cross-sectional themes.

THERAPIST: I see you were able to use this worksheet to record examples of your thoughts over the past week. Thanks for doing this. Was this easy or hard to do?

MARK: It was OK.

THERAPIST: All right. Let's look together at what you wrote to see whether the automatic thoughts you collected give us any new ideas about what triggers or maintains your low mood.

MARK: Well, it is the same as before. Lots of times my mood gets worse when I think about work and mistakes I have made there.

THERAPIST: OK, so that seems pretty consistent. Did you notice anything new?

MARK: Well, I think a lot about how I am such a failure and cannot do anything right.

THERAPIST: OK, I see several thoughts in your examples related to this idea, "I'm a failure," "I always make mistakes," "I'm useless … a waste of space."

MARK: Yes, I realize that about myself in lots of situations.

THERAPIST: When you think about yourself as useless and a failure, do those thoughts lead you to avoid doing things?

THOUGHT RECORD

Situation	Moods Rate 0–100%	Automatic Thoughts (Images)	Actions What did you do to help manage your feelings?
In the line at the store, thinking about work on Saturday.	Sad 90%	I am always thinking about something else; I can't even pay attention to my daughter. I am such a failure as a dad.	Cried, went home, and went to bed for the rest of the day.
I was at home thinking about my work.	Low 75%	I always make mistakes. I cannot do this job anymore.	I tried to watch TV, but kept thinking about work. I stayed up really late watching bad TV.
I was at work and was asked to come to the weekly update meeting.	Anxious 80% Low 90%	I am useless—I've not done anything since last week. What a waste of space I am. It is only a matter of time until I get sacked.	Went to the meeting, but kept very quiet about what I had done.
At home getting ready to visit my mother.	Anxious 90% Worried 90%	I may have left the stove on.	Went back to check four times, then got Clare to check it last.
Saturday, at home. I saw John take his son Michael out to play football.	Sad 90%	I am useless as a Dad. John does so much more than I ever do—I never do anything with my daughter.	Went and worked on the garden to distract myself.

Figure 6.8. Examples of problematic situations Mark gathered as homework.

MARK: Sure. What's the use of doing things if I'm going to make mistakes and fail anyway?

THERAPIST: And then when you avoid doing things as a dad or husband and doing things at work, what effect does that have on your thoughts about yourself as useless?

MARK: Well, it makes things worse. I can see that. Because when I do less then I feel even more like a waste of space.

THERAPIST: Let's draw these ideas on the model we've been working with. What if we replace "thinking about work" with these automatic thoughts that give us more information about the types of thoughts that come up over and over again? This makes our model more general to all situations whether they involve work or Clare or the kids.

MARK: OK.

THERAPIST: Now, if we want to make this model general to *both* work and home, what should we write instead of "avoid work"?

MARK: Avoid work, Clare, and the kids?

THERAPIST: All right. Why don't you write that on the model? (*Watches quietly while Mark writes this on the model.*) Now, how can we show this idea that thinking you are a failure leads you to avoid doing things, and then avoiding doing things confirms you are useless and a failure?

MARK: (*Silent for a minute.*) We should draw some arrows.

THERAPIST: Why don't you do that? (*Watches while Mark completes the revised model shown in Figure 6.9.*) Mark, can you think back to any earlier work that we have done that would help us understand how this hits home with you so much?

MARK: It is the same as with work, isn't it? My theme song is failure. If I make a mistake or am not doing everything well then it shows I am useless.

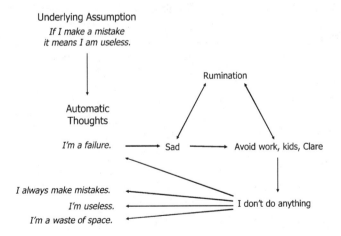

Figure 6.9. Addition of central automatic thoughts to Mark's model of triggers and maintenance factors for low mood.

Adding more specificity about Mark's thoughts clarifies the cognitive dimension of his conceptualization and leads to a more comprehensive understanding of Mark's low mood. His thoughts that he is useless and a failure contribute to his avoidance. In turn, his avoidance maintains these thoughts by providing evidence that he is not contributing at work or home. Similarly, rumination's role in maintaining his problems is clear. Mark's therapist suspects there is an underlying assumption driving the rumination along the lines of, "If I want to be seen as competent, I must do everything well," or "If I don't do everything well, I will be seen as incompetent." These underlying assumptions could explain why he checks over the day's events in his mind and focuses on mistakes or slips that otherwise may have gone unnoticed. Similarly, the therapist is curious about Mark's views of his own father because these may be relevant to understanding Mark's concerns about being a good father. She decided to flesh these points out in a subsequent session because there is not sufficient time remaining in this session.

At this point, the therapist does not know whether Mark is realistic in his interpretations. If further examination of the evidence supports Mark's conclusions that he is a poor father, husband, and worker then therapy will target improvement in his contributions. On the other hand, if Mark's thoughts are overly critical misinterpretations of his performance, he and his therapist can work to develop more balanced self-appraisals. In either case, once specific thoughts are identified, Mark and his therapist can examine the links between Mark's thoughts and behavior patterns that trap him in an unhelpful cycle of self-criticism and avoidance.

The central role of Mark's self-critical thoughts fits with Beck's theory (Beck, 1976) and research, which shows that a negative view of oneself is a key feature of depressive thinking (Clark et al., 1999). The therapist can help Mark learn to evaluate his negative automatic thoughts by drawing on the extensive literature designed to help therapists (Beck et al., 1979; J. S. Beck, 1995; Padesky & Greenberger, 1995) and clients (Burns, 1989; Greenberger & Padesky, 1995) successfully use Thought Records and behavioral experiments for this purpose. The goal of these interventions is to help the client develop explanations of experience that account for all aspects of experience, both positive and negative. If the current conceptualization is correct, more balanced thinking achieved via Thought Records and behavioral experiments will lead Mark to experience improved mood and more functional coping responses to mistakes and shortcomings.

When people cope resiliently they tend to construe events positively, including objectively challenging events. Clients are often not aware of these positive automatic thoughts. Conceptualizations of resilience bring these interpretative biases into awareness so clients have choices about how to respond during challenging times. The therapist can remain alert to times when Mark's automatic thoughts contribute to his resilience. As on the day when Mark's mood was robust throughout the workday, Mark is able to identify positive automatic thoughts when prompted.

Mark's revised explanatory conceptualization added a new set of interventions to the treatment plan. Over the next several weeks, Mark became more aware of his frequent self-criticism. With the help of the client manual *Mind over Mood* (Greenberger & Padesky, 1995), his therapist taught Mark to use thought records to test his self-evaluations that he was "useless," "a failure," and a "waste of space." When he looked at all the evidence from his week, Mark realized his global self-condemnation neglected to take into account many positive things that he was doing both at work and at home. As Mark developed skills to test out his negative thoughts, his mood noticeably improved. The results of these interventions helped Mark and his therapist evaluate the "fit" of the revised conceptualization. His positive response to cognitive interventions targeting self-critical automatic thoughts provided strong support for the revised explanatory conceptualization shown in Figure 6.9.

Discussion of one of Mark's thought records led him to reflect on the first onset of his low mood in adolescence. His therapist listened to Mark's description of this first episode of depression with interest to see whether their current working conceptualization fit his experiences during this time period as well. Mark described a period around the age of 17 when he prepared for school exams. His mother was preoccupied with his father's health problems, so Mark independently tried to organize his study schedule. When he failed several of the exams, his own disappointment was exacerbated by criticism from his mother. Her response contributed to his growing sense of hopelessness.

Mark began to see himself as useless and impotent. These beliefs strengthened as his despondency grew. He found it difficult to recover or even do daily homework and activities. It was several months before he reengaged academically and socially. Mark's first experience with depression closely matches the themes, triggers, and maintenance factors evident in his cross-sectional conceptualization for his current depression. This provides powerful support for the importance of these themes. Chapter 7 considers how these historical bases of Mark's depression can inform a longitudinal explanatory conceptualization in order to help Mark work more proactively with predisposing and protective factors to ensure his continued mental health and build resilience.

This chapter so far has illustrated how Mark and his therapist identified triggers and maintenance factors to form explanatory conceptualizations of his low mood and also his resilience on days when his mood is robust. However, it is also apparent that Mark is deeply concerned about "worries," especially related to his checking behavior and worries about contracting HIV. Thus Mark and his therapist followed the same four steps to develop explanatory conceptualizations for these additional presenting issues.

AN EXPLANATORY CONCEPTUALIZATION OF OBSESSIONAL WORRIES

Step 1: Gather Examples of Obsessional Worries

Mark's presenting issues list prioritized three sets of obsessive worries: concerns about neglecting to lock doors or leaving on the stove or lights, rumination about mistakes at work, and health worries that centered on fears of contracting HIV. These worries also showed up on Mark's thought records as shown earlier in this chapter (Figure 6.8). Mark raises these issues in one of his therapy sessions:

MARK: My mood seems to be getting better. I was hoping today we could talk about my worries, like worrying about HIV and checking everything before I can leave the house.

THERAPIST: I think that's a good idea. I notice one of the thought records you brought in covers one of those experiences. Would it be a good idea to start there? (*Indicates the fourth example on the thought record in Figure 6.8.*)

MARK: Yes, that is a good example. We were getting ready to leave the house to visit my mother. It can be quite hectic organizing the kids and all their stuff. Clare asked me to get their shoes on and help remember everything we had to take. It was a bit chaotic and I got a little stressed. As I was locking the house I thought about the stove being on, so I went back to check and it was OK. But every time I went to lock up I kept getting the thought that the gas might be on and, even though I had already checked, I had to keep going back. I was there about 10 minutes, so Clare got out of the car to see what was up. In the end I made her check while I got in the car with the kids.

THERAPIST: Is this a typical example of what happens?

MARK: Yes, it is usually the stove and the lights, but sometimes it can be the locks on the door or an appliance or the water faucet. I just get stuck checking over and over again.

THERAPIST: Let's see if we can figure out what gets you stuck and how you might get out of it. Let's start at the beginning. You said you were a bit stressed locking up, and as you did so a thought came into your mind that the stove could be on. So what would you describe as the trigger?

MARK: Leaving the house, but it can be locking up at night as well.

THERAPIST: Do you get these concerns at any other times?

MARK: Actually, I do sometimes, even when I am sitting at home.

THERAPIST: What does that tell you about the trigger?

MARK: Maybe it is not so much the time of day or situation but when a certain thought comes into my mind. I start to worry I've left the stove or lights on.

THERAPIST: OK, so the common trigger seems to be a thought about the stove being on, or the lights. Let's write that down. Tell me, on that day when you and your family were leaving the house, what were you afraid would happen if the stove was on?

 INSIDE THE THERAPIST'S HEAD

Here Mark's therapist considers whether these are intrusive thoughts characteristic of OCD. If so, the therapist expects themes of responsibility and the need to be in control (Frost et al., 1997).

MARK: Then the gas would build up in the kitchen. It would only take a spark and boom! Our house would burn down.

THERAPIST: When you thought this, did you have a picture or image in your mind of this happening?

MARK: Yes, exactly. (*Looks relieved to be understood.*) In my mind I saw the explosion and then the house on fire.

THERAPIST: Now I understand why you felt so worried. Let's write this down on a diagram. You had the thought the stove could be on and then an image of an explosion and the house burning down. This led you to become very anxious and worried. What did you do then?

MARK: I went back in the house and checked the stove.

THERAPIST: And once you checked it, how did you feel?

MARK: Better, but every time I left the house I got the same feeling that the gas could be on, even though I had just checked. It was like once I had checked, if it did burn down it would be my fault because I had checked and it had still happened. So it seemed to make it worse. Every time I wanted to leave, I had to go back and check the stove. I was acting crazy.

 INSIDE THE THERAPIST'S HEAD

Mark's thoughts seem typical of OCD. The therapist also notes Mark's view of himself as "crazy" and takes the opportunity to introduce information about OCD to help normalize Mark's experiences.

THERAPIST: I can see why it seemed crazy to you. Actually, we all sometimes have thoughts that don't make sense and yet we can't shake them. Therapists call these "intrusive thoughts." Research shows everyone has intrusive thoughts sometimes.

MARK: I've never known Clare to have thoughts like this.

THERAPIST: Her intrusive thoughts may be different than yours. And most of the time for most people, they are not much of a problem. Like when we can't stop thinking about all the things we have to do the next day.

MARK: But worrying about the stove and lights even after I've checked them a number of times just seems weird.

THERAPIST: When you keep checking things like you do and can't get these types of intrusive thoughts out of you mind, it sounds like what we call obsessive–compulsive disorder, or OCD. Have you heard of that?

MARK: I read about that on Internet when I was trying to figure out what was wrong with me. It sounded like me. Can you help me with that? The website said it could be treated.

THERAPIST: Yes, it can. To start, let me tell you how we understand OCD and see whether it fits with your experience. The first important idea is that a thought pops into our heads and triggers distress. These are often unwanted, unpleasant thoughts that we call intrusive thoughts. Yours often seems to be about the stove being on. Is that right?

MARK: Yes, most days.

THERAPIST: I have written this intrusive thought down [Figure 6.10]. As I said before, everyone get these types of thoughts but only some people are distressed by them. The meaning you make of this thought seems to determine how distressing it is. You said you feared there could be an explosion and the house would burn down and it would be your fault. Have I got that right?

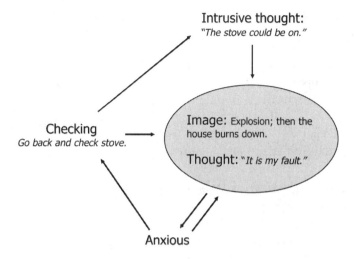

Figure 6.10. A model of Mark's OCD concerns.

MARK: Yes. It would be awful.

THERAPIST: Let me add this information to our model. (*Adds this information on Figure 6.10.*) What do you make of this so far?

MARK: Yeah, that is what it is like for me. It would be awful if the house burned down and it would be my fault.

 INSIDE THE THERAPIST'S HEAD

Here the therapist notes that Mark talks again about it being his responsibility, which is one theme identified as central in OCD (Frost et al., 1997).

THERAPIST: Sure. And what would be the worst part from your point of view?

MARK: It would be my fault that the kids did not have a home and that we had nowhere to live. People would think I was incompetent for not even checking the stove.

As demonstrated in this dialogue, explanatory conceptualizations can develop quite fluidly. As Mark's therapist begins to gather examples of Mark's obsessional worries there appears to be a very close match to the diagnosis of OCD, for which evidence-based theories exist. Thus the therapist begins to teach Mark about OCD and asks probing questions to assess whether the expected cognitive aspects of OCD (e.g., responsibility) map onto his experience. This discussion leads Mark and his therapist to tentatively consider that his worries about the stove might meet criteria for OCD. Prior to this session, the therapist had already noted examples in the assessment information Mark provided and his thought records that fit the pattern of OCD. Thus, instead of gathering additional examples in this session, Mark's therapist proceeded directly to the search for triggers and maintenance factors.

Step 2: Identify Triggers and Maintenance Factors of Obsessional Worries

THERAPIST: You say checking the stove helps but also makes it worse because if something happens after you check that makes it even more your fault. Let's write that down because it helps us understand the reaction you had to this intrusive thought. Do you think your actions have any impact on keeping this problem going?

MARK: Well, I know that the more I check the worse I feel, but I feel I have to check.

THERAPIST: So to show that checking both helps and makes it worse, we can draw one arrow that shows you check when anxious and another arrow that shows the more you check the more you feel it is your fault. Is that right?

MARK: Yes, if I check and then something bad happens it makes me look even worse.

THERAPIST: You said in the end you asked Clare to check. Is that right?

MARK: Yes, if she checks last then I feel OK.

THERAPIST: How does that help?

MARK: Well, it's odd, really, because I am not that certain she really checks. She is quite laid back about things. But it helps because then, if something did happen, it would not be my fault.

INSIDE THE THERAPIST'S HEAD

Here the key issue of responsibility emerges again, reinforcing the selection of the disorder-specific OCD model.

THERAPIST: So it sounds like the notion of who is to blame or who is at fault is really central. What makes it so important to you that it is not your fault?

MARK: Well, as a father, as the man of the house, it is my responsibility to make sure everyone is safe. I am the responsible one.

THERAPIST: OK, that is helpful to know. When we looked at your low mood we discovered that some behaviors like avoidance and rumination can actually make a problem persist even when it seems like they help in the short run. In this example of checking, do you think any of your behaviors can help us understand what keeps this worry going?

MARK: (*Looks interested.*) I think two things are key. The first is I do go back and check again and again, which does not help. It is like my ruminating about work. The more I check the more things there are to find are wrong. The other is I try to avoid being the last one out of the house. I see if I can get Clare to leave after me. There is that word "avoid" again. I do it here, too.

THERAPIST: Those are helpful observations. Let's write down on our model all the ways you try and manage this experience. (*Mark and therapist construct Figure 6.11.*)

This developing understanding of Mark's OCD identifies the trigger as a normal intrusive thought, "The stove is on," that resonates with his underlying assumptions about responsibility. His anxiety is maintained by the steps he takes to reduce his anxiety. Whereas rumination and avoidance maintain Mark's low mood, checking behaviors and avoidance of responsibility appear to maintain his OCD. To treat OCD it is vital to elicit all the behaviors that serve to neutralize anxiety. These can be overt compulsive behaviors and also covert behaviors such as mental rituals. Treatment is usually effective only when all maintenance behaviors stop (Abramowitz, 1997; Emmelkamp et al., 1988; van Oppen et al., 1995; Salkovskis, 1999).

Common to most CBT models of OCD is the idea that the person experiences an intrusive thought with particular personal resonance that causes high levels of distress (Frost et al., 1997). This leads to anxiety. The person is motivated to reduce the distress by acting to "neutralize" it (van Oppen & Arntz, 1994). This process of neutralizing the anxiety, if repeated, is expressed in the form of compulsions. Hence, the therapist can compare Mark's experiences to a very specific theoretical model.

The conceptualization that emerged helps Mark understand that his assumptions about responsibility are central to the problem, as are

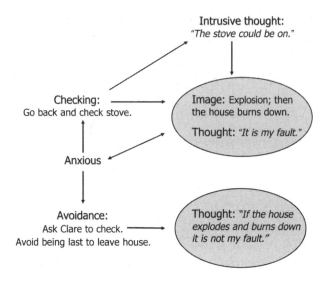

Figure 6.11. An elaborated model of Mark's OCD concerns.

his maintaining behaviors (checking and avoidance). As his avoidance behaviors make clear (see bottom section of Figure 6.11), Mark's anxiety is more closely linked to the idea he is responsible and to blame than it is to the fear of his house burning down. His anxiety is reduced if Clare is responsible for the disaster. This conceptualization is a close "fit" with cognitive-behavioral models of OCD (Emmelkamp et al., 1988; van Oppen et al., 1995).

Step 3: Select Interventions Based on the Explanatory Conceptualization of Obsessional Worries

Mark checks the stove, door locks, lights, appliances, and faucets repeatedly. Once again, Mark's therapist adds knowledge of theory and research to the crucible by accessing the research literature on effective treatments for OCD and specific methods of intervention for OCD concerns (Abramowitz, 1997). The integration of Mark's personal experiences with CBT theory and research guided his therapist to three vital areas for intervention: (1) intrusive thoughts, (2) an inflated sense of responsibility, and (3) the maintenance behaviors of checking and avoidance. The nature of these interventions is briefly outlined here.

The goal of OCD treatment is not to stop intrusive thoughts but to recognize these thoughts as normal phenomena made worse by attempts to control them. The OCD treatment literature emphasizes the importance of eliciting and examining every behavior that occurs in response to intrusive thoughts. People engage in a variety of safety-seeking behaviors that can range from very overt behaviors, such as checking or cleaning compulsions, to very discreet, almost unnoticeable behaviors, such as not touching the therapist's door handle on the way into the office (in order to prevent contamination), to covert or mental neutralizations, such as counting or thinking positive thoughts. Because people with OCD believe each of these responses can help prevent the feared catastrophe, each must be identified and added to the conceptualization. An important part of treatment is to stop all maintaining behaviors in order to learn that the feared outcome will not happen in the absence of these safety behaviors. In addition, the client learns to accept and cope with a reasonable amount of responsibility when bad events do happen. Mark's therapist decided his checking behavior was well suited to standard CBT interventions for OCD, including education regarding the CBT model, exposure and response prevention, and cognitive evaluations of responsibility beliefs (van Oppen & Arntz, 1994).

The first stage of this therapy was to normalize the occurrence of Mark's intrusive thoughts. Although lists of intrusive thoughts and self-help materials can help normalize these experiences, it is far more compelling if the client can discover for him- or herself that these thoughts are common and can be experienced in the absence of distress. For this reason Mark and his therapist devised a "survey" whereby Mark asked people he trusted whether they ever experienced intrusive thoughts. This homework assignment drew on Mark's identified strength of having a close and supportive family and friendships. As described below, the results of this intervention reduced Mark's distress and enhanced the utility of the case conceptualization:

THERAPIST: Thanks for the update as to how you have been. What would you like to put on the agenda for today?

MARK: Well, I want to let you know what I found out from my survey.

THERAPIST: I'm curious to hear about it. (*Builds the rest of the agenda.*) Shall we begin with your survey? (*Mark nods eagerly.*) Tell me what you found out.

MARK: Even though last week you gave me a list of intrusive thoughts that other people have reported, I was not really sure whether people I know have these kinds of thoughts. So we agreed I would ask people I trusted whether they ever had odd or unusual thoughts.

THERAPIST: That's what I remember, too. What did you learn?

MARK: Well, I was a little embarrassed, but I asked Clare and my friend John.

THERAPIST: Good for you! What did you find out?

MARK: Well, I was really surprised. I never thought Clare had these sorts of thoughts, but she told me that when Jessica was very young, Clare used to think she would let go of the stroller on a hill and Jessica would crash. She was worried that thought meant she wanted it to happen, and so she used to tie a strap to her wrist and the stroller so it could not roll away. I never knew that.

THERAPIST: That does sound similar to some of your thoughts.

MARK: Yes. And then John told me he sometimes gets this thought in his head about saying something really rude in church, especially when it is really quiet. He is really religious, and it surprised me he would think about that. He says he tries not to think about it when it happens and he prays when the thought is strong.

THERAPIST: I am really impressed with what you found out. What do you make of it?

MARK: Well, it is like we discussed. Odd thoughts seem to be common, but what bothers one person may not bother another. I would not be bothered about saying anything in church, for instance.

THERAPIST: How does that fit with our understanding of your difficulties?

MARK: Well it really fits, doesn't it! It is not the thought itself but my reaction to it that really matters.

THERAPIST: How does that make you feel?

MARK: Well, a little better to know I am not the only one who has thoughts like this. I'm not sure I know how to do things differently, but I don't feel so different!

Step 4: Review and Revise Conceptualization of Obsessional Worries

Mark's survey results normalized the occurrence of intrusive thoughts. At the same time, his survey helped evaluate the conceptual validity of their working conceptualization. Clare's and John's responses supported the idea that other people have unwanted and intrusive thoughts. In addition, their responses provide tentative support for the importance of responsibility. Clare's example coincided with her new sense of responsibility for a young child. John felt a religious responsibility to control the language he used. Mark and his therapist used a number of additional methods to understand how responsibility appraisals influenced the meanings placed on intrusive thoughts and to reduce the responsibility Mark felt for negative events. For example, pie charts were drawn to consider all the factors or people that share responsibility when particular negative events occurred (Greenberger & Padesky, 1995). This notion of responsibility is given further consideration in Chapter 7 because it proved to be an important predisposing factor for Mark. The third key element in the conceptualization of Mark's obsessive worries was avoidance and checking behavior. This was tackled with good success using exposure and response prevention for the range of behaviors identified.

To check the fit of the emerging conceptualization of Mark's OCD, he and his therapist considered whether it could explain the onset of his difficulties. Mark did not think his OCD had an onset with discrete episodes. Rather, it emerged when he was a young teen and had been a feature of his life since. His OCD varied in its intensity, but Mark saw himself as someone who always had checked things. The focus of his concerns had changed over time from checking the time on his watch so he would not be late and checking homework assignments in school to checking faucets, stoves, and doors, but the pattern was the same. Mark described how he first noticed he checked repeatedly when he became anxious in his teenage years. During this time, he was given more responsibility for his brother David in order to help his mother care for his father, who had periods of poor physical health and difficulties as a result of his bipolar disorder. Although there is no specific onset event in Mark's account, the theme of responsibility is present from the beginning and one that is evident very much in the here and now.

Mark's HIV Worries: OCD or Health Anxiety?

The OCD model proved a close "fit" for Mark's worries about the stove and his checking behavior. It was therefore natural for Mark and his therapist to see whether this same model applied to Mark's concerns about contracting HIV. However, the guidelines for generating a good-enough conceptualization (Box 2.2) emphasize the importance of regarding a conceptualization as provisional and actively entertaining alternative conceptualizations. With this principle in mind, Mark's therapist considered whether Mark's HIV worries were better explained by health anxiety models (Salkovskis & Warwick, 2001).

Health anxiety and OCD share many similarities, such as frequent checking behavior. They differ in that people with OCD focus on responsibility for negative events, while those with health anxiety typically fear they have an illness that is life threatening in the short or medium term. In addition, people with health anxiety commonly seek reassurance that they are healthy and request medical tests and interventions to search for evidence of illness. Like those with health anxiety, Mark did seek reassurance from Clare. He also took HIV tests. When the test results were negative his anxiety would decrease for a short time. However, Mark perceived the risk of contamination as high, so it was not long before his anxiety about HIV was activated again. These observations fit with health anxiety.

On the other hand, Mark told his therapist that the most upsetting aspect of being diagnosed with HIV would be the perception of others that his behavior was immoral and irresponsible. This observation fits best with the OCD spectrum of disorders rather than a health anxiety, in which the worst aspect would be loss of life. Once again Mark and his therapist reviewed the onset of his worries to help establish whether responsibility was a key issue in the development of his HIV concerns.

Mark described how his HIV worries began nearly 20 years earlier when he was a young man in his first serious relationship with a woman. He was unfaithful to her one night when he had unprotected sex with another woman. It was at a time when education regarding HIV and AIDS was high. Public health campaigns were encouraging safer sex practices. There were public predictions that many people would develop AIDS. Also at that time there was a presumptive association between AIDS and promiscuous homosexual behavior or drug use. His concerns about HIV had persisted for two decades despite his monogamous sexual relationship with Clare for the past 14 years. Whenever Mark saw blood, a stain, or any material that could contain bodily fluids he had an intrusive thought that he could acquire HIV from physical contact with it.

Mark's experiences seemed to partially match a diagnosis of OCD and partially match a diagnosis of health anxiety. Although diagnosis is helpful to the case conceptualization process, it is important to remember that diagnosis and conceptualization serve compatible but nevertheless different functions. Like overlapping Venn diagrams, health anxiety, OCD, panic disorder, social phobia, and even conditions like generalized anxiety disorder overlap to some extent and share common features (Beck et al., 1985). Each of these disorders is marked by vigilance for and misinterpretation of normally occurring phenomena such as intrusive thoughts or bodily sensations. Mark's HIV worries thrived on vigilance and overestimation of risks. At the same time, his worries incorporated both the reassurance seeking common in health anxiety and neutralization processes common in OCD.

Therefore, Mark's therapist considered theory and research regarding both the OCD and health anxiety literatures in the construction of a conceptualization model for Mark's HIV worries. Using the steps outlined in this chapter, they developed an understanding of triggers and maintenance factors for Mark's HIV concern. During the conceptualization process it helped that Mark could recognize that his concern was not constant over the years but varied in terms of conviction and distress. This observed variability following on the heels of conceptualizations already formed for his low mood and OCD suggested to Mark that his thoughts and behaviors probably played a role in determining his degree of anxiety about contracting HIV.

Mark acknowledged early in discussions that his anxiety was not primarily linked to fears about the physical dangers of HIV. He recognized that, even if he developed HIV, he had access to medications that would make the disease manageable. Instead, he was afraid people would think he had been unfaithful to his wife and consequently think poorly of him. The threat was to his moral values and his standing in the community. Mark described how his own father had been unfaithful at times when he experienced periods of elation and mania. Mark knew that this was, in part, a feature of his dad's bipolar disorder, a condition he did not share. Even so, Mark remembered how much it hurt his mother when his father had sexual relationships with other women. Mark believed he should have learned from this experience to never act irresponsibly. To bolster the point that he did not want to be seen by others as sexually irresponsible, Mark was not concerned about catching hepatitis C or another blood-borne infection because these did not have the same stigma attached to them.

As shown in Figure 6.12, Mark's HIV worries were triggered by a variety of events ranging from red marks on a cup to swimming in public pools. Once triggered, Mark found it hard to cope with the anxiety caused by the fear of having acquired HIV and the underlying assumption, "If I have HIV then other people will think I have been unfaithful to Clare and think badly of me." He employed the same strategies of avoidance and checking behavior that characterized his OCD. His checking behavior included seeking reassurance from Clare that he had not contracted HIV and scanning his body for signs of infection or ill health. He recognized that he was alert and vigilant for blood and bodily fluids in the environment around him, often avoiding situations where he might come into contact with these. A negative HIV test would temporarily neutralize his anxiety until the cycle started again.

The conceptualization of Mark's HIV concerns was so similar to ones formed for Mark's low mood and OCD that it surprised him. He thought his health worries were completely distinct from his other presenting issues. The similarity of this model to those formulated earlier in therapy helped this conceptualization serve a useful function of acting as an alternative explanation in the treatment of his HIV worries.

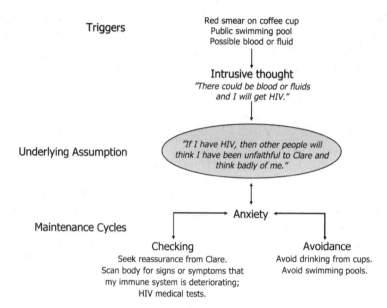

Figure 6.12. A conceptualization of Mark's HIV concerns.

Salkovskis (1999) describes the futility of trying to prove to someone that a feared future outcome will not happen. Even an HIV test did not stop Mark from worrying; it only temporarily relieved his anxiety. Salkovskis described the usefulness of building an alternative theory (theory B) to test against the person's distressing explanation (theory A). For Mark theory A, "You have acquired HIV," can be evaluated against the conceptualization, theory B, "You are only worried about acquiring HIV and being socially judged." The costs of maintaining the original theory A were emphasized by Mark's therapist, who used a range of metaphors and analogies (Blenkiron, 2005) to help him see that his best efforts to keep himself safe actually maintained the problem and exacted a huge cost in time, money, distress, and reduced quality of life. This approach helped Mark begin to appreciate that theory B, the conceptualization in Figure 6.12, was an adequate and less demanding view of his experiences.

Mark was able to see parallels between the intrusive thoughts that triggered his HIV concerns and those that triggered his OCD checking behavior. Discussions with his therapist helped him reappraise HIV infection as not reflecting on immorality or irresponsibility. Mark recognized that people could acquire HIV in a variety of different ways, and this helped reduce the negative evaluation he attached to acquiring HIV, reducing his anxiety about it. Standard exposure and response-prevention methods were used to expose Mark to perceived potential risks such as coffee cups and the public swimming pool. Mark also stopped other maintenance behaviors such as seeking reassurance from Clare and taking HIV tests.

CONSIDER HOW THE PRESENTING ISSUES ARE LINKED

Whenever possible, conceptualizations should highlight commonalities between presenting issues. Mark and his therapist noticed common features in operation across Mark's presenting issues of low mood, OCD, and health concerns. Each had triggers that centered on themes of mistakes or risk for negative outcomes. These triggers elicited themes of failure and responsibility that increased Mark's low mood and anxiety. Mark attempted to cope with distressing moods, whether depression or anxiety, through avoidance, checking, and rumination. As a result of these similarities, Mark and his therapist constructed a more generic conceptualization of his emotional distress as shown in Figure 6.13. This general model highlights the common triggers, beliefs, and maintenance factors for Mark's depression and anxiety. In Chapter 7 Mark and his therapist link these explanatory conceptual models to predisposing and

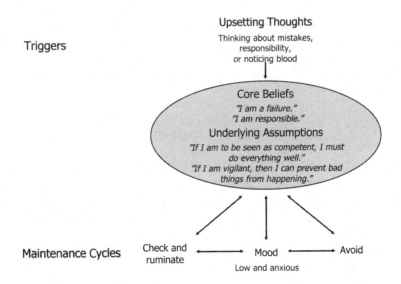

Figure 6.13. A unified conceptualization of Mark's low mood, OCD, and HIV worries.

protective factors, helping Mark understand why he is vulnerable to these particular issues.

Some readers may wonder why Mark's therapist did not begin with a unified conceptual model similar to that shown in Figure 6.13. There are several reasons. First, case conceptualization is a process that typically starts with simple descriptive models and evolves over time into more elaborated explanatory models. Early in therapy, an experienced therapist may well see the outline of an elaborated explanatory model that includes beliefs, triggers, and maintenance factors common to several presenting issues. However, by developing the conceptualization over time using a collaborative and empirical approach the client participates fully in the process. Active client participation ensures that checks and balances are in place on therapist heuristic errors at each level of conceptualization (Chapters 2 and 3).

Second, if theory and research about a specific disorder map onto a client's presenting issues, the disorder-specific model has primacy due to its empirical support. Only by taking the time to describe the presenting issues (Chapter 5) and develop simpler explanatory models of the main presenting issues can the therapist establish which disorder-specific models fit. As illustrated in this chapter, because these explanatory models were derived from Mark's own observations, he considered their implications with an open mind. While looking at mood, checking behavior, and HIV fears, Mark and his therapist were able to test the fit of three disorder-specific models and Mark was motivated to follow their companion treatment plans. We argue that the collaborative and empirical step-by-step conceptualization of triggers and maintenance factors is more important than the speed or generality of the model chosen. Conceptual models can be revised; they are means to an end, not an end in themselves.

OUTCOMES OF THE CRUCIBLE PROCESS

According to our thesis, the two fundamental purposes of case conceptualization are to alleviate distress and build resilience. To what degree did the explanatory conceptualizations derived by Mark and his therapist foster these goals? First, consider reductions in his distress. At the conclusion of this work on triggers and maintenance cycles, Mark and his therapist reviewed his presenting issues list. They noted improvements in mood, reduced OCD checking behaviors, and reduced concerns about HIV. Mark told his therapist he believed he had achieved some of his short- and medium-term goals, especially in relation to low mood (see Box 5.5). He rated his mood as 5 or 6 most of the time. Mark reported reduced avoidance and rumination and generally more effective work performance. He also commented on an increased range and number of rewarding activities during his week. Mark reported similar improvements in relation to his checking and HIV concerns. This was corroborated with repeat administration of the BDI-II and BAI at each session, indicating a reduction in depression to 12 and on the BAI to 14 by session 15. Measures of OCD introduced at session 10 (e.g., Padua Inventory; Sanavio, 1980) also demonstrated the impact of OCD interventions.

In terms of resilience, Mark reported increased use of coping methods linked to resilience, such as more active problem solving, acceptance of difficulties and mistakes as a "normal part of living," and a greater appreciation of his capacity to contribute to his family and workplace. Mark's growing conviction in the disadvantages of avoidance, rumination, and checking gave him new resolve to learn alternative approaches to manage his distress. The extent to which he succeeds in these efforts will strengthen his future resilience.

It may be tempting to end therapy at this time. For many clients, especially those with more recent onset of problems, explanatory conceptualizations are sufficient to achieve a positive therapy outcome and ensure a low risk of relapse. However, Mark reports chronic difficulties in these areas and a propensity to relapse after a period of feeling better. For these reasons, his therapist believes Mark can be helped further and perhaps stay well longer if they consider additional questions. First, what led to these issues developing in the first place; that is, what predisposed Mark to these issues? Second, can Mark meet his longer-term goals, remain well, and show greater resilience in the future? The following chapter shows how Mark and his therapist investigate these important issues.

Chapter 6 Summary

- Explanatory conceptualizations answer the question "Why does this keep happening to me?"
- Explanatory conceptualizations generally emerge from a four-stage process:
  —Gather and describe several specific examples.
  —Identify specific triggers and maintenance factors by collaboratively looking for themes and commonalities among these examples. Eval-

uate triggers and maintenance factors in the light of existing evidence-based models for the presenting issue and "fit" to subsequent client experiences.

—Select interventions based on the explanatory conceptualization.

—Review and revise the conceptual model based on observations of the effects of chosen interventions. Does the model "fit," and do the interventions help as expected?

• These four steps are repeated for additional presenting issues. Therapist and client consider whether the presenting issues are linked by common triggers and maintenance factors.

• The triggers and maintenance factors are considered in relation to the onset of the presenting issues to determine whether the themes present in the here and now were evident at the onset.

• Ultimately the value of an explanatory conceptualization is judged in terms of whether it leads to interventions that reduce client distress and increase client resilience.

Chapter 7

"Does My Future Look Like My Past?"

Longitudinal Explanatory Conceptualizations

MARK: I'm doing better. That sense of feeling low all the time has mostly passed; it's made a real difference, especially at work. (*Half smiles*.)

THERAPIST: You've made real progress, Mark, and that's due to the hard work you have put into therapy. I am pleased for you because improving things at work was a high priority for you when we started working together. (*Smiles encouragingly and then, picking up on Mark's nonverbal communication, says*:) I'm sensing a "but" in what you are saying.

MARK: (*Pauses, half smiles again, and then begins to look hopeless*.) Yeah, last Saturday morning we had a blowout at home that shook me, particularly after it seemed like I was making real progress.

THERAPIST: Tell me what happened and let's see what we can learn from it.

MARK: I'd had a tough week at work, and mostly I handled it well. But when I woke up on Saturday morning I immediately started to worry, you know all those familiar thoughts about "I didn't do that report as well as I should," "My boss noticed that I was late to the staff meeting and thinks I am not up to my job," and so on ...

THERAPIST: So, how did you handle the worry?

MARK: (*cutting in*) I'm not done yet. My daughter, Jessica, came into the bedroom. She and I had agreed to go swimming first thing on Saturday morning. (*Looks up.*) We've been doing that as a father–daughter routine these last few months. Anyway, she came in all bright eyed and (*looking ashamed*) I pretended to be asleep. I just didn't feel up to it. I just lay there thinking, "I can't do it today."

INSIDE THE THERAPIST'S HEAD

The therapist observes that Mark is identifying a stream of automatic thoughts—"I didn't do that report as well as I should," "My boss noticed that I was late to the meeting and thinks I am not up to my job," and "I can't do it today"—that are consistent with the underlying assumption "If I want to be seen as competent then I must do everything well" and core beliefs related to the themes of failure and responsibility previously identified (see Chapter 6). She also notes that Mark has started going swimming with his daughter on Saturday mornings, providing evidence that he has made progress on his goal "Go swimming with my children at the public pool" (see Chapter 5). Given Mark's progress and the fact that this is a session in a later stage of therapy, she chooses to see whether Mark is able to transfer the skills he has developed previously in CBT to cope resiliently with this situation at home.

MARK: (*after a pause, continuing*) And that's not the end of it. After 10 minutes Clare comes in and she blows her top. She says, "Mark, you promised Jessica you'd take her swimming. This means a lot to her. Get out of bed and stop feeling sorry for yourself. This isn't OK." I lay there, I felt like such a waste of space (*looking really dejected now*), but as hard as I tried I couldn't bring myself to get out of bed and I asked Clare to leave me alone. That didn't go down too well. She stormed out of the bedroom saying, "I've had enough of you feeling sorry for yourself. I'll take the kids swimming myself, but by the time we get back I want you to have pulled yourself together." Then she went out, slamming the bedroom door on her way out. (*Half smiles.*)

THERAPIST: How come you're smiling?

MARK: Because I feel so lucky to have Clare. She was right; she helped me get out of that funk.

THERAPIST: (*noting the resilience embedded in Mark's statement and wishing to encourage his growing self-efficacy*) Great, so what did you do to get out of the funk?

MARK: I waited for them all to leave. And then I got out of bed and completed a Thought Record, which was sort of reassuring because it was all there, the same old thoughts, and I was able to respond to them. When they came back I was out of bed and we had a good family day afterwards. I distracted myself, sort of. Here's the Thought Record. (*Gets out the Thought Record, Figure 7.1.*)

THERAPIST: OK, let's look at this together. (*Mark holds the Thought Record while the therapist reads through it.*) What did you mean when you said "I distracted myself, sort of" just now?

MARK: Two things, really. First, I was kind of worried because I was used to having these kinds of thoughts about work, but not so much about my family. Home seemed like a good part of life, and it wasn't good to have these useless thoughts in relation to Clare and the kids.

THERAPIST: And the second thing?

MARK: Well, you can see when I came up with the responses to my negative thoughts, I didn't actually believe all my responses as much as the negative thoughts. (*Looks miserable.*)

THERAPIST: Mark, at this stage in our work together I would like to suggest that whenever you have these setbacks you look for what you can learn from them. Setbacks provide chances for us to find out whether the skills you have learned so far can help you to cope with setbacks in the future. (*Mark nods.*) What you are saying is that this thought, "I can't even get things right at home, Clare thinks I'm useless," was a bit like your thoughts at work, and you believed this thought more than the response on your Thought Record (*looking at the form together*), "She thinks I am a good father sometimes," which you rated 50% compared with 95% for the negative automatic thought. Have I understood you right?

MARK: Yeah. You know, the feeling I couldn't shake off was "I'm a waste of space." (*pauses*) Worse than that, "I'm a waste of space at work and at home!"

THERAPIST: So beneath this thought on the Thought Record, "I can't even get things right at home, Clare thinks I'm useless," was a more all-encompassing thought, "I'm a waste of space."

MARK: That's right.

THERAPIST: I think it's great you managed to use the skills you have learned so far to get out of your funk during the weekend. And I notice you did successfully answer your worry thoughts about work (*pointing at the Thought Record, Figure 7.1*) enough to have a good

THOUGHT RECORD

Situation Who, what, when, where?	Moods Specify Rate 0–100%	Automatic thoughts (Images)	Evidence that supports my hot thought(s)	Evidence that does not support my hot thought(s)	Alternative/Balanced Thoughts Rate how much I believe this: (0–100%)	Rate moods now 0–100%
I was at home on Saturday morning and couldn't get out of bed.	Anxious 70%	I didn't do that report as well as I should. 90%	I did the report quickly before the meeting.	The report was routine and didn't require anything special.	This worry is nonproductive; I will work hard on Monday when I have a chance to do my job right. 95%	Anxious 20%
	Sad 80%	My boss noticed that I was late to the staff meeting and thinks I am not up to my job. 75%	My boss looked up when I walked into the room.	I don't know what my boss thought. He didn't act upset.	Same as above. 95%	Sad 60%
	Ashamed 60%	I can't even get things right at home, Clare thinks I'm useless. 95%	I promised Jessica we'd go swimming. Clare told me she is fed up with me.	Yesterday I took care of the kids while Clare went shopping and did an OK job.	She thinks I am a good father sometimes. 50%	Ashamed 55%

Figure 7.1. Thought Record completed by Mark showing summary of three hot thoughts with evidence. Seven-column Thought Record copyright 1983, 1994 by Christine A. Padesky (*www.padesky.com*). Adapted with permission.

time with your family. Also, it sounds like you've been getting to the pool with Jessica these last few weeks. That's progress. Would you like to spend some time working on this "waste of space" idea since it seems to be something you are finding difficult to deal with using the skills you have learned so far?

MARK: Yeah, I need to do that.

Mark has made real progress in his ability to respond to automatic thoughts using Thought Records. He is able to identify when ruminative thinking starts and, for the most part, has learned to step out of non-productive thinking patterns about work. Despite this progress, Mark remains more vulnerable to setbacks than his therapist expects based on his improvement on mood measures (see end of Chapter 6) and reduction in his OCD and health anxiety symptoms. When therapy focused on Axis I problems does not progress as expected it may be that enduring underlying assumptions and core beliefs are implicated in the presenting issues. The dialogue above illustrates the pervasiveness of the underlying assumption, "If I want to be seen as competent then I must do everything well," that underpins both his mood problems and anxiety (Chapter 6). It affects other parts of his life as well, including his views of himself as a husband and father. Mark also identifies a thought, "I'm a waste of space," which has occurred in various domains of Mark's life and elicits such strong emotions that it appears to be a core belief.

Thought Records are designed to help clients test automatic thoughts, not underlying assumptions or core beliefs. Therefore it is understandable that Mark's attempts to cope using a Thought Record were only partially successful. The behavioral experiments Mark has completed to date in therapy addressed specific worries and OCD-related beliefs such as "If I don't check the stove, a disaster will happen and I will be responsible" and "If I make a mistake, others will criticize me." He has not yet used behavioral experiments to test out "If I want to be seen as competent, I must do everything well." Further forward movement in Mark's therapy may require another level of understanding.

In this chapter Mark and his therapist use longitudinal conceptualization to explore how key developmental experiences led to the underlying assumptions and core beliefs that threaten to derail his progress. This higher level of conceptualization seeks to understand the links between Mark's developmental history, core beliefs, underlying assumptions, behavioral strategies, and his vulnerability to setbacks. By incorporating strengths into Mark's longitudinal conceptualization, his therapist helps Mark construct a model of resilience that can help maintain his progress in the future.

WHY USE A LONGITUDINAL CONCEPTUALIZATION?

CBT's focus on goals and emphasis on the present are often cited as basic principles (e.g., J. S. Beck, 1995, pp. 7–8). If CBT is present focused and goal oriented, why use a longitudinal conceptualization? When CBT based on a cross-sectional conceptualization is sufficient to achieve clients' goals, it is not necessary to extend therapy to include longitudinal conceptualization. In fact, unless there are pervasive and enduring problems, for example, in people with personality disorders, we suggest that longitudinal conceptualization is not typically necessary to achieve CBT's goals of alleviating distress and building resilience. However, even Axis I difficulties sometimes show a very slow response to CBT. Other times, positive therapy responses achieved for Axis I problems seem fragile and highly vulnerable to relapse. In these instances, longitudinal conceptualizations can help decipher the underlying assumptions and core beliefs that interfere with more enduring positive outcomes.

How will a focus on the past help Mark move forward toward achieving his goals? By their very nature, underlying assumptions and core beliefs tend to persist across situations and time. They are often learned through key developmental experiences (Beck, 1976). People learn paired core beliefs (e.g., "I'm a waste of space" balanced with "I'm worthwhile"), with one of these paired beliefs activated at a time, depending on a person's moods and life circumstances. When a core belief is activated most of the time, regardless of mood and situation, this can signal that a paired alternative belief is either very weak or missing. In this circumstance, it is often necessary to employ therapy methods designed to build and strengthen new core beliefs (Padesky, 1994a). Similarly, underlying assumptions that persist across multiple life circumstances are unlikely to shift unless tested directly via behavioral experiments.

During the opening dialogue of this chapter, Mark's therapist wonders:

- Why are Mark's gains not sticking?
- Why is Mark being drawn back into old patterns?

Longitudinal conceptualizations offer answers to these questions. Longitudinal conceptualizations:

- Explain why there has been limited or short-lived progress with cross-sectional conceptualizations based on triggers and maintenance factors.
- Explain why problems persist across situations and time by sug-

gesting how key developmental experiences shaped client core beliefs, underlying assumptions, and coping strategies.

• Predict similar future client reactions, thus recommending therapy foci on resilience as well as relapse prevention and management.

Consistent with our principle that higher levels of explanation emerge over the course of therapy, a longitudinal conceptualization typically evolves from a cross-sectional one. It is often a feature of middle and later stages of therapy. Thus, the conceptualizations of triggers and maintenance factors for Mark's presenting issues (Chapter 6) serve as the starting point for constructing a longitudinal conceptualization of how his beliefs and strategies developed. In fact, longitudinal conceptualizations can be viewed as a special form of cross-sectional explanation in which the conceptualization is viewed through the lens of a client's developmental history. Longitudinal conceptualizations ask, "How were these core beliefs, underlying assumptions, and coping strategies learned? Why are some issues more potent triggers than others? What factors contributed to maintenance patterns? How did the person's strengths prevent the presenting issues from being worse?"

By providing an understanding of how presenting issues developed over time, the longitudinal conceptualization provides guidance to devise interventions that can break up pervasive beliefs and behavioral patterns connected to distress and build resilience.

HOW TO CONSTRUCT A LONGITUDINAL CONCEPTUALIZATION

Longitudinal conceptualizations move iteratively through two phases. First the therapist and client construct a conceptualization that uses cognitive-behavioral theory to link the client's presenting issues with his or her developmental history. Next, this conceptualization is used to design interventions that can help break up the pervasive beliefs and behavioral patterns that maintain presenting issues. In addition, interventions are often designed to strengthen beliefs and behavioral patterns that are more functional for the client. Intervention outcomes and the learning these prompt provide feedback for the conceptualization, either confirming or suggesting modifications for it. As shown in Figure 7.2, therapy moves between these two phases of (1) longitudinal conceptualization and (2) conceptualization-based intervention. Each phase is informed by therapist and client answers to the question, "How well does the conceptualization fit?"

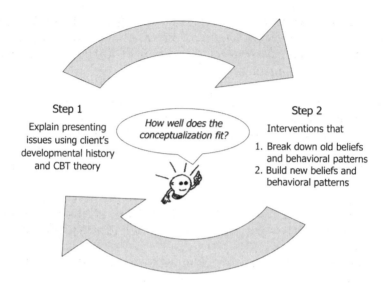

Figure 7.2. Steps in constructing a longitudinal conceptualization.

Step 1: Use CBT Theory to Link Presenting Issues with the Client's Developmental History

Mark made good progress toward his therapy goals through the middle phases of therapy using traditional CBT approaches (Chapter 6). However, as we saw in this chapter's opening dialogue, his mood and anxiety problems resurfaced one Saturday morning along with familiar distress-related beliefs ("If I want to be seen as competent, I must do everything well" and "I'm a waste of space") and strategies (rumination and withdrawal). These experiences fit with the transdiagnostic conceptualization Mark and his therapist derived to explain the maintenance of his presenting issues (Figure 6.13). Therefore his therapist chooses to use this model and add a developmental overlay to it. She asks Mark to add the core belief "I'm a waste of space" in the Core Beliefs section of Figure 6.13. If Mark and his therapist had not yet developed a unified model of his presenting issues, they could do so now by reviewing his cross-sectional conceptualizations, highlighting shared thematic content in triggers, beliefs, and maintenance strategies.

Based on his developmental history (see his Aid to History Taking Form in Appendix 5.1 and initial assessment information summarized in Chapter 5), the therapist can form hypotheses about the developmental origins of his current issues. Mark has described several experiences that may account for his beliefs and behavioral strategies and his therapist is curious about the meanings Mark ascribed to each of these experiences. The therapist is open to reviewing Mark's entire developmental history to answer the following questions:

- Mark has a long history of depression. What triggered his first depressive episode in late adolescence?
- Mark's excessive health worries began about the same time. Did anything happen at age 18 beyond the unprotected sexual experience he described (see Chapter 6) that might explain how Mark's health anxiety developed and persisted?
- Mark's father suffered from bipolar disorder and attempted suicide when Mark was 8 years old. This placed considerable financial and emotional strain on the family. Mark's relationship with his father is complex (Chapters 5 and 6). How did this affect Mark, and what did he learn about himself, others, and the world?
- While he grew up, Mark's mother could be quite critical and was sometimes rather preoccupied with Mark's father's mental health. Even now she is quite critical of Mark and Clare. What beliefs and strategies did Mark learn from his relationship with his mother?
- Mark's brother, David, is quite a few years younger. Sometimes Mark's mother asked him to assume more of a parental than a sibling role toward David. What did this mean to Mark? What did he learn about himself, others, and the world?
- Mark had an important relationship with his grandfather, who was a role model and supported Mark during difficult times, including the months following Mark's father's suicide attempt. What impact did this relationship have on Mark?
- Music has been an important and enjoyable activity for Mark throughout his life. How does this positive interest inform a longitudinal conceptualization?
- Are there any additional life experiences not yet mentioned that were seminal in Mark's development?

In summary, his therapist is curious how Mark's early experiences shaped his more enduring core beliefs, underlying assumptions, and ways of coping.

A Developmental View of Mark's Core Belief "I'm a Waste of Space"

To derive a longitudinal conceptualization, Mark's therapist begins with a direct inquiry into the developmental origins of the core belief that is in the foreground of Mark's mind: "I am a waste of space." A central and emotional memory emerges that is consistent with themes in Mark's Thought Records.

THERAPIST: Mark, you said this belief, "I'm a waste of space," is something you can't shake off. This idea has come up more than once on your Thought Records and in our sessions. It sounds to me like it might be a core belief for you, a belief that is central to how you think about yourself.

MARK: Yes, I think it is. (*looking dejected*) I often feel like a waste of space.

THERAPIST: How long would you say you have thought of yourself this way? Can you remember when you first thought you were a waste of space?

MARK: (*without hesitation*) Yes, vividly, I remember a particular day. (*Therapist invites him to elaborate.*) I guess I was about 8 and my brother, David, he was a lot younger. Anyway, we were staying at my grandfather's house. It was after my father tried to kill himself. We had been at my grandfather's for a few weeks and we didn't know what was going on. (*Looks distressed as he describes this memory; he seems to be reliving the scene.*) I didn't get it, I just didn't get what was going on. I didn't know if I was going to lose my dad, I didn't know what he had done. What had I done? I just didn't know. (*On the verge of tears, but pulls himself together to continue.*) My mother came to visit, and obviously I really wanted to know what was happening. She didn't like to be questioned; you never knew when she might go off. At the visit she was pretending like nothing had happened. My grandfather read the situation; he knew David and I wanted to know how Dad was, so he asked. Well, the look that came over her face, I can just see it now. (*His face and posture seem to collapse.*)

THERAPIST: What was the look? Can you put it into words?

MARK: (*Struggles to find the words.*) It was like a flash of anger, followed by a look of blame. (*At this stage he visibly clams up and shakes his head.*)

INSIDE THE THERAPIST'S HEAD

Mark's therapist notes shifts in Mark's affect and posture that communicate important information about the activation of this memory. Mark begins to clam up and visibly shake when he interprets his mother's look as anger and blame. The therapist hypothesizes that Mark's struggle to find appropriate language indicates he is feeling and thinking like an 8-year-old and reexperiencing the event as if it were happening now. She is mindful to communicate openness, support, and caring because Mark's negative core beliefs about himself and others are likely to be activated along with this memory. In this moment he is particularly prone to see himself as useless and others, including the therapist, as critical.

THERAPIST: Mark, can you look at me? (*He does.*) This memory is upsetting, I know, but if we can understand this a bit better it might help us make progress. Can you say what you are feeling in this scene?

MARK: (*struggling to find the right words*) Guilt? Ashamed, I think.

THERAPIST: And what is going through your mind?

MARK: That it was my fault, that somehow I was responsible. I was supposed to look after David, help my mother with chores, tell my mother if I noticed anything wrong with my dad, and I never seemed to do it right. (*Starts crying.*)

THERAPIST: (*empathically*) What's going on right now?

MARK: I just felt so useless, so impotent. I wanted to run away and hide.

THERAPIST: It's OK, take your time. It hurts to reconnect with these feelings. (*There is a period of silence as they sit quietly. Mark's breathing settles and he regains his composure.*) Is this something you experienced at other times growing up?

MARK: I often felt like I could never quite get things right, what I did was never good enough for my mother. (*pauses*) And that I had to be responsible for noticing my dad's moods ... that somehow his suicide attempt was my fault.

THERAPIST: This sense of being useless, impotent, like you want to disappear—is this something you experience now, as an adult?

MARK: Oh yes, every time I feel down and stay in bed this is exactly what I am feeling. On Saturday morning when Clare came in, it is *exactly* how I felt. I lie there feeling caged by my thoughts and feelings, unable to get out of the funk. That's why I kind of close down and hibernate.

THERAPIST: It takes real courage to face these feelings and memories. If I understand you correctly, this belief about being a waste of space dates back to at least when you were 8 and the sense that you could never do enough in your family to get things right, to keep your dad well? (*Mark nods.*) And now, as an adult, when things seem overwhelming at work or at home, perhaps both, you get in touch with very similar thoughts and feelings and you can't easily step out of them—you feel caged by them. This seems to be what happened on Saturday morning and may help us explain why the Thought Record helped with your worry thoughts but only helped a bit with your thought about Clare seeing you as useless.

MARK: (*more animated*) Then I get angry with myself for being like that; you know, I used to see my father when he was low and the way it affected the family. I don't want to be like that! (*more gently*) I don't want to affect my family the same way.

THERAPIST: I can understand that.

MARK: (*Nods again; his posture improves.*) What can I do about this?

THERAPIST: Perhaps you could start by writing something in your therapy notebook to record what we are talking about. (*Mark writes "waste of space" and "impotent" in his notebook and then draws a cage around the thoughts.*) I can see how you feel caged by these old patterns of thinking. Is that a helpful way of drawing it?

MARK: Yes, except I want to be different.

Mark's persistent mood problems are underpinned by beliefs that are thematically linked to past experiences. When his core beliefs that he is "useless" and "a waste of space" are activated, the intensity of Mark's reactions often appears mismatched with current situational triggers. However, his reactions make perfect sense in the context of his past. An 8-year-old who believes his mother holds him responsible for his father's mental health understandably might think of himself as useless when he finds he is unable to influence his fathers fluctuating moods. Discussions like the one above normalize core beliefs by placing them within their original context. At the same time, they lay the groundwork for Mark to differentiate his adult experiences from childhood ones. He states emphatically that he doesn't want to behave like his father. By writing his core beliefs down and drawing a cage around them he begins to see these beliefs and behaviors from a different vantage point.

A Developmental View of Mark's Maintenance Strategies

Mark also examined his maintenance strategies through the lens of his developmental history. Functional analyses and Thought Records (Chapter 6) revealed the intended coping value of rumination for Mark:

he ruminated to manage feelings of anxiety and sadness. When linked to early childhood experiences, Mark appreciated that rumination developed as an adaptive coping strategy. The demands placed on him by his family sometimes outpaced his developmental capacities. Mark recalled his mind-set as a boy: "I thought if I worried it would help me be better prepared. If I could anticipate problems, I could prevent things from getting worse. Every day without a disaster convinced me it worked."

Mark and his therapist added his relevant developmental experiences to the conceptualization of his maintenance cycle previously shown in Figure 6.13. The resulting longitudinal conceptualization links Mark's beliefs with his early experiences and is shown in Figure 7.3. This marks the beginning of understanding Mark's beliefs and strategies through the lens of his developmental history. As research (Chadwick et al., 2003; Evans & Parry, 1996) and clinical papers (Padesky, 1994a) emphasize, this process can be emotional and sometimes difficult for clients. It is important that therapists ensure it is a constructive process. Therapists do this by fostering client self-compassion and incorporating client strengths.

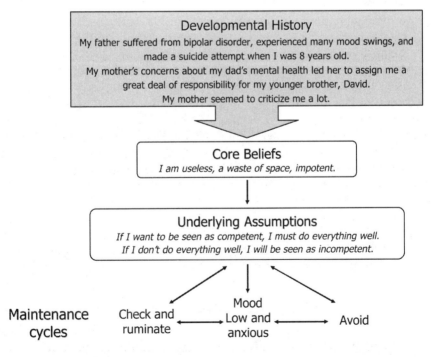

Figure 7.3. A preliminary longitudinal conceptualization for Mark.

Fostering Clients' Self-Compassion

One of the reasons for developing longitudinal conceptualizations is to help clients understand the origins of their beliefs and see that they make sense in their developmental context. Even when beliefs are clearly false (e.g., "It is my fault my father tried to kill himself"), it can be therapeutic for the client to see how these interpretations might seem logical to a young child's mind.

The high levels of responsibility expected from Mark, the roller coaster of his father's moods, the shock of his father's suicide attempt, and his mother's preoccupation with her husband were realities of Mark's childhood. Mark's recollection that his mother held him responsible to some degree for family difficulties is consistent with current statements his mother makes to him. It is apparent how Mark's underlying assumptions ("If I want to be seen as useful, I must be responsible and do everything well") and his strategies (work to a high standard, take on a lot of responsibility) were adaptive in Mark's family when he was a child.

The processes of collaborative longitudinal conceptualization offered Mark perspective so he could understand and normalize his reactions as a child:

> "I see my children, Jessica and James, and how much Clare cares for them, how much we both care for them. When I think how much I was holding everything together as a kid on my own, the responsibility for my brother and myself ... kids aren't equipped to hold that much responsibility. It's a miracle how resilient I was and that I didn't just give up."

The longitudinal conceptualization helped change Mark's perspective from seeing himself as useless to seeing himself as resilient in the face of challenges that children do not ordinarily face. Moreover, his therapist used compassionate language to communicate the earlier functionality of his beliefs and strategies—for example:

- "It makes sense to me that in these circumstances you would think/practice [belief/strategy]."
- "I can see how you feel caged by these old patterns of thinking."

These reflections help clients shift to a more self-compassionate perspective.

Incorporating Client Strengths

Another way to ensure that longitudinal conceptualization is constructive is to incorporate client strengths. If Mark and his therapist look at the problem-focused conceptualization in Figure 7.3, important information about Mark is missing and the emergent conceptualization is unhelpfully one-dimensional. Active inquiry into Mark's childhood strengths and positive supports led to critically important information that had not yet emerged in therapy.

His therapist learned that Mark accompanied his grandfather on camping trips in the wilderness as a boy. His grandfather skillfully taught Mark to be resourceful and confident in these circumstances. Mark's resourcefulness and can-do attitude generalized to other areas of his life as he matured. These strengths are now valued by his colleagues, friends, and family and are a foundation for many of Mark's successes.

Unlike many boys in his school, Mark's sports participation was restricted by asthma. As a result, he had extensive time for music and developed friendships with other students who shared this interest. He became an accomplished piano player, talked for hours with friends about music, and played in a band during his teenage years. Mark credits the protective strategies he developed as a teenager with helping him establish a loving marriage, build an adult network of good friends, and parent his own children well. The elaborated conceptualization in Figure 7.4 highlights values and strengths that give Mark's life positive meaning and help him cope resiliently.

By incorporating Mark's strengths, his therapist maintains a balanced view of Mark that can be enlisted in planning interventions. If the conceptualization at this stage does not incorporate client strengths, this can indicate that the therapist is not focusing on strengths as much as may be ideal. In later stages of therapy it can help to have a conceptualization of client resilience that specifies the core beliefs, underlying assumptions, and strategies that underpin the client's resilience in the face of adversity. This is illustrated later in this chapter as Mark's longitudinal conceptualization is elaborated during the final stages of his therapy.

Protective or Predisposing?

Notice the titles on the left and right of Figure 7.4. It is important for therapists and clients to discern whether elements of a longitudinal conceptualization are protective, predisposing, or some combination of both. Similar strategies can serve different functions and be driven by different beliefs. Just as it is important to identify the core beliefs and underlying assumptions that drive them, skillful conceptualization involves understanding the function of strategies.

For example, while conscientiousness can be a strength, Mark's tendency to feel overly responsible can create difficulties. Thus for Mark, conscientiousness functions more often as a predisposing factor than a

PROTECTIVE FACTORS	PREDISPOSING FACTORS
Developmental History	
Grandfather a good role model Always enjoyed music Strong friendships around music Stable and supportive marriage Care for and love my family Success in my career and work	Father's bipolar disorder and suicide attempt Mother's preoccupation with dad's mental health led her to assign me a great deal of responsibility for my younger brother, David Frequent criticism from my mother
Core Beliefs	
I am creative, capable, "can-do." I am loving, others love me.	I am useless, a waste of space, impotent.
Underlying Assumptions	
When I take care of my family and friends, it helps them flourish. When I have a productive week at work, I learn that I have a lot to offer. If I am playing music, I lose myself in it and enjoy myself.	If I want to be seen as competent, I must do everything well. If I take responsibility for my family's safety, they will stay safe. If my responsibility for my family's safety slips up, something terrible will happen to them.
Strategies	
Resourcefulness: "can-do" approach Nurture relationships with family and friends All aspects of music	Rumination Work to a high standard vs. avoid challenges Overresponsibility vs. abdicating responsibility Withdrawal: "hibernation" Avoidance Checking behavior (conscientiousness)

Figure 7.4. Longitudinal conceptualization for Mark incorporating strengths.

protective one. Another example is Clare's support, which can enhance their relationship and soothe Mark's distress. However, the same behavior can reinforce Mark's tendency to withdraw for long periods of time. As Mark notes in the opening dialogue of this chapter, Clare's impatience with him motivated Mark to use some of the skills he had learned in CBT. However, if Mark had been more severely depressed, Clare's behavior might have fueled his core belief he was useless and exacerbated his depression.

Understanding the Onset of Mark's Presenting Issues

One of the reasons for developing a longitudinal conceptualization is to better understand the onset of clients' presenting issues. Therapist and client want to ensure that the longitudinal conceptualization maps the past well before they use it to inform interventions that shape the future. So far Mark and his therapist have identified the context in which Mark learned his beliefs and strategies. How does this fit with understanding Mark's first onset of depression, OCD, and health worries?

The First Onset of Mark's Depression

The events surrounding Mark's first episode of depression are described in Chapter 6. Recall that when he was 17 Mark withdrew from his band to prepare for university entrance exams. His mother was preoccupied with his father's health problems during this time. When Mark did poorly on his exams, his mother's criticism underscored his own sense of uselessness. His father, due to his own mental health problems, provided no support or alternative perspective. Mark, copying the strategies he had seen his father use, withdrew socially and academically. He recalled that this was his first experience of long-term avoidance, or "hibernating" as he thought about it at the time. Using his longitudinal conceptualization as shown in Figure 7.4, Mark now understood this time period as follows:

> "When I didn't do well on the exams, I decided this was just more proof I was useless. Since I couldn't perform to a high standard, I decided to withdraw and avoid all challenges. I'd seen it work for Dad. But the more I hibernated, the more useless I felt. The left side of this chart (*pointing to Figure 7.4*) shows what pulled me out of it. It was my friends and my music. After a few months one of the band members called me up to say they needed me back because the other fellow who filled in for me just was not as good. Once I started playing again my mood lifted a bit; I started to think I had

something to contribute. In the new school term I found it possible to start studying again, too."

The First Onset of Mark's Health Anxiety and OCD

What about the first onset of Mark's difficulties with OCD and health worries? As already discussed, Mark began to develop beliefs and strategies regarding responsibility in adolescence, "If I want to be seen as useful, I must be responsible and do everything well." It was functional within his family for Mark to adopt a high level of responsibility for his brother and himself. These beliefs and strategies generalized to his early relationships with peers. When he had unprotected sex at a party at age 18, Mark condemned his behavior as irresponsible. His judgment was consistent with the prevailing standards of that time and was exacerbated by knowing that his father had been sexually irresponsible in the context of manic episodes. In the ensuing months he was consumed with worry that he had contracted HIV. His worry and physical anxiety were mutually reinforcing, leading to the development of checking and rumination strategies as described in Chapter 6. Mark believed his rumination and checking kept his anxiety from spiraling out of control. Mark's reliance on rumination and checking to manage anxiety had first appeared in childhood and by early adulthood it was overlearned and self-maintaining.

The onsets of Mark's presenting issues make sense in the context of his longitudinal conceptualization (Figure 7.4). These discussions with his therapist increased Mark's self-compassion. He now understood how his presenting issues became pervasive over time.

Step 2: Select Conceptualization-Based Interventions

A primary function of conceptualization is to help therapists and clients devise interventions that ameliorate clients' distress and build resilience. A therapist uses the conceptualization as a rationale for interventions, asking, "Does this make sense? Are you willing to [observe/make a change in one or more elements] and see how it works out?" A good conceptualization clearly suggests particular interventions such as behavioral experiments designed to test the functionality of client strategies (Bennett-Levy et al., 2004).

Using Longitudinal Conceptualizations to Generate Alternative Beliefs and Strategies

Mark's predisposing core beliefs and underlying assumptions are activated in a range of situations. Can his longitudinal conceptualization help Mark learn alternative ways of thinking and behaving? Cognitive-behavioral texts are rich with strategies that can be used (J. S. Beck, 1995; J. S. Beck, 2005) to generate alternative thoughts and behaviors. Mark's therapist decided to use a contemporary approach for working with intrusive memories (Wheatley et al., 2007). The aim was to reframe the meanings embedded in Mark's emotive memory of the encounter he described with his mother and grandfather following his father's suicide attempt. His longitudinal conceptualization guides the therapist to focus on Mark's grandfather in the image, because Mark's grandfather is identified as protective in his longitudinal conceptualization.

THERAPIST: (*being careful to communicate curiosity, not blame*) I want to understand better this situation when your mother came to your grandfather's house. You said you felt so useless, so impotent, like you wanted to disappear. I'm curious what might happen if we look at this situation from another perspective. For example, can you put yourself in your grandfather's shoes? (*speaking slowly*) Take a moment to shift your perspective so you see this scene through your grandfather's eyes, so to speak … seeing your 8-year-old grandson, your younger grandson David, and their mother, your daughter … what might be your perspective as you think back on it? Are you able to do that?

MARK: (*after a moment*) Yes. It must have been so difficult for my mother, she must have been scared, overwhelmed, confused. … Seeing it from my grandfather's perspective I want to do what I can to help her, it's an awful situation for her.

THERAPIST: Staying with your grandfather's perspective, what do you think about Mark and David?

MARK: (*Takes a moment to think about it.*) It is quite possible he realized my mother didn't have the capacity to really think about us, her head was so full up with what happened to Dad. (*pauses*) I guess he must have felt really protective toward us. I remember feeling that from him. That fits with how he was toward us generally, like a big protective grizzly bear. I felt safe with him.

THERAPIST: How does your grandfather's perspective compare with what you felt and thought as an 8-year-old?

MARK: (*Looks sad.*) I can really feel for my mother. (*Seems to brighten.*) I was lucky to have my grandfather. As an 8-year-old, particularly as a bit of a worrier, I was prone to take it very personally. You know as a boy, like we said before, I just wasn't equipped to deal with all this.

THERAPIST: Your reaction as a boy is quite understandable; as you say, it fits with the degree of responsibility you sometimes were given in your family. How much can you believe your grandfather's view on what was going on for your mother in that situation?

MARK: Oh, 100%.

THERAPIST: And from this perspective, how much do you believe that your mother thought you were useless?

MARK: If I think about my kids, Jessica is about that age. There is no way she takes anywhere near that responsibility. I think my mother was all over the place. I guess I don't believe that in that moment she was thinking I was useless.

THERAPIST: So how much can you believe this alternative perspective—that your mother was all over the place and not having space to think about you?

MARK: One hundred percent intellectually, but I also feel angry and sad about it.

This interchange illustrates how using imagery to shift perspectives can help develop alternative meanings for a seminal memory. This reconceptualization of what occurred with his mother is more functional and provides Mark with seeds for new core beliefs ("I am capable") and underlying assumptions ("If something is out of my control then it is not my fault if it goes wrong"; "If others are lost or upset, it may have nothing to do with me"). The dialogue above shows only how Mark's therapist began this work with him. Interestingly, Mark's reframing introduces a new emotion, anger. The therapist would explore Mark's anger with him. It is beyond the scope of this chapter to outline the full range of possible cognitive strategies that can be used to develop new beliefs and strategies, but interested readers are directed to relevant texts and articles (J. S. Beck, 1995, 2005; Padesky, 1990; Padesky, 1994a; Padesky & Greenberger, 1995).

Using a Longitudinal Conceptualization to Prevent Relapse and Build Resilience

Mark's difficulties are long-standing. His core beliefs, underlying assumptions, and strategies are likely to be triggered again in the future. His longitudinal conceptualization (Figure 7.4) can help Mark and his therapist predict what circumstances might trigger his predisposing beliefs and strategies. They hypothesize that multiple simultaneous demands, criticism, serious mistakes, and threats of harm (e.g., flood, fire) or illness affecting family members might reactivate Mark's vulnerability to depression, OCD, and worries. Given the likelihood of one or more of these occurring, the therapist asks Mark to use his longitudinal conceptualization to create a "coping card" (J. S. Beck, 1995, 2005). She invites him to make a card that summarizes the most important things he has learned that can help him stay resilient when these triggers occur. She explains that the coping card can be a quick reminder for Mark when things became stressful.

Mark drew two images on his coping card along with summaries of key ideas he had learned in therapy. The first image was of a bear in a cage, representing Mark caged by his predisposing beliefs. The second image reminded Mark of his grandfather. It was a grizzly bear, holding a list of protective beliefs and strategies (Figure 7.5). As the following dialogue reveals, Mark's imagery-rich coping card promotes his resilience.

MARK: The grizzly bear represents all the ways my grandfather taught me to be. He is active and figures things out and uses a lot of creativity and a "can-do" attitude. This bear in the cage just lies down and gives up.

THERAPIST: That really is a choice! Why don't we road-test this coping

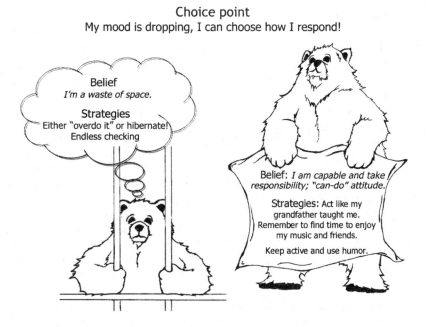

Figure 7.5. Mark's "coping card" conceptualization of his vulnerability and resilience.

card? Is there a situation coming up that is likely to affect your mood, the sort of situation where you really need to access the grizzly bear?

MARK: (*Pauses to think.*) Christmas is always a really bad time because my retail work gets really busy and Clare and I have to think about my mother. It's a stressful time.

THERAPIST: That sounds like a good example. Imagine a difficult situation that could come up and describe it to me as if it were happening right now.

MARK: Let's see. (*Takes a moment. When he has thought of an example he begins.*) My mother is staying with us and at breakfast she makes some critical remarks about how Clare and I are doing things—no, she doesn't say anything, she just looks as if she thinks we are doing everything wrong. Clare looks upset and the kids are acting out. I get into work, and there is just too much to do, and my boss says he is overwhelmed with work and he wants to delegate some of his projects to me.

THERAPIST: What you are feeling? What is going through your mind?

MARK: I feel like the bear in the cage (*points to the coping card*), depressed, I want to hibernate, close out the world for a long while!

THERAPIST: What else is happening for you? What is happening in your body?

MARK: I feel overwhelmed, tightness in my shoulders and chest, breathing more quickly. I want to look at my coping card. (*He does.*) OK, yes, it's all there: the waste of space and the desire to hide away. So, I'm taking a deep breath and saying to myself, "I have a choice about how I respond!" Seeing the strong grizzly bear helps. (*Reads from the card.*) "I have a lot to offer." (*Pauses to think about this.*) "What would my grandfather do here?" (*pauses*) He would make a joke about the situation, say something to my boss like, "You'll have to pay me a big Christmas bonus," and then say, "I want to help but if I do the annual marketing report then the routine e-mail will have to wait until after Christmas, is that OK?" (*Looks up at the therapist and smiles.*)

THERAPIST: Good! As you do this, what's running through your mind?

MARK: You know, when I give myself this space it allows the thought to pop into my mind, "My boss trusts me at this busy time to lean on me. He respects my work!" What else? I think I would make sure I had some time out with Peter, my friend, maybe go and see some music, you know, recharge the batteries. Perhaps on Christmas Eve

I could get out of the house for a bit. There's a good local band that traditionally plays on Christmas Eve. I used to go every year before the kids were born, once I even got up and jammed with the band. (*His demeanor and posture visibly improve as he speaks.*)

☀ INSIDE THE THERAPIST'S HEAD

The therapist uses moments like this to get Mark to notice activated functional beliefs and strategies. Mark is naturally very tuned in to beliefs and strategies when on a downward trajectory, and it is important that he learn to notice beliefs and strategies when he is on an upward trajectory as well. The coping card he has developed is proving helpful in activating functional beliefs and strategies at just the right time.

THERAPIST: What is running through your mind and what are you feeling?

MARK: You know what? I feel good, stronger: like that grizzly bear! (*Points to the coping card.*) I can handle this. If I can pace myself through to New Year's it will be OK. As my grandfather would say, "If you encounter a bear, just give it lots of space. It just wants to get on with its life in peace." He was a great one for seeing the good in situations. (*Smiles fondly.*)

While Mark uses his coping card well in the scenario above, his therapist wonders what would happen if Mark was already somewhat depressed? Also, what if his wife does not want him to leave the family on Christmas Eve? And how could his grizzly bear respond to his mother's continued criticism? Together they decide to rehearse further scenarios, including ones in which Mark's mood is progressively worse. These imagination exercises and role plays led Mark to add "keep active" and "use humor" to his coping card.

Difficulties can either sensitize a person and increase their vulnerability (Monroe & Harkness, 2005) or, like small doses of a virus, immunize a person and increase their resilience (Rutter, 1999). In the session above, the therapist uses small, escalating doses of stress to inoculate Mark so he can handle future real-life stressors without collapsing. Role plays and imagination exercises allow Mark to practice self-efficacy and alternative beliefs and strategies. Each stressful event Mark negotiates is an opportunity to elaborate the conceptualization so it becomes a better support to prevent and manage future relapses.

Client Values and Resilience

Therapy that includes a focus on values and longer-term goals helps move people from a reactive mode to responsive and proactive modes. Jon Kabat-Zinn makes the distinction between reactive and responsive modes. He describes the difference between reacting automatically to stimuli and responding with awareness of the stimulus, its effects, as well as associated beliefs and actions (Kabat-Zinn, 2004). Initially, Mark was overwhelmed by problems. As expressed in the opening dialogue of this chapter, although Mark understood his presenting issues better by the middle stages of his therapy he was still highly reactive to triggering stimuli when he experienced downturns in mood.

Being proactive means articulating and working toward goals that are grounded in values (Addis & Martell, 2004). As he described in the opening dialogue, some days Mark feels unmotivated when he wakes up. Whenever he and his therapist move from a sole focus on vulnerability to an emphasis on resilience as well as vulnerability, the odds increase that Mark will be able to use his values and goals to responsively and proactively manage periods of low motivation. Each time he behaves proactively, Mark reinforces constructive beliefs and strategies that strengthen his resilience.

In his final weeks of therapy, Mark reflected on the longitudinal conceptualization he and his therapist had devised and articulated the following values: "If I want to be seen as capable in my work then it is important to be responsible and work hard at what I do. At the same time, I know I will make mistakes, and when I do, it is acceptable to acknowledge these and move on" and "If I take responsibility for my family then it is a sign I love them. Clare can share this responsibility because she loves me and the children." These positive values about work and family describe the life he aspires to lead rather than a life within which he feels trapped (as drawn in Figure 7.5).

These values help Mark get out of bed when he feels unmotivated because they uncouple responsibility and perfectionism. Mark's values link the benefits of responsibility with the flexibility of accepting mistakes and asking for help when necessary. When Mark acts on these values even when his motivation is low it provides evidence in support of a new core belief, "I am capable and take responsibility." In turn, such proactive behavior demonstrates his preferred strategy to "act like my grandfather." Values-based behavior is highly reinforcing. When Mark gets out of bed, showers, and goes to work or takes his daughter swimming on low-energy days he experiences mastery from having acted on his values rather than on his low mood.

The therapist also encouraged Mark to engage in enjoyable activities that lifted his spirit and highlighted his strengths. Music had been important to Mark throughout his life and seemed an important interest for him to continue. During a scheduled follow-up session a few months after therapy ended, Mark told his therapist he had bumped into the singer from his former band and they were going to perform at a local bar during an open-mic evening. Mark laughed when he said they were calling their new band the "Grateful Bears." Repeat administration of the BDI-II and BAI during this follow-up meeting suggested Mark was almost completely symptom free. Repeat administration of the WHO-QOL-BREF measure showed he was now scoring in the normative range in each of the four domains: physical, psychological, social, and environmental. Mark credited his continued improvement to having more enjoyable things in his life as well as living by more flexible standards.

Does the Conceptualization Fit?

Throughout the iterative steps of developing and applying longitudinal conceptualizations therapists test their fit using collaborative empiricism. Some of the questions asked to ensure a good fit are:

- Does the conceptualization make sense? Is it coherent and logical?
- Have the client and therapist developed the conceptualization collaboratively? Does the client fully agree with the conceptualization?
- Do different sources of information "triangulate"?
- Does a supervisor or consultant think the conceptualization makes sense?

Each of these questions is considered in turn in relation to the longitudinal conceptualization derived by Mark and his therapist.

Does the Conceptualization Make Sense?

The first test of a conceptualization's fit is whether it makes sense. Do the developmental history, core beliefs, underlying assumptions, and strategies cohere in a logical way? Does the conceptualization add explanatory power? Client presenting issues and goals can be mapped explicitly onto the conceptualization as a test of its utility. Ideally, the conceptualization links and explains the list of presenting issues. By doing so, it will often speed progress toward therapy goals.

Mark's cross-sectional conceptualization highlighted Mark's core beliefs about himself as "useless" and "impotent." These drive a conditional assumption, "If I want to be seen as useful, I must be responsible and do everything well." The maintenance strategies for his presenting issues flow from this assumption and rule. How does his developmental history as summarized on the longitudinal conceptualization help explain the origins of these core beliefs, underlying assumption, and each of Mark's presenting issues? Recall Mark's descriptions of what he learned from key developmental experiences. As a child, he felt "useless" and "impotent" when he could not fulfill the responsibilities he thought were assigned to him: to monitor his father's moods and watch after his younger brother. He frequently perceived his mother as critical. Now when Mark fails to meet his own high standards or he does not fulfill his responsibilities at work or home, these perceived shortcomings resonate with his experiences growing up. His core beliefs are activated and his mood drops.

Mark then overcompensates by withdrawing, just as he learned to do in adolescence from watching his father's response to depression. Withdrawal from his family and work duties provides ample opportunity for worry and rumination, which maintain his low mood. Worry and rumination are part of a self-perpetuating cycle in which Mark continually scans for information consistent with his negative core beliefs (e.g., "Am I doing this right?" "Do people think I am a waste of space?"). Mark's decision-making difficulties can be linked to his high standards and low self-confidence, both experienced in early childhood when he was given high levels of responsibility and yet received low levels of parental support.

While theory-driven models of hypochondriasis and OCD provide good explanations for how Mark's checking behavior is maintained, his longitudinal conceptualization helps explain what predisposed him to these particular problems. Mark's attempts in early childhood to be highly responsible, coupled with catastrophic beliefs about what would happen if he failed to carry out his responsibilities, generated a lot of anxiety for him. As a child, he managed this anxiety by checking. This strategy generalized and strengthened over Mark's lifetime. Finally, Mark's impatience and anger with colleagues at work can be viewed as similar to the frustration he feels toward himself when his high standards are not met.

In summary, the longitudinal conceptualization derived by Mark and his therapist seems to account well for all of Mark's presenting issues, not just those that were part of his active therapy focus. His memories of childhood and adolescence reveal the probable origins of beliefs and strategies that made sense in the context of his early experiences and were functional for him within his family context. This same conceptualization makes sense of Mark's current emotions, beliefs, and strategies across a number of presenting issues. Even so, therapists committed to collaborative empiricism remain open to alternative conceptualizations. At each point during therapy, Mark's therapist actively seeks additional perspectives. She encourages Mark to notice and report experiences that do not fit this conceptualization.

Have the Client and Therapist Developed the Conceptualization Collaboratively?

The second criterion is whether the client has actively participated in the development of the conceptualization and endorses its fit. Of the three levels of conceptualization, longitudinal conceptualization involves the greatest amount of inference because it hypothesizes explanatory mechanisms based on client history rather than making deductions from current, readily observable life events. Collaborative empiricism is therefore necessary to minimize thinking errors and maximize a conceptualization's fit to both past and present client experiences.

Each of the dialogues with Mark illustrates this process. At every step the therapist actively pursues Mark's ideas, memories, and observations. The longitudinal conceptualization is written in Mark's own words. Each inference is summarized and Mark is asked, "Does this make sense to you?" or "Are there ways this does not fit your experience?" Mark writes the conceptualization in his therapy notebook and observes whether it fits well with his subsequent experiences.

Do Different Sources of Information "Triangulate"?

Does information from different sources converge, or "triangulate"? Various methods for developing a longitudinal conceptualization can be used to triangulate an evolving conceptualization. For example, Mark completed the Personality Belief Questionnaire (PBQ; Beck & Beck, 1991) in an early therapy session. The PBQ assesses how strongly a client holds beliefs that are consistent with various personality disorders. Mark endorsed items from the avoidant (e.g., "Other people are potentially critical, indifferent, demeaning, or rejecting"; "If others criticize me, they must be right") and obsessive–compulsive (e.g., "I am fully responsible for myself and others"; "If I don't perform at the highest level, I will fail") clusters, but not at a level to suggest he fully expressed a personality disorder. These beliefs are consistent with his conceptualizations derived in session.

With client permission, additional sources of information can include family members, friends, other health providers, written records, questionnaires, other mental health instruments, and even coworkers.

For example, in the case of Zainab in Chapter 4 her therapist sought the active participation of Zainab's husband, Muhammad, to help construct useful conceptualizations of Zainab's vulnerability and resilience.

Does a Supervisor or Consultant Think the Conceptualization Makes Sense?

A fourth check on the fit of a conceptualization comes from discussion with experienced colleagues or, in the case of therapists in training, in supervision. Supervision or consultation with another CBT therapist can help clarify conceptualizations and highlight areas that require further development with the client. Furthermore, supervision/consultation is a good opportunity to practice making comprehensive summary conceptualizations as shown in Figures 7.6 and 7.7. These figures show how the presenting issues can be understood alongside one another in terms of triggers, maintenance, and predisposing or protective factors. Note that while the conceptualization of Mark's presenting issues has closed maintenance cycles (Figure 7.6), crucially, the conceptualization of Mark's resilience shows the breakup of these cycles (Figure 7.7).

Summary conceptualizations such as these are rarely helpful to clients. We do not recommend that therapists show summary conceptualizations to clients unless the client is keenly interested in circuit board drawings! Consider an analogy with computer software. The software "user interface" is as simple as possible, readily understandable and easy to use. Conceptualizations developed with clients are as simple as possible, readily understandable, and inform CBT interventions. However, in supervision or consultation it can help to make explicit the full "programming code" of the conceptualization in order to check the conceptualization's fit. The underlying programming code is much more elaborate and complex. Making the detail of conceptualizations explicit and searching for links among presenting issues can inform treatment decisions and also help uncover problems with clinical decision making (see Chapter 2).

SUMMARY

This chapter illustrates how a longitudinal conceptualization helped Mark better understand his difficulties in the later phases of therapy. This conceptualization was used to design interventions that could build Mark's resilience as well as help him prevent or successfully manage relapse. The cycle of longitudinal conceptualization–evaluation–intervention–evaluation is repeated as often as necessary to help clients

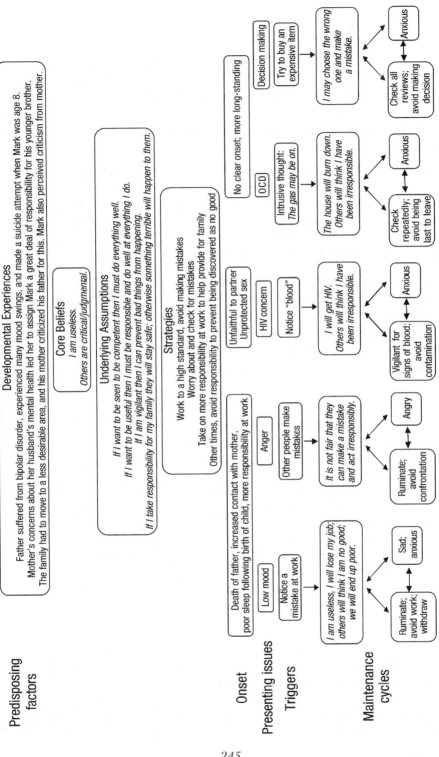

Figure 7.6. A summary conceptualization of Mark's vulnerability.

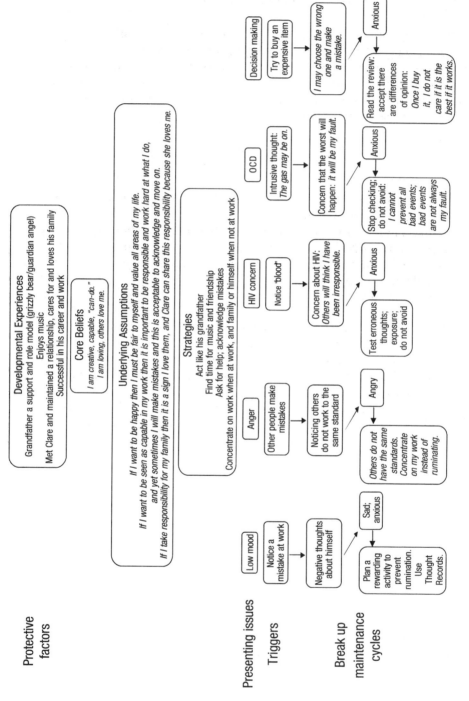

Figure 7.7. A summary conceptualization of Mark's resilience.

achieve their therapy goals. This phase of therapy increasingly emphasizes helping clients use their emerging resilience to become their own CBT therapists. As is so often true in successful therapy, Mark's experiences illustrate the principle: "The things that go right in our lives do predict future successes and the things that go wrong do not damn us forever" (Felsman & Vaillant, 1987).

Chapter 7 Summary

- Longitudinal conceptualizations link client history, presenting issues, and cognitive-behavioral theory.
- Longitudinal conceptualizations are only necessary when explanatory cross-sectional conceptualizations prove insufficient to achieve client goals. As such, these conceptualizations usually emerge in later stages of CBT and normally only when the focus of therapy is treatment of personality disorders or clients report chronic, multiple, and overlapping problems.
- Longitudinal conceptualization involves a cycle of formulating a developmental understanding of client presenting issue(s) and using this model to design interventions, evaluating the conceptualization's fit after each step. The cycle repeats as often as necessary to help clients achieve their therapy goals.
- Longitudinal conceptualizations can be used to predict future relapses and plan how the client can prevent and/or successfully manage these. Used in this way, they help build resilience.

Chapter 8

Learning and Teaching Case Conceptualization

"I followed what Mark's therapist did in the last three chapters with interest. I might have handled things differently in a few places, yet overall the conceptualization and treatment plan made good sense. I'd like to teach this approach to my students. Where do I start?"

—ADVANCED CBT THERAPIST

"I wish my case conceptualization and treatment skills were on a par with those of Mark's therapist. While everything in the past three chapters made sense to me, I'm not sure I would have helped Mark construct his conceptualizations so clearly or carried out the treatment plans so well."

—INTERMEDIATE CBT THERAPIST

"How long did it take Mark's therapist to learn all those theories? Do I really have to know research findings to help clients construct CBT conceptualizations? I've got a lot to learn. Where do I begin?"

—NOVICE CBT THERAPIST

Readers of this text are likely to have reactions similar to one or more of the therapists' above. How does a therapist develop the knowledge and skill necessary to capably construct useful conceptualizations with clients? Once one has these skills, how can they be conveyed to other therapists in supervision, consultation, classrooms, and workshops?

This chapter presents a model for learning and teaching case conceptualization. We recommend specific steps to therapists of all skill levels (novice to advanced), designed to help them acquire and refine the core skills and knowledge embedded in our collaborative case conceptualization model. Some steps can be taken independently, and others can be done with peers or with the guidance of a more experienced supervisor, teacher, or consultant. For advanced CBT therapists who are instructors or who provide supervision or consultation to other CBT therapists, we offer a framework for teaching the information in this book to peers.

CONCEPTUALIZATION: A HIGH-LEVEL SKILL

Case conceptualization is a high-level skill. Figure 8.1 shows a model of therapist competence articulated by a working party of CBT experts involved in treatment development, training, and supervision (see Figure 8.1; Roth & Pilling, 2007). Applied to case conceptualization, this model suggests that there are layers of knowledge and skill therapists need to master to develop competency. First, therapists need to draw on

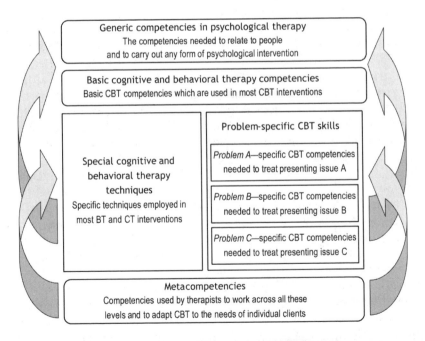

Figure 8.1. Roth and Pilling's (2007) model of CBT competencies.

the generic CBT theory (described in Chapter 2) and relevant disorder-specific CBT theories, and to collaborate with clients to apply these to client experiences. Next, therapists need to be able to deliver evidence-based cognitive and behavioral interventions (see Box 1.3), using conceptualization as a springboard for these interventions. As CBT evolves for particular disorders and expands to consider new applications, the array of possible interventions in which therapists need to be competent grows (Beck, 2005).

In addition to these basic competencies, CBT therapists benefit from various metacompetencies that enable them to integrate different knowledge bases and skills (Roth & Pilling, 2007). Metacompetencies emphasized in this text include collaborative empiricism, working at the appropriate level of conceptualization for a given client at a particular time in therapy, and incorporating client strengths so there can be a balance of problem-focused and resilience-focused work. Mark's therapist demonstrated these competencies and metacompetencies while helping him conceptualize his issues in Chapters 5 through 7. Mark's therapist showed evidence of a broad and deep knowledge base. Furthermore, she was able to translate this knowledge flexibly at each level of conceptualization within an actively collaborative therapy relationship. She drew out Mark's strengths at each phase of therapy. By its conclusion, she and Mark had developed a conceptualization not only of his problems but also of his resilience that he can use to prevent relapse and achieve his longer-term goals.

Therapists with these basic and metacompetencies in case conceptualization are more able to shift rapidly between descriptive and more inferential levels of conceptualization. Such flexibility may prove to be a key variable that predicts differences in therapy outcomes. Some therapists consistently attain above-average outcomes with clients, and a small minority apparently produce deterioration in their clients (Okiishi, Lambert, Nielsen, & Ogles, 2003). In CBT, the more competent therapists have better client outcomes (Kuyken & Tsivrikos, in press). We speculate that therapists' conceptualization skills and the ability to link conceptualizations iteratively to treatment methods explain some of the relationship between therapists' competence and therapy outcomes. A therapist who can *collaboratively describe a person's presenting issues using cognitive-behavioral theory and make explanatory inferences about causes and maintaining factors to inform interventions* (our definition of case conceptualization in Chapter 1) provides clients with pathways to successful change.

A skilled therapist continually monitors therapy progress, adapting the case conceptualization and therapy methods in response to client feedback. To illustrate this point, let's look at how one therapist adapted to working with a client, Lionel, who entered therapy with complaints of procrastination and frequently did not complete his homework. His therapist held a provisional hypothesis that Lionel's homework noncompletion was a form of procrastination driven by fear of criticism. When Lionel reported difficulty completing a job application, his therapist took the opportunity to test out the "fear of criticism" hypothesis. The therapist asked Lionel to write down his automatic thoughts every time he procrastinated on filling out the job application:

THERAPIST: I'm curious as to what you learned this week about your procrastination, Lionel. Were you able to capture some automatic thoughts about your job application?

LIONEL: I didn't do it very much, but I made a few notes on the chart you gave me. (*Gets the paper out of his pocket.*) Let's see. OK (*pauses*), last Wednesday I sat down to fill in the application and then got up to clean the kitchen.

THERAPIST: So what went through your mind as you sat down to fill in the application form?

LIONEL: Nothing, really. (*Appears a bit evasive.*) I just felt really bad and started to sweat and have heart palpitations. (*Gets visibly anxious and distressed.*)

INSIDE THE THERAPIST'S HEAD

The therapist begins to question the working conceptualization that Lionel's procrastination is linked to automatic thoughts about perceived inadequacy or expectations of criticism. Automatic thoughts about inadequacy often lead to avoidance but are unlikely to lead to sweating and heart palpitations. The therapist thinks, "We might be using the wrong conceptualization." He decides to search for what else might be going on.

THERAPIST: (*leaning forward toward Lionel*) It looks like you feel upset just thinking about this. (*Lionel makes eye contact and half-nods.*) So when you sat down to do the application you noticed a lot of physical anxiety in your body, but not many thoughts. Can you say what happened just when you decided to fill out this form and then felt all these physical sensations?

LIONEL: I sometimes get these pictures in my head, and I got this particularly horrible picture. (*Appears more anxious and distressed.*)

> **INSIDE THE THERAPIST'S HEAD**
>
> Lionel may be experiencing anxious imagery or he even may be having a trauma memory right now. If it is a trauma memory, research suggests this memory may seem real and imminently dangerous (Ehlers & Clark, 2000). The therapist thinks, "As I test out this hypothesis, I want to keep in mind that Lionel may need extra support while we discuss this."

THERAPIST: You look upset as you remember this. It could help us to find out why this picture is getting in the way of you completing the job application. Are you willing to tell me a bit more about it? What you see?

LIONEL: OK. What do you want to know?

THERAPIST: (*with a very steady and supportive nonverbal stance*) Describe to me what you see, like you are seeing it right now.

LIONEL: It's more like a video than a picture. This group of guys is coming at me from different directions and they take turns pushing me from different sides, until I go to the ground and I feel and hear their boots kicking me. I hear these voices saying things like "loser" and laughing.

> **INSIDE THE THERAPIST'S HEAD**
>
> This "video" is described largely in the present tense, without much meaning or context provided. This provides some evidence to support the hypothesis that Lionel is experiencing a trauma memory, which is often visual, visceral, and not integrated as a higher-order episodic memory (Brewin, Dagliesh, & Joseph, 1996).

THERAPIST: That sounds awful.

LIONEL: Yes, toward the end of my time in the military I used to get pretty badly bullied, you know, humiliated and beaten by this group of men. By the end I was a mess, just a real mess. (*Tears begin to roll down his cheeks.*) This video plays off in my head; however hard I try to stop it, it comes back. It's horrible, it's like I'm right back there.

THERAPIST: It sounds like you went through an awful time, and you felt humiliated. (*Lionel nods.*) And applying for a new job brings back these pictures or images these experiences during your military service? (*Lionel nods again. After a pause.*) And you are afraid to apply for a new job because ... (*Pauses so Lionel can fill in the end of this assumption.*)

LIONEL: I'll get bullied again.

THERAPIST: That really explains why it has been so difficult for you to fill out your job application. Thank you for describing this video that plays in your head. It helps me understand much better what you are struggling with. I have a guess about why you see these videos in your mind.

LIONEL: (*Looks up at the therapist with tearful eyes.*) Why?

THERAPIST: It seems to me these videos might be what we call traumatic memories. The good news is, if you are willing, we can work on these memories to stop them coming into your mind with so much distress. Would you like to learn how to work with these upsetting images so you can come to terms with your memories of what happened to you?

This interchange illustrates how a skilled therapist can use homework noncompletion as an opportunity for further assessment and conceptualization. By remaining curious and encouraging Lionel's ongoing self-observation, the therapist turns a potential therapy roadblock (incomplete homework) into a rich therapeutic opportunity to reevaluate and revise the current case conceptualization. Instead of automatic thoughts about inadequacy, Lionel and his therapist discover that imagery related to traumatic memories triggers his procrastination. All the competencies shown in Figure 8.1 are displayed. How do therapists develop these high-level conceptualization skills? We address that question next.

HOW THERAPISTS LEARN CASE CONCEPTUALIZATION SKILLS

Over the last few decades several models of CBT therapist learning have been proposed. These models describe mechanisms by which therapists learn and how different aspects of therapist skill (e.g., engagement, conceptualization, attending to problems in the therapeutic relationship) relate to one another. Below, we adapt James Bennett-Levy's model (Bennett-Levy, 2006) to offer a framework for understanding, teaching, and developing case conceptualization skills. As shown in Figure 8.2, Bennett-Levy articulates three related aspects of learning: declarative, procedural, and reflective.

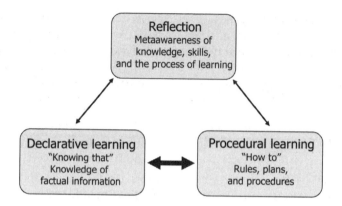

Figure 8.2. Bennett-Levy's (2006) model of CBT therapist learning.

Declarative Learning

Declarative learning is concerned with *acquiring relevant knowledge* such as CBT theories, treatment protocol stages, and understanding in principle how to structure a CBT session. It is concerned with "knowing that" (Bennett-Levy, 2006). Early in training, therapists learn theories related to common diagnoses as well as the functions of assessment and case conceptualization. Declarative knowledge can include both relatively simple models and ideas (e.g., the cognitive model of panic; rationale for case conceptualization) and deep comprehension of complex models and ideas (e.g., modes in personality disorders; transdiagnostic processes). Declarative learning about case conceptualization includes: learning the definition and functions of case conceptualization (Chapter 1); the generic CBT model as well as disorder-specific CBT models (Chapter 1; Box 1.3); cognitive–emotional–physiological–behavioral patterns in particular disorders (Chapter 5); diagnostic markers of different disorders; and the steps involved in case conceptualization (Chapters 5 through 7). It also applies to knowing *in theory* about the principles and processes integral to CBT case conceptualization (Chapters 2 through 4). In the case of Lionel it refers to knowing models of procrastination (Burns, 1989; Burns, Dittmann, Nguyen, & Mitchelson, 2001) and PTSD (Brewin et al., 1996), as well as how to work with trauma imagery (Ehlers, Hackmann, & Michael, 2004; Ehlers et al., 2005; Wheatley et al., 2007).

Therapists with advanced declarative knowledge demonstrate knowledge of simple and complex models in CBT and, crucially, this knowledge is well structured so she or he can easily navigate this knowledge base (Eells et al., 2005). There is also evidence that therapists with a more highly developed knowledge base use higher-order principles to organize the knowledge they possess (Eells et al., 2005). For example, therapists with an advanced understanding of conceptualization might more readily collaborate with clients to ensure there is a check and balance on the fit between an empirical knowledge base and client experience.

Procedural Learning

Procedural learning is concerned with *skill acquisition* and "how-to" conduct CBT (Bennett-Levy, 2006). Examples include being able to ask questions that gather information about a client's presenting issues or complete a functional analysis of a presenting issue (Chapters 3, 4, and 5). Procedural learning refers to principles, plans, and steps involved in carrying out therapeutic skills. It includes nonverbal skills (e.g., noticing subtle changes in clients' emotional state), interpersonal skills (e.g., ensuring genuine collaboration), and technical skills (e.g., teaching clients to use Thought Records). Procedural learning is when "declarative understandings become actualized in practice and refined" (Bennett-Levy, 2006; p. 64).

Broad areas of procedural learning are required for effective case conceptualization including skills in collaboration, empiricism, implementation of each step in each level of conceptualization described in Chapters 5 through 7, and being able to balance incorporation of difficulties and strengths. Therapists need to develop procedural competence in building a strong therapeutic relationship, engaging clients in collaborative investigations, and all the other micro skills involved in psychotherapeutic work generally and in CBT specifically. For example, procedural learning might involve developing the skills to collaboratively develop a descriptive conceptualization of the client's presenting issues using the five-part model (Chapters 3 and 5). Lionel's therapist needs to know how to communicate that he understands Lionel's distress, collaboratively switch the focus of the session, maintain a therapeutic alliance when working with strong emotion, and describe relevant CBT models in language Lionel can understand.

Therapists possess advanced procedural competencies when they can carry out most CBT interventions with relative ease, including collaborative case conceptualization. For example, in Chapters 5 through 7 Mark's therapist illustrated mastery of procedural learning in CBT because she was able to help Mark conceptualize his various concerns, incorporate strengths at each level of conceptualization, and deftly navigate among CBT protocols, even blending protocols when Mark's conceptualizations suggested that his concerns shared common triggers and maintenance factors.

Reflective Learning

Reflective learning describes what goes on when therapists stand back from their clinical practice and observe what has happened in order to improve knowledge, skills, and therapeutic behavior. Self-observation, analysis, and evaluation are required; reflection can either be in the moment or after the fact (Bennett-Levy, 2006). Reflection occurs in the moment when a therapist notes and responds to something as it is happening. The therapist in the dialogue earlier in this chapter demonstrated reflective learning when he noticed Lionel's strong autonomic reactions in session and reconsidered his original hypothesis about the meaning of Lionel's incomplete homework.

While in training, CBT therapists are commonly asked to record and review therapy sessions. Reflective learning takes place during these review sessions. Therapists have the time and space to observe elements of therapy sessions that may have been difficult to reflect on fully in the moment. For example, in the session with Lionel, a novice therapist might respond with frustration, "It is important you do the homework if you want to make progress. You don't need to do it perfectly." Review of a session recording allows the therapist to observe his or her automatic reactions and reflect on their impact as well as consider alternative responses that might be more therapeutic. Other examples of reflection might involve reviewing a recording of a session to assess how well collaborative empiricism was employed and to consider how to do it better in future sessions. A supervisor or consultant can guide this reflective process.

Reflective learning regarding case conceptualization includes evaluating a conceptualization's fit, paying attention to what needs to be learned, and noticing whether therapy is progressing as expected. Reflection is apparent in session when the therapist notices a mismatch between his or her own enthusiasm or curiosity regarding a conceptual model and the client's. Outside of session, therapist reflections often identify missing or misplaced elements in a conceptualization. Throughout this book we use "Inside the Therapist's Head" boxes to capture therapist reflective processes. As Mark and his therapist try to make sense of how his history shaped his beliefs and strategies in Chapter 7, the therapist asks herself "Does this make sense? Does this fit?" and decides there are problems of fit that require further exploration.

There is evidence that more advanced therapists have better-developed self-monitoring skills than less-skilled therapists: "They are more aware of when they make errors, why they fail to comprehend, and when they need to recheck their solutions" (Eells et al., 2005, p. 587). Even so, more can be learned at every stage of professional development.

Learning at Every Stage of Professional Development

Collectively, the authors have experience teaching case conceptualization to therapists at every level from senior-year undergraduates to CBT therapists who have been practicing for many years. Psychology undergraduates typically find case conceptualization fascinating because it provides an opportunity to move from theory to an understanding of real clinical applications. At this early stage, learning tends to be almost entirely declarative, although the quality of undergraduates' critical thinking and questions can be superb. Their declarative knowledge serves these students well when they watch a video recording of a therapist and client engaged in collaborative case conceptualization. However, if they are asked to role-play collaborative case conceptualization they discover that doing it requires a different set of skills (procedural knowledge). Consequently, undergraduate student role plays are typically awkward.

Graduate students invited to do the same role play attempt to synthesize what they know (declarative knowledge) with developing therapy skills (procedural knowledge). Graduate students can also be stilted in role plays because this synthesis is challenging. Asked to reflect on what has happened in a role play, graduate students are capable of insightful and elegant discussions because they have an opportunity to consider their experience of uniting theory and skills *in vivo*.

At the other end of the continuum, highly experienced CBT therapists often have developed such well-practiced and reflexive skill sets that they need to reflect a minute before they can describe the rationales that underlie their choice of conceptualization and intervention. Advanced therapists may no longer consciously notice therapy choice points because therapy patterns become so rehearsed they operate outside awareness. Instead, they sometimes reflect at higher-order levels such as combining various conceptual frameworks with their experience of similar clients and therapeutic issues.

For example, when it became clear that Lionel had not done the homework, his therapist noted Lionel's visible anxiety in session. Based on experience, he intuited that Lionel's extreme anxiety was unlikely to result from automatic thoughts about inadequacy. Lionel's therapist knew from theory and experience that the ideal time to identify central anxious thoughts and images is when anxiety is highly activated. Thus he decided to use Lionel's distress as an opportunity to empathically inquire about upsetting imagery in the hope that this would guide them to alternative hypotheses. If asked what rules of thumb he used to make choices about intervention and conceptualization in this session, Lionel's therapist may not be able to immediately articulate these; he may say his choices were "intuitive." And yet reflection on these processes could help him identify useful or biased operating principles in his clinical practice. This is necessary if he wants to identify what is working and what can be improved in his clinical practice. It can also help him be a better teacher or supervisor.

STRATEGIES FOR DEVELOPING CASE CONCEPTUALIZATION EXPERTISE

In order to collaboratively develop case conceptualizations as described in Chapters 3 through 7, therapists must acquire specific skills and learn to artfully combine them in different ways depending on clients' needs and strengths. On the following pages we integrate Bennett-Levy's learning processes into a four-stage learning cycle (see Figure 8.3) designed to develop case conceptualization expertise. The four stages are (1) assess learning needs; (2) set personal learning goals; (3) participate in declara-

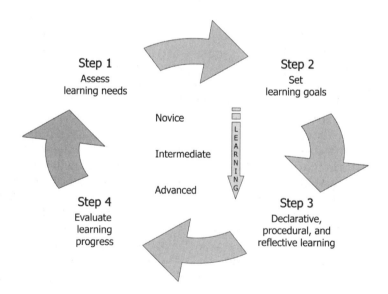

Figure 8.3. Four steps of therapist learning.

tive, procedural, and reflective learning processes; and (4) evaluate learning progress to determine further learning needs (cycling back to step 1). We discuss this learning cycle for each of the principles emphasized in this text: collaborative empiricism, levels of conceptualization, and incorporation of client strengths. As implied by the term "cycle," this learning model can extend throughout a career and be used by therapists of all expertise levels to improve case conceptualization practice. It can guide therapist self-study as well as CBT supervision, consultation, and instructional programs. The sections that follow describe in detail how therapists can use this learning framework to improve their case conceptualization skills.

Step 1: Assess Learning Needs

General Issues

For each of our three principles, we recommend that therapists make a self-assessment of their knowledge, skills, and learning needs. To aid this assessment process, we have made specific recommendations regarding the knowledge and competencies therapists need to conduct collaborative case conceptualization. These are organized into three boxes (Boxes 8.1, 8.2, and 8.3) summarizing what a CBT therapist is expected to master for each of our three principles. Each box groups competencies into novice, intermediate, and advanced levels of expertise. By novice we refer to therapists who are either still acquiring the most fundamental knowledge sets described (via declarative learning) or who have limited experience successfully implementing this knowledge (procedural skill). Note that years of experience do not dictate level of therapist knowledge and competency regarding case conceptualization. Therapists may have many years of experience and still be novices in some of the principles outlined in this text.

Therapists are rarely equally skilled in the application of each of our three principles. For instance, a therapist may be highly skilled in collaborative empiricism and yet a novice in the incorporation of client strengths into case conceptualization. These summary boxes are intended to help therapists and supervisors identify gaps in knowledge and design appropriate plans for focused study. Mastery of each knowledge area or competency listed in these boxes requires both declarative knowledge and procedural skill. Usually declarative knowledge is acquired first and then procedural skill develops with experience. As a reflection of this developmental progression, we recommend that therapists rate their skills for each item in each summary box on the following 5-point scale:

0 = an absence of declarative knowledge
1 = minimal declarative knowledge
2 = good declarative knowledge but little procedural skill
3 = good declarative knowledge with moderate procedural skill
4 = good declarative knowledge and good procedural skill with many but not most clients
5 = thorough declarative understanding integrated with flexible procedural skill

We have described what we regard as a typical developmental progression. However, therapists may discover that their own learning shows a different pattern of development in knowledge and competency. Areas of relative weakness can be targeted in self-study, peer consultation, supervision, or consultation using methods outlined in step 3 below. Some therapists will give themselves moderate or higher scores on items in more than one level (novice, intermediate, advanced) of these lists. This is to be expected because learning can develop in many different patterns. Consider whether these strengths can help in areas where there are knowledge gaps. Also, depending upon the ratings, therapists may follow novice guidelines for learning some topics and intermediate or advanced guidelines for other areas of study.

Assessing Learning Needs Regarding Collaborative Empiricism

To establish and maintain collaboration with clients during case conceptualization, therapists rely on both generic therapy competencies and those specific to case conceptualization. As shown in Box 8.1, generic therapy competencies essential to collaboration include novice abilities such as learning to establish a therapy alliance and to listen accurately and empathically. Advanced generic therapy competencies include the ability to collaboratively navigate conflict and negotiate therapy impasses. In addition, collaborative empiricism requires competencies specific to case conceptualization that allow the therapist to create conversational bridges between client observations and empirically derived models. These include intermediate-level skills such as flexibility in use of language and metaphor in order to adapt empirically derived models to a particular client experience and recognition of client experiences that fit or contradict a particular conceptualization. As therapists become more advanced, they are able to exercise these skills in a relaxed, conversational manner and engage clients in an active search for links between different aspects of experience. In addition, it is helpful for a therapist to possess and model qualities of curiosity, compassion, and open-mindedness.

Box 8.1. Recommended Knowledge Base and Competencies to Employ Collaborative Empiricism in Case Conceptualization

---

Therapist Skill Level	Recommended Knowledge Base and Competencies
Novice	• Know how to form and sustain a positive therapy alliance.

• Communication skills
—can communicate ideas clearly.
—can listen well and understand client communications.
—verbal and nonverbal expressions are congruent.

• Understand the role of collaboration in CBT and how to collaborate to accomplish common tasks (e.g., agenda setting).

• Recognize the importance of therapy structure, including knowledge of how to negotiate tasks within the therapy hour (e.g., time spent on various topics).

• Understand how to use functional analysis and/or the five-part model.

• Have basic familiarity with explanatory conceptualizations for common disorders such as depression, specific anxiety disorders, and other common presenting issues in the clinician's practice.

• Know methods to identify and rate emotions, thoughts, and physiological phenomena.

• Understand how to engage clients in behavioral observation.

• Know the four stages of Socratic dialogue.

• Have knowledge of cultural variations.

• Know basics of how to set up and debrief behavioral experiments.

• Know how to use Thought Records, prediction logs, and other written methods to observe and test beliefs.

• Understand how to use relevant questions to gather the information necessary to form a case conceptualization.

Intermediate   **All knowledge at novice level plus:**

• Know how to adapt therapist language and metaphor to educational level, culture, and personal interests of client.

• Recognize client experiences that fit with and contradict particular conceptual models.

(cont.)

Box 8.1 (*cont.*)

- Can engage clients so they actively search for links between different aspects of their experience (e.g., thoughts and feelings) outside of therapy sessions and report these to the therapist verbally and/or in writing.

- Has clear understanding of cognitive conceptualizations for depression, anxiety disorders, and other problems common to the clinician's practice.

- Aware of features that differentiate between similar presenting issues.

- Is able to incorporate cultural factors into conceptualizations.

- Can use Socratic dialogue to effectively test beliefs.

- Can maintain objectivity and genuine curiosity about client experience; can flexibly adapt conceptualization to client feedback.

- Can present evidence-based models to client that fit with client-reported experiences.

- Can construct individualized conceptualizations that incorporate relevant evidence-based models.

- Can make predictions and employ behavioral experiments to evaluate case conceptualization.

Advanced   **All knowledge at novice and intermediate levels plus:**

- Can navigate conflict and collaboratively work through therapy impasses.

- Is able to attain and maintain collaboration with most clients, including those who have great difficulty collaborating in relationships.

- Can create natural conversational bridges between client observations and empirically derived models.

- Is alert to subtleties in similarities and differences between client reports of experience and empirically supported models.

- Can use and/or seek data from client to reconcile differences between empirically supported models and client's personal experience.

- Is able to weave empirical methods seamlessly into the fabric of therapy.

- Can readily use case conceptualization to navigate therapy impasses, evaluate treatment options, and plan for relapse management.

- Is able to reflect on and identify personal biases that interfere with empirical processes.

Empiricism sometimes means linking client experiences with empirically supported models of a particular disorder. Other times, empiricism refers to derivation of a conceptualization from careful observations of client experience integrating many different sources of client data. There is evidence that more advanced therapists are better able to see and use large patterns in data, perhaps because their knowledge base is highly organized and they are more skilled in navigating their knowledge base (Eells et al., 2005).

Therapists, supervisors, and CBT instructors can use Box 8.1 to guide assessment of core strengths and knowledge gaps in collaborative empiricism. Novice, intermediate, and advanced therapists are expected to attain different levels of competency and breadth of knowledge. A novice in collaborative empiricism needs to master foundational competencies and knowledge such as how to establish and maintain a positive therapy alliance and accomplish basic collaboration tasks such as setting a session agenda. In addition, novice therapists need knowledge specific to case conceptualization, such as how to elicit the client observations necessary to construct a conceptualization. Intermediate-level therapists are able to fulfill these basic tasks with greater skill, across a wider variety of client presenting issues, and with greater individualization to client needs.

Novice therapists often struggle to apply knowledge, whereas intermediate therapists put knowledge to competent use, often individualizing it to particular clients. The following therapist statements illustrate the differences between novice and intermediate use of language during case conceptualization:

NOVICE: Let's see if we can draw a picture to show how your thoughts and feelings link up to each other. (*same words used with virtually every client*)

INTERMEDIATE: You mentioned earlier that you like to tinker with motorcycles. When you do that, is it important to know what connects to what? (*Client nods.*) Maybe we can use your motorcycle skills to learn to tinker with your moods a bit. First let's see if we can figure out what is connected to what.

Intermediate therapists also acquire a broader knowledge base than novice therapists regarding empirically supported models for conceptualizing common problems. In addition, they have an awareness of features that overlap and differentiate between similar models. Intermediate therapists are often more attuned than novice therapists to culturally based variations in experience and know how to incorporate cultural factors into conceptualizations. Therapists can spend many years at an intermediate level of case conceptualization skill.

Advanced competency in collaborative empiricism is marked by the ability to elicit collaboration and client engagement under challenging circumstances and also to collaboratively reconcile conflicts between empirically supported models and client observations. At this level, case conceptualizations are readily used to navigate therapy impasses, evaluate treatment options, and plan for relapse management. Advanced therapists are also expected to be highly reflective about how their beliefs and values affect the case conceptualization process.

Assessing Learning Needs Regarding Levels of Conceptualization

Mark's extended case example (Chapters 5 through 7) illustrates how case conceptualization can evolve over time from description (e.g., functional analysis and the five-part model), to cross-sectional explanation (e.g., triggers and maintenance factors), to a longitudinal understanding of the predisposing factors that contribute to client vulnerability and the protective factors that serve as a platform for building resilience. We call this progression "levels of conceptualization" (see Figure 2.1). In order to use levels of conceptualization, therapists need to acquire the knowledge base and competencies summarized in Box 8.2.

As noted in Box 8.2, novice therapists need to learn theory and research on particular disorders, rationales, and methods involved in particular conceptualization frameworks (e.g., the five-part model), and fundamental therapy processes such as constructing a presenting issues list and setting goals. Therapists with intermediate competencies regarding levels of conceptualization acquire knowledge with greater depth and breadth of application. Advanced therapists are able to cross-fertilize ideas from theories and research and understand much more thoroughly how to integrate client difficulties and resilience within conceptualizations at each level. In addition, advanced therapists are better judges of the appropriate level of conceptualization for a particular client at a particular point in therapy.

Mark's therapist displayed an advanced level of skill and knowledge regarding levels of conceptualization. She skillfully completed all necessary tasks at each level of conceptualization, recognized and highlighted themes that connected Mark's presenting issues, capably implemented and coordinated several treatment protocols, and identified and integrated Mark's resilience throughout therapy. A therapist with less knowledge and fewer competencies is unlikely to have accomplished so much with Mark in the time available. Consider how Mark's therapy might have proceeded with a less knowledgeable or competent therapist.

Box 8.2. Recommended Knowledge Base and Competencies to Employ Levels of Conceptualization

Therapist Skill Level	Recommended Knowledge Base and Competencies
Novice	**Descriptive level** • Can differentiate thoughts, moods, physical reactions, behaviors, and situational aspects of client experience. • Understands purposes and rationale for presenting issues list. • Understands principles and processes of functional analysis. • Understands principles and processes of five-part model. • Familiar with one or two evidence-based conceptualization models (e.g., panic disorder, OCD). • Understands goal-setting processes. **Explanatory level (triggers and maintenance)** • Can identify automatic thoughts, underlying assumptions, and core beliefs. • Understands generic cognitive model (see Chapter 1). • Can identify triggers and maintenance factors. • Recognizes safety behaviors. • Knows research regarding etiology, maintenance, and treatment for one or two common diagnoses. **Predisposing and protective factors** • Knows CBT theory of personality development (Beck et al., 2004). • Knows at least one model for understanding resilience. • Understands rationale for linking developmental history, presenting issues, and relapse management.
Intermediate	**All knowledge at novice level plus:** **Descriptive level** • Familiar with evidence-based diagnostic models for all common disorders in one's practice.

(cont.)

Box 8.2 (cont.)

Explanatory level

- Actively follows research regarding etiology, maintenance, and treatment for many common disorders in one's practice.

- Recognizes recurring themes across situational client examples.

- Possesses knowledge of a wide repertoire of CBT interventions and understands how to select these based on the conceptualization.

- Familiar with expected treatment length and outcomes based on knowledge of relevant research with various clinical populations.

Predisposing and protective factors

- Aware of personality types as well as common underlying assumptions and core beliefs associated with each.

- Understands how to elicit metaphors, stories, and imagery from client that are linked to key themes and presenting issues.

- Understands how to formulate a longitudinal conceptualization for both presenting issues and also for client resilience.

- Able to identify possible risk factors for future relapse based on client longitudinal conceptualization.

Advanced   **All knowledge at novice and intermediate levels plus:**

Descriptive level

- Recognizes recurring themes in evidence-based models (e.g., rumination) and can identify themes that link client presenting issues.

- Able to provide clinical rationale for when to use each level of conceptualization with a particular client.

- Understands the rationale and methods for incorporating resilience at each level of conceptualization.

Explanatory level

- Regularly updates knowledge to integrate research findings from various CBT approaches and across many disorders.

- Recognizes triggers and maintenance factors that are common to multiple client presenting issues.

Box 8.2 (*cont.*)

- Knows how to modify CBT interventions to match peculiarities of a client conceptualization or to adapt to treatment barriers.

Predisposing and protective factors

- Understands interview modifications that enhance CBT with various personality disorders (Beck et al., 2004).

- Knows how to integrate predisposing and protective factors within a longitudinal conceptualization.

A novice therapist working with Mark might have understood the necessity of each therapy task and yet struggled with its implementation. In addition, novice therapists might have experience treating depression or OCD or health worries, but are less likely to have experience with all three issues. Thus novice therapists frequently struggle with how to link conceptualization and treatment methods, especially with multiproblem clients. The breadth of knowledge required is either absent or the therapist has declarative knowledge without procedural skill. Furthermore, novice CBT therapists often are so attentive to client distress that they forget the benefits of simultaneously working with client resilience.

How might Mark's therapy proceed if he is matched with a therapist with intermediate skill in levels of conceptualization? An intermediate level therapist is more likely to know CBT conceptual models and a treatment for each of Mark's presenting issues. Intermediate skill level typically spans a long learning period. Thus while some intermediate therapists are akin to very experienced and highly skilled novices, others practice at a level similar to advanced therapists. Unlike novice therapists, intermediate therapists experience only occasional gaps in knowledge and skill. When they do encounter gaps, most intermediate therapists know how to acquire the requisite knowledge and skill, whether through study of the relevant literature, consultation with another therapist, or personal reflection. Unlike advanced therapists, intermediate-level therapists are less likely to adeptly integrate client difficulties and resilience at each level of conceptualization. They are also less likely to use higher-order principles in solving therapy dilemmas such as when Mark's therapist integrated OCD and hypochondriasis models to address Mark's health worries (see Chapter 6).

Assessing Learning Needs Regarding Incorporation of Client Strengths

Throughout this text we illustrate the benefits of incorporating client strengths into case conceptualizations. Box 8.3 summarizes the knowledge base and competencies that help therapists do this. Therapists who do not currently incorporate strengths into case conceptualizations first need to develop a conviction that this is desirable. Knowledge of the literatures of positive psychology and resilience (see Chapter 4) can help therapists appreciate the benefits of practicing strengths-focused CBT. These knowledge bases also help therapists develop a broad theoretical and empirical understanding of the links between client strengths and mental health and resilience.

Box 8.3. Recommended Knowledge Base and Competencies to Incorporate Client Strengths

Therapist Skill Level	Recommended Knowledge Base and Competencies
Novice	• Understands relevance of client strengths for case conceptualization.
	• Knows questions for eliciting client strengths (cf. Chapter 4).
	• Can employ guided discovery methods to help clients identify strengths.
	• Able to observe unspoken strengths at least some of the time.
	• Knows positive psychology literature and understands empirical bases of a strengths focus.
Intermediate	• Knows the resilience literature (see Chapter 4) and is familiar with diverse areas of strengths.
	• Understands how to incorporate strengths into conceptual models.
	• Able to observe unspoken strengths.
Advanced	• Able to integrate strengths and difficulties seamlessly throughout each level of case conceptualization.
	• Recognizes pathways to change within identified strengths.
	• Observes and infers unspoken strengths and can facilitate client awareness of these throughout each stage of therapy.
	• Integrates both strengths and resilience into treatment plans.

Novice therapists are expected to be able to ask questions that identify client strengths and understand the relevance of strengths for case conceptualizations. As therapists reach an intermediate level of competency in incorporation of client strengths they begin to naturally observe client strengths and incorporate these into case conceptualizations with relative ease. An advanced level of competency is associated with incorporating strengths throughout each stage of therapy and level of conceptualization. In addition, advanced therapists actively integrate client strengths and resilience into treatment plans.

Clarissa: A Case Example in Assessing Learning Needs

Clarissa is a CBT therapist working in a community mental health center. She rates herself on the knowledge base and competencies listed in Boxes 8.1, 8.2, and 8.3. On all novice knowledge and skills she rates herself a 3 to 5; 4 is her most common novice rating. On intermediate knowledge and skills she rates herself 2 through 5, with most ratings at 2 through 4. On advanced skills she rates herself 0 through 5, with most ratings in the 1 to 3 range. These ratings indicate that, for most areas of knowledge and competency, she is at an intermediate level. Her most advanced ratings are in the incorporation of client strengths into case conceptualization. The community mental health center where she works emphasizes building on client strengths, so she is at ease assessing and incorporating client strengths into most conceptualizations and treatment plans. In addition, Clarissa recognizes that her own strengths lie in collaborating with clients and using collaborative empiricism with depression and anxiety diagnoses. These strengths are supported by a solid understanding of CBT theory and treatments for depression and anxiety.

Clarissa decides she wants to expand her knowledge regarding CBT theories and practice beyond depression and anxiety disorders. Many of the clients in her clinic experience auditory hallucinations as part of psychosis. Clarissa discovers there is a rich area of CBT theory and research regarding psychosis and decides CBT with psychosis, especially for clients with auditory hallucinations, is an area of knowledge she wants to improve.

Step 2: Set Personal Learning Goals

Just as Clarissa has done, readers are encouraged to review their knowledge and competency ratings in order to choose and prioritize areas for more learning. Consider the clients you serve and the types of clinical issues you face. Choose one or two areas for improvement that you think would benefit you and your clients the most. Therapists can make this decision on their own or with the help of a supervisor or consultant. It is best to set a learning goal that can be accomplished in a few weeks' or months' time. It is easy to feel overwhelmed if you decide to work on too many areas for improvement all at once or if you set learning goals too high. It is much better to target one or two areas for improvement at a time.

Once areas are chosen for learning, form personal goals related to these. It is helpful to identify your goals in specific, objective, and measurable terms. Clarissa sets learning goals to (1) learn a CBT model for understanding auditory hallucinations, (2) work with two or more clients who hear voices and see how this model fits with their personal experiences, and (3) use these clients' language and personal metaphors to collaboratively construct a conceptualization of their voices that makes sense to them. These goals are specific and objective.

Clarissa decides to measure her progress on each of these three goals in the following ways: (1) ask a colleague to role-play a client and rate the clarity of her explanation of a CBT model of auditory hallucinations, (2) listen to her session recordings and self-rate how well she elicits descriptions of her clients' auditory hallucinations that can provide evidence for fitting or varying from the CBT model, and (3) ask her clients to rate how much the conceptualization they co-construct fits with their personal experience. She will decide that she has successfully met her learning goal when ratings in each of these areas are 3 or above on the 5-point scale recommended in this chapter. Notice Clarissa's goal is not perfect expertise. A rating of 3, which indicates "understanding with moderate skill," is quite an achievement when learning something new. It is not necessary to attain greater mastery than this before moving on to new areas of learning. With continued practice, competence will increase over time.

This process for setting personal learning goals is the same whether goals are set in the area of collaborative empiricism, levels of conceptualization, incorporation of client strengths, or some combination of these three principles. Keep in mind when setting goals that there are interactions among the areas of learning listed for each principle. For example, collaboration can be enhanced when therapists have a good understanding of CBT theory because the theory guides the therapist to ask questions regarding themes central to a client's presenting issues. Thus a client is more likely to perceive a knowledgeable therapist who can help, and this can enhance the client's interest in collaborating with that therapist. Similarly, there are interactions among areas of knowledge across our three principles. For example, therapists who incorporate strengths at each stage of conceptualization may also achieve greater collaboration with clients. Thus progress on a single learning goal benefits not only that particular area but also broader therapist competency.

Step 3: Participate in Declarative, Procedural, and Reflective Learning Processes

Once learning goals are set, therapists will choose how to best achieve these. Common learning modes include reading, workshop attendance, role play, structured clinical practice, and recording sessions for self-review or consultant feedback. As an overview, Box 8.4 summarizes these learning modes and links them to Bennett-Levy's declarative, procedural, and reflective learning processes. Bennett-Levy's model is a helpful framework for organizing a learning plan. It often makes sense to begin with declarative learning methods and next employ procedural methods to learn how to put into clinical practice what has been learned. Reflective processes are helpful throughout the learning process to evaluate how learning is proceeding, notice areas where new learning applies or is a mismatch, and identify therapist beliefs, experiences, and interpersonal processes that enhance or impede learning progress.

Declarative Learning Processes

The primary declarative learning processes are reading, attending classes, and workshops. These are the best starting points for most learning goals, whether a therapist's knowledge is at the novice, intermedi-

---

Box 8.4. Matching Types of Learning to Primary Learning Modes

Type of learning	Primary learning modes
Declarative: "knowing that"	Reading; observation of clinical demonstrations; class and workshop attendance (live or listening to recorded workshops)
Procedural: "knowing how"	Role-play practice with feedback; clinical work; recorded clinical sessions with feedback from a consultant or supervisor; teaching or demonstrating skills to others
Reflective: meta-awareness of knowledge, skills, and the process of learning	Collaborative empiricism in session; reflective clinical practice (e.g., self-review of session recordings); self-practice of CBT methods; reflective supervision; reflective reading/writing; personal therapy; personal/professional retreat experiences; identification and testing of relevant therapist beliefs

Note. After Bennett-Levy (2006).

ate, or advanced level. Therapist knowledge of the empirical literature is best attained by reading books and articles that summarize empirically supported models (see Box 1.3). Empirical knowledge continually advances. As research progresses, our understanding of the etiology and maintenance of common presenting issues is modified and improved. Thus therapists of all levels are well advised to regularly update their knowledge base by reading CBT journals, participating in peer study groups, and attending CBT conferences and empirically based clinical workshops. Therapists who don't have ready access to live workshops can obtain audio recordings of workshops as well as observe DVD demonstrations of CBT in action (e.g., Padesky, 2008). Websites that feature information about recorded programs include *www.beckinstitute.org, www.octc.org*, and *www.padesky.com*.

Procedural Learning Processes

Procedural learning commonly occurs through role play or clinical practice followed by self-review of session recordings as well as feedback from peers, clients, supervisors, or a consultant. Therapists at all skill levels can practice specific conceptualization tasks in both role plays and therapy with the intent of following the principles outlined in this text. Consider a therapist who wants to learn or fine-tune a skill set such as making a presenting issues list along with impact ratings and prioritization. Many therapists find it helpful to review the principles involved and make a reminder note of the steps they intend to follow in session. Therapists are more likely to follow procedures when steps are written on an index card or a notepad. In addition, a written reminder frees the therapist to attend to the client and issues of collaboration rather than constantly searching for mental reminders of the next step she or he wants to take. Written step-by-step reminders of how to accomplish conceptualization tasks also may help therapists learn the steps and offer an opportunity to consider why the steps are ordered as they are.

Therapists who are self-conscious about checking notes during session are encouraged to make this a collaborative process by telling clients they are following notes, giving a rationale for doing this, and seeking client input. For example, a therapist might say:

> "I've made a few notes for today's session to make sure I gather all the information I think is important. You may see me checking my notes from time to time to help me stay on track. If you think we are getting off track, encourage me to check my notes. (*Offers a warm smile.*) I also encourage you to make notes inside and outside of session to make sure we stay on track to meet your therapy goals."

Feedback from peers, a consultant, or a supervisor is invaluable while learning various conceptualization tasks. Therapists are encouraged to record sessions or role plays and review these in detail with colleagues (once appropriate client permissions are received, of course). Therapists at all skill levels experience some anxiety when they demonstrate their clinical skills to others. Thus we recommend that therapist feedback always begin with a review of what he or she did well. Just as clients respond well when their strengths are incorporated into therapy, therapists find it easier to hear and incorporate constructive feedback when strengths are also acknowledged. Just like clients, therapists may not be aware of their strengths. Highlighting these may help therapists use strengths even more productively in therapy.

The following dialogue is between Karen and Erik, intermediate-level CBT therapists who work in the same clinic. They have just finished a role play in which Karen took the role of a client with social anxiety; Erik worked with her to derive a conceptualization of triggers and maintenance factors. Now Karen is about to give Erik feedback.

ERIK: Whew! I wasn't sure for awhile that I could get you to identify your maintenance processes, but we got there. How do you think I did?

KAREN: Let's start with positive feedback. What do you think you did well?

ERIK: It's a bit easier to say what I don't think I did well. (*Karen remains silent with an encouraging smile on her face, so Erik continues after a short while.*) Well, I think I explained social anxiety to you in a pretty clear way. And we identified your triggers right away. (*laughing*) I hope you experienced me as warm and genuine.

KAREN: Actually, I did. One of the things I really liked about this interview is that you looked at me a lot ... not with an examining attitude that might have made me uncomfortable, but with a real sense of caring. When I was role-playing this woman, that attitude of caring really would have helped me talk about these very uncomfortable things.

ERIK: Thanks.

KAREN: I also think you did a good job in picking up on my use of the phrase "I feel trapped." When you kept using that language it kept me in my experience. And when you asked me if I had any images attached to this feeling ... that really burst through my barriers because the images were so powerful. If you had used different words or not looked for the images, I think we would have gotten off track. (*Offers a few additional positive observations of Erik's interviewing skills.*)

ERIK: OK. I'm ready. Where do I need to improve?

KAREN: I did get a bit lost when you introduced the idea of maintenance processes. Everything seemed very conversational up to that point, and then you seemed to get very professorial and formal in describing maintenance to me. If I was really this client I think I might have become a bit frightened ... like your serious tone meant you were about to deliver some bad news.

ERIK: Hmm, that's interesting. I wasn't aware I came across that way. I do struggle a bit more with how to talk about maintenance factors, so maybe that is why I became more academic at that point.

KAREN: Maybe if we listen to that point in our session recording, you'll hear what I mean. Do you think it would help to talk about different ways you might have made this transition?

ERIK: Yes, I would like to do that. I really struggle with introducing maintenance. Maybe you can switch roles with me and show me how you talk about maintenance.

KAREN: Sure. You did so well up to that point. I was really with you and felt you were my ally in figuring all this out. If you can figure out a way to introduce and look for maintenance factors that keeps you in the same conversational and concerned mode, I think your sessions will go better. We could role-play that part of the session a few more times until you find a better way to introduce this information.

ERIK: Let's do it. I'll find the spot on the recording.

Notice that Karen gives Erik very specific feedback about his therapeutic manner. Her language is objective, commenting on specific behaviors, rather than judgmental. As is often the case, Karen notes aspects of Erik's performance that are out of his awareness. Although he recognizes that he struggles more with the identification of maintenance factors, he is not aware that his tone shifted at this point in the interview and that his more professorial tone might have a negative impact on his clients. Erik listens to and considers Karen's feedback. It is clear in this interchange that Karen and Erik respect each other as therapists and both of them value learning. Rather than simply talking about these issues, Erik and Karen show a willingness to do additional role plays to experiment with various options that could improve Erik's competence.

This brief example of peer consultation and feedback following a role play provides a good model for readers to follow. Prior to entering into consultation with each other, therapists are encouraged to discuss the learning focus, format (e.g., specific objective comments, positive feedback first), and roles (e.g., will therapists take turns giving and getting feedback?) that will characterize the interaction. At each level of therapist skill, the more familiar a skill becomes in role play the easier it will be to express it in therapy sessions.

Case discussions and listening to session recordings with colleagues can also help hone case conceptualization skills. It is important during each of these activities to keep empiricism in mind. At times, clinical case discussions wander into personal conjecture and anecdotal musings based on personal experience or history with other clients. Although these ideas sometimes lead to fruitful hypotheses, it is important for therapists to look for evidence in the current client's experience and to value empirically based findings more highly than single-case anecdotes. It is also important to remember that conceptualizations developed collaboratively with clients have greater utility than those generated by therapists only, no matter how expert the therapists.

Reflective Learning Processes

In the preceding peer consultation dialogue, Erik indicated that he was not aware he adopted a more academic tone with Karen in the middle of the interview. In order for reflective learning to occur, therapists need to develop a reflective awareness of their own thoughts, behaviors, emotions, and physical reactions in and outside of therapy. For example, it is important that therapists strive to become aware of their own biases that may interfere with case conceptualization (Chapter 2). Some therapists favor particular conceptual models so strongly that they are blind to objectively hearing divergent client experiences. In a similar vein, therapists can become so enamored of particular therapy methods that they apply these interventions regardless of their relevance to the case conceptualization.

Sometimes biases that interfere with case conceptualization are more closely linked to a therapist's personal issues rather than general cognitive heuristic errors. Personal therapy for the therapist can be an important part of reflective learning, especially when this therapy is done with a CBT therapist. Whether in therapy or not, it is beneficial for therapists to conceptualize their personal issues in CBT terms. Therapists can compare conceptualizations of personal difficulties with existing cognitive models, looking for both similarities and differences. As part of a reflective learning process, therapists can gather additional data from their own lives to resolve ambiguities in the conceptualization.

Use of empirical methods such as observation, evaluation of

thoughts, and behavioral experiments with oneself increases therapist confidence in using these methods with clients (Bennett-Levy et al., 2001). Many therapists report self-observational exercises among the most valuable to heighten awareness of links among different aspects of human experience. Bennett-Levy conducted research (Bennett-Levy et al., 2001) in which therapists learning cognitive therapy participated in self-practice exercises guided by the client workbook *Mind over Mood* (Greenberger & Padesky, 1995). Therapists who used this workbook as a guide to practice cognitive therapy methods on themselves reported greater understanding of the rationale and purposes of cognitive therapy as well as improved ability to explain and guide clients in the use of these methods. Many graduate class instructors and CBT supervisors encourage self-practice of CBT, and this has been recommended as an important part of learning (Padesky, 1996).

Review of session recordings enables reflective practice for therapists of all skill levels. With appropriate written client permission (as required by professional codes of practice), these recordings can be reviewed independently, with a supervisor/consultant, or in collaboration with a peer therapist group. Therapists can use session recordings as stimuli to identify their own automatic thoughts and underlying assumptions that interfere with case conceptualization. For instance, some therapists have an internal clock that tells them how fast therapy "should" be occurring. When this timetable is exceeded, these therapists may become overly didactic in order to speed the pace of therapy. Padesky (2000) teaches therapists to use such impasses and difficulties as a prompt to identify their own underlying assumptions. She shows therapists how to devise behavioral experiments in and outside of therapy sessions to test these interfering assumptions.

It is helpful for therapists to stay alert for instances when emotions, beliefs, and behavioral patterns present in therapy parallel those in the therapist's personal life. Each instance in which this occurs is a good opportunity to identify and rate thoughts, emotions, behaviors, and physical responses and compare these observations with relevant cognitive models. Therapists can use these occasions and observations to conceptualize their own therapy reactions using methods taught in this text, as shown in the following example.

Theresa: A Case Example of Therapist Reflective Practice

Theresa noticed that she frequently felt tired when she met with a particular client, Joe, even though this reaction was not present in her sessions before and after her appointments with him. While attending to feelings of fatigue in session, Theresa tried to perk herself up only to feel sluggish again a few minutes later. She reflected on her sessions with Joe over several weeks, looking for triggers of her fatigue. She realized her energy deflated as soon as she saw Joe's name on her appointment calendar. In order to understand these reactions, Theresa decided to attend to her thoughts, feelings, behaviors, and physical reactions related to Joe. She used the five-part model as shown in Figure 8.4 to link her observations and conceptualize her fatigue in session with him.

Theresa noticed that Joe's vocal tone and patterns of complaint evoked images of her older brother, Pete. Theresa had tried throughout her lifetime to help Pete cheer up and tackle his problems rather than avoid them. As a child, Theresa felt quite tense in the face of her brother's distress. She responded to this tension by emotionally distancing herself. A favorite method of coping was to allow her body to go limp like her favorite rag doll. This image helped her disengage while her brother raged against life's difficulties. In recent years Theresa distanced herself from Pete out of frustration; he persisted in complaining rather than coping with challenges.

Theresa realized that her client Joe's perceived similarities to Pete provoked irritation with this client during the intake interview. Not rec-

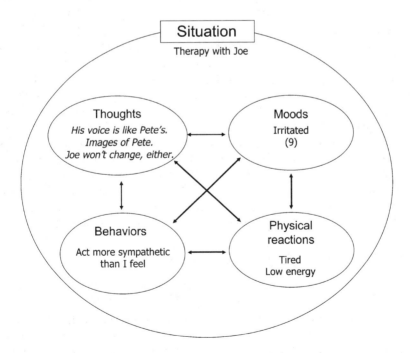

Figure 8.4. Theresa's conceptualization of her reactions to a client, Joe.

ognizing at the time that he evoked memories of Pete, Theresa felt guilty about her irritation with this new client. She held an underlying assumption, "If I feel irritated with a client then I cannot do good therapy." Thus she covered her irritation with overly kind and sympathetic responses to his complaints. Her hopelessness that this client would change (just as Pete had not changed) and her feigned sympathy created tension, which Theresa countered by becoming as tired as she felt in childhood when mimicking her limp rag doll.

Once Theresa completed this five-part model conceptualization of her reactions to Joe, she understood more fully what was causing her fatigue in sessions. This conceptualization guided her to look for similarities and differences between Pete and Joe so she could consider Joe's presenting issues on their own terms. Theresa asked a colleague to consult with her regularly while she treated Joe to help her process her personal reactions and also to ensure that she stayed engaged and active in devising treatment plans that were likely to be effective. This consultant helped Theresa role-play ways to directly and therapeutically talk with Joe about how his patterns of complaint and avoidance curtailed progress toward his goals. Theresa's energy and alertness in session with Joe immediately improved when she implemented these changes. This response validated the pertinence of her conceptualization. She monitored fatigue throughout her course of therapy with Joe and other clients as a warning sign that her personal history might be intruding on her therapy.

Theresa experienced a number of ineffective therapy sessions with Joe before she realized she needed to reflect on what might be causing difficulties in his therapy. As therapists advance in knowledge and skill, they often naturally engage in spontaneous reflective learning processes during and immediately after each session. Learning becomes more integrated for therapists when they reflect on processes central to CBT conceptual models in relation to their own life experience. Therapists also spontaneously think about treatment dilemmas outside of therapy sessions. When doing so, therapists are encouraged to reflect on these dilemmas in light of relevant case conceptualizations.

Processes for Learning Collaborative Empiricism

Basic texts on CBT usually address collaborative empiricism and provide clinical examples of it in action (cf. J. S. Beck, 1995; Westbrook et al., 2007), as do books on special topics such as the use of behavioral experiments in CBT (Bennett-Levy et al., 2004). As therapists develop competence in collaborative empiricism, learning includes more nuanced study of these processes related to case conceptualization. Appendix

8.1 includes a variety of learning exercises that help promote clinical expertise in collaborative empiricism for therapists at novice, intermediate, and advanced levels of clinical expertise. These sample exercises are offered as a resource for CBT instructors who offer training courses in case conceptualization. Individual therapists may also find it helpful to scan these exercises, looking for those that can help achieve personal learning goals.

Therapists develop empiricism by careful study of the empirical literature and also through clinical practices that foster objective observation and analysis of client self-reports. Thus therapists need to be both empirically informed and empirically minded. Once therapists understand and value this approach, it often takes months of practice to comfortably blend collaboration and empiricism. Novice CBT therapists often find it difficult to maintain both a collaborative and an empirical stance with clients while mastering basic procedural tasks. Therapists learning CBT may appreciate the importance of empiricism and yet get lost in the "data" of client reports of thoughts, moods, and behaviors. Therefore it is helpful for therapists new to CBT case conceptualization to listen to session recordings, either alone or with a supervisor, to organize client data and link it to evidence-based models. Information organized between sessions can then be discussed with the client during subsequent meetings. As therapists gain experience, it becomes easier to maintain an empirical stance during sessions.

The focus of learning shifts as therapists become more adept in the use of collaborative empiricism during case conceptualization. For example, a novice therapist might role-play with a peer practicing micro skills such as accurate summaries of client presenting issues and gathering client information relevant to a conceptualization. Intermediate therapist role plays might focus on methods for evoking relevant client observations in session and linking these to empirically supported conceptual models. Advanced therapists may want to role-play collaboration challenges or methods for integrating conflicting client observations within a coherent case conceptualization. Intermediate and advanced therapists can use session recordings to evaluate their use of collaborative empiricism and seek feedback on how to improve these aspects of case conceptualization.

Clarissa: A Case Example for Learning Processes Regarding Collaborative Empiricism

Earlier in this chapter we met Clarissa, a therapist who set goals to learn a CBT model for understanding auditory hallucinations and to use this model with psychotic clients in her community mental health center. She already has intermediate CBT competence in collaborative empiricism, and so she sets a further goal to use these clients' language and personal metaphors to collaboratively construct a conceptualization of their voices that makes sense to them. What learning processes does Clarissa follow to reach these goals?

First she identifies several books on CBT for psychosis that include helpful theory, research, and clinical information on how to understand and conceptualize auditory hallucinations (e.g., Morrison, 2002; Wright, Kingdon, Turkington, & Basco, 2008). Over a 2-week period, Clarissa reads relevant sections of these books until she understands the theory and clinical methods commonly used. She is able to attain this knowledge fairly quickly because Clarissa realizes as she reads these books that the CBT competencies she has developed in treating depressed clients are exactly the same skills employed by therapists in the psychosis treatment manuals. Thus, as often occurs once someone reaches an intermediate level of knowledge and competency, Clarissa's new learning builds on existing skills.

Next, Clarissa asks a colleague who works with clients with psychosis to meet with her to role-play conceptualization of auditory hallucinations. This colleague is not a CBT therapist, but he is very knowledgeable about psychosis, so Clarissa thinks he can give her helpful and realistic feedback on how clients might respond to her collaborative empirical style. She records this interview so she can listen to it later. During her review of the recording, she first makes note of what she does well. As is typical for her, she observes that she collaborates well and makes good use of guided discovery in the interview. Next she searches for areas that need improvement. Although she stumbles a bit in some sections of the role play, Clarissa thinks she has done a fairly good job of conceptualizing the "client's" voices and she believes she merits at least a 3 on the 5-point rating scale. This self-assessment matches the feedback from her colleague. Therefore she decides she is ready to accept a client with auditory hallucinations into her caseload.

Given that there are more aspects to psychosis than hearing voices, Clarissa asks another CBT therapist to consult with her while she treats this first client. From her reading, she has a reasonable understanding of the treatment foci in working with psychosis. She also has an appropriate level of CBT competence from her long-standing work with depression and anxiety to undertake this new type of therapy application. She meets with her consultant every other week to review portions of her recorded therapy sessions. Her consultant offers Clarissa valuable feedback, such as noting when Clarissa misses nonverbal indications that the client may be hearing voices in session.

Clarissa also regularly reflects on her therapy with this new client.

After one session she realized she was so keen to conceptualize her client's voices that she was pushing the client to do this even when he clearly stated he wanted to discuss pressing problems with his roommate. Once she recognized this break in collaboration, she put her learning goal in the background until a more appropriate time. When she and the client finally were able to conceptualize his voices, she was pleased that she was able to incorporate one of his metaphors into the conceptualization. The client told her he believed the model they developed fit his experiences 75%, which Clarissa thought was a strong endorsement.

By using these various learning methods, Clarissa was able to achieve all three of her learning goals over a 15-week period. Although she was by no means expert in working with clients who heard voices, she felt more confident that she could, with occasional consultation, work with these clients. Given that her clinic experienced a shortage of clinicians who had experience working with psychosis, her new knowledge and skills benefited many clients.

Processes for Learning Levels of Conceptualization

Review of the relevant chapters in this book is a first step toward strengthening competency in levels of conceptualization. Descriptive (Chapter 5), cross-sectional (Chapter 6), and longitudinal (Chapter 7) conceptualizations are each illustrated in detail. In addition, there is a succinct summary of the generic cognitive model (Chapter 1) and references, which are good starting points for learning the theory and relevant research regarding common presenting issues (Box 1.3).

In addition, therapists of all levels can benefit from reading other texts on case conceptualization and attending classes or workshops on this topic. Many CBT journals include case reports that can be read as case conceptualization samples. Most journal articles, whether clinical or empirical in focus, provide succinct summaries of cognitive theory and research regarding particular client issues. Thus therapists of all levels are encouraged to subscribe to CBT journals and read one or more articles per month to stay updated on new theory and research that can inform each level of conceptualization.

Appendix 8.2 suggests a variety of learning exercises that help promote clinical expertise in levels of conceptualization for therapists at novice, intermediate, and advanced levels of clinical expertise. For example, observations of expert clinical demonstrations (live or recorded) often help clarify how particular conceptualization tasks at each level appear in actual practice. Novice therapists can watch these demonstrations to learn the fundamental skills. Intermediate therapists can try to identify what client information is sought and what important information is missed in these demonstrations. Advanced therapists can consider when and why particular client information is or isn't useful at particular points in the therapy. Peer groups can view clinical demonstrations of case conceptualization and discuss what happens in terms of a "levels of conceptualization" framework.

Procedural knowledge regarding levels of conceptualization includes (1) learning how to co-construct each level with the client and, also, (2) acquiring the clinical wisdom (intuition informed by clinical experience and evidence-based research) to choose which level may be best at a particular point in therapy. The first skill set can be attained with repeated practice and supervision. The second skill set is of a higher order and benefits from clinical experience as well as solid knowledge of empirical developments in CBT. Thus novice and intermediate therapists develop and improve skills required to co-construct each level of conceptualization. Therapists with advanced skill develop clinical wisdom as to how to be most efficient in applying these skills.

Provision of a more structured format for conceptualizations improves the quality of conceptualizations, at least for novice and intermediate therapists (Kuyken, Fothergill, et al., 2005; Eells et al., 2005). In this text we provide a step-by-step structured format for each level of conceptualization, from the descriptive conceptualizations (Chapter 5) to CBT models that help therapists and clients make theory-driven inferences about underlying beliefs and strategies (Chapters 1 and 7).

Research summarized in Chapter 2 suggests that the reliability and quality of CBT conceptualizations deteriorate as therapists move to more inferential levels (Kuyken, Fothergill, et al., 2005). To avoid this decay in quality of conceptualization, therapists need commensurately greater declarative knowledge, procedural skills, and reflective capacity as they move to higher levels of conceptualization.

Processes for Learning Incorporation of Client Strengths

Therapists novice in strengths-focused therapy are encouraged to review Chapter 4 and the sections of Chapters 5 through 7 that discuss the importance of including client strengths in case conceptualization. To learn more about strengths, therapists can read books and journal articles in the fields of positive psychology (cf. Snyder & Lopez, 2005), the psychology of strengths (cf. Aspinwall & Staudinger, 2002), and resilience (cf. Davis, 1999). These are rapidly developing fields, and therapists are encouraged to attend conferences that include these perspectives. In addition, some CBT workshop instructors frequently incorporate client strengths into treatment approaches and clinical demonstrations. Workshop brochures are likely to highlight whether this is the case.

Appendix 8.3 provides a variety of exercises that can help develop competencies necessary to incorporate strengths into case conceptualizations. For example, therapists can practice identifying client strengths while viewing clinical demonstrations. When a therapist explicitly searches for strengths in a demonstration, viewers can notice what therapist nonverbal behavior, questions, and statements facilitate or hinder this goal. Even when a demonstration therapist does not search for strengths, viewers can practice looking for strengths and discuss how bringing these into client and therapist awareness might or might not be therapeutic.

Novice CBT therapists often struggle to balance all the elements of case conceptualization—collaborative empiricism, levels of conceptualization, and incorporation of client strengths—while also learning micro and macro interviewing and conceptualization skills. For them, it is helpful to practice searching for client strengths as the main goal of a role play. When first learning an approach, it is easier to practice skills that are pared down to their essence. Therapists who are more intermediate in CBT case conceptualization and yet who rarely incorporate client strengths can add a strengths focus to existing conceptualization skills. Those who are more advanced in their CBT conceptualization skills can challenge themselves to search for unidentified strengths, incorporate strengths into case conceptualizations on a regular basis, and consider with their clients how existing strengths can assist progress toward therapy goals.

Client strengths can be incorporated into every level of case conceptualization. Initially, therapists may learn to do this as an "add-on," listing strengths parallel to a problem-focused conceptualization. At an intermediate skill level, therapists begin to incorporate strengths within case conceptualizations as illustrated in Chapters 4 through 7 of this text. Advanced skill in this area is evident when cognitive therapists are equally attuned to strengths and difficulties throughout each stage of therapy, recognizing that a strengths awareness often reveals an easier path to positive therapy outcomes. Thus therapist learning begins as a skill in searching for strengths, gradually evolves into a skill of integrating strengths and difficulties, and ultimately progresses to become a holistic perspective on understanding human functioning.

Therapists who look for client strengths in every session find it much easier to incorporate strengths into case conceptualizations. Novice CBT therapists can practice different ways of asking about strengths and also practice looking for unspoken strengths. Prototypical questions are listed in Chapters 4, 6, and 7. For example, one therapist noted that an extremely depressed woman came to each therapy session nicely dressed with coordinating accessories. One session the therapist commented that it must be difficult to dress so well when she felt so depressed. The client stated that she believed it was important to dress well no matter what her mood and revealed that she actually made all her own clothing because she was living on a limited income. In this brief interchange, this therapist learned that the client's fashionable dress revealed multifaceted strengths. She possessed special expertise in design, color, imagination, as well as sewing and fiscal management. Identification of these strengths led to fruitful incorporation of these skills as well as fashion metaphors into subsequent case conceptualizations.

Typically clients are not aware of all their strengths and thus may not readily report them to the therapist. Thus therapists can practice active searches for client strengths using observation and inference. Observation involves noticing things about the client and client activities that reflect strengths. The example above regarding the depressed woman who arrived at sessions impeccably dressed is an illustration of therapist observation followed by a search for client strengths. Searching by inference means considering the client's life and activities while imagining what strengths might be embedded in the fabric of that life story. For example, a client with low income who cares for five children must have a variety of strengths in order to house and feed her family. Therapists are encouraged to use guided discovery methods (Padesky, 1993; Padesky & Greenberger, 1995) to boost client recognition of these silent strengths.

Therapists are often attuned to strengths in certain areas, such as problem-solving or emotion-management skills, and relatively blind to strengths in other areas of a client's life. For example, many therapists do not assess religious or spiritual faith issues, even though these areas may be a powerful source of strength for clients. Thus it is helpful for therapists to identify blind spots regarding client strengths. Ask:

- "What areas of strength am I most likely to overlook?" (e.g., cognitive, moral, emotional, social, spiritual, physical, behavioral)
- "What domains of a client's life do I most often neglect in interviews?" (e.g., work, family, friends, hobbies, sports, music, volunteer activities, intellectual interests, media involvement)

Fostering an awareness of the rich diversity of clients' lives outside their presenting issues is a necessary learning step toward incorporating strengths into case conceptualizations.

Even therapists who are dedicated to identifying client strengths and incorporating these into case conceptualizations sometimes skip doing this with particular clients. It can help to do a caseload review to identify any clients for whom only a few strengths have been identified. Consider how you might search for additional strengths with these clients. Questions listed in Chapter 4 can serve as a guide. It also may be relevant to reflect on whether you hold any beliefs that interfere with a search for strengths within particular client types. For example, one therapist confided in consultation that he did not think people who had been on social service support for more than 6 months were motivated to participate in CBT or any other therapy that required effort. He thought these clients were "lazy and unmotivated." He had not done a strengths review with any of these clients on his caseload. Although this example is extreme, therapists sometimes hold "low-expectation" beliefs regarding clients with particular diagnoses or of certain ages or cultural groups. Therapists who hold low expectations for clients are less likely to wholeheartedly search for strengths.

This is not to say that all clients have an equal number of strengths. Some clients have fewer strengths; others have strengths that are barely developed. Therapists can reflect on whether they take a different therapeutic stance toward clients with varying degrees of strength. Some therapists are more engaged with clients who are perceived as more vulnerable and possessing fewer strengths. Others work harder with multistrength clients who more easily tackle therapy tasks. Consider whether any differences in therapeutic stance make sense in light of the case conceptualizations for these clients or whether they merely reflect therapist bias. Also reflect on how what you do with these different types of clients might promote or inhibit further strengths development.

When therapist reflective learning processes focus on client and therapist strengths, new dimensions of understanding often result. For example, most therapists initially dread listening to themselves on therapy session recordings. This reluctance increases when therapists find they have a keener ear for "errors" and "omissions" than they do for strengths. The following example from a training course illustrates this point.

John: A Reluctant Review

John took a weeklong training course for intermediate CBT therapists and hoped to receive feedback on his therapy skills. On the second day of the course, he approached the instructor, who suggested he bring to class the next day a 10-minute segment from one of his recorded therapy sessions for which he had client permission to do so. The class would listen and offer feedback. In addition, the instructor told John to write down two or three specific questions regarding areas in which he wanted feedback. The following day, John told the instructor he had changed his mind about playing the recording. John had listened to it the night before and concluded it was just too horrible an example to play in front of the group. The instructor listened to John's self-disparaging comments and then gave John an assignment to listen to the recording again that evening. While he listened, John was asked to make a list of everything he noticed that he did well as a therapist in those 10 minutes.

John returned to class the following day with his recording. Before John played the recording, the instructor asked him to tell the group the positive things he had written down the night before. John read an extensive list of positive comments about his therapy. He commented with a shy smile, "You know, this session was much improved over when I first listened to it." Then he played the recording and asked for feedback regarding his consultation questions. Many hands shot into the air as classmates vied to give John feedback. However, the instructor suggested that John first try to answer his own questions drawing on what he had been learning in the course that week. Classmates could then fill in the points that John missed. After a pause John began to talk about therapy principles that could help him with his case dilemmas. He also noted areas where he had not used his therapy skills to full advantage and suggested things he might do differently when he next saw this client. The instructor asked John's classmates for their additional ideas. Not a single person spoke other than one woman who commented that John had made an excellent summary of the week's learning.

As this example shows, it is just as important for therapists to notice and reflect on their own strengths as it is for clients to do so. When John listened to his recording searching for what was wrong, he concluded it was a terrible therapy session. When he listened the next evening searching for what was right (i.e., his strengths), the same session seemed quite good to him. Any therapy session can be improved, but if therapists only listen and watch for problems in their recordings, many sessions will appear as abysmal as John's session initially seemed to him.

Therapists are encouraged to develop a reflective learning habit of observing strengths and positive qualities first, whether they are offering or receiving consultation. When strengths and positive qualities are acknowledged, it is easier to be open and receptive to new learning as well as to apply knowledge one already possesses. Rather than accept this statement at face value, readers of this book are encouraged to do the following reflective exercise:

1. Make a session recording and choose 10 minutes of it for review.
2. Listen to the recording with the intention of noticing every flaw, weakness, and error. Imagine how a more skilled therapist might sound in this same session.
3. Listen to the recording a second time and write down anything you do well as a therapist. Notice relationship factors ("Am I

genuine? Warm?"), general therapy skills ("Am I listening accurately? Is the pacing appropriate to the client?"), CBT skills ("Am I following the agenda? Noticing important thoughts, feelings, and behaviors?"), and case conceptualization skills ("Am I collaborating? Are we using a level of conceptualization appropriate to the client at this point in the therapy? Did I notice or acknowledge any client strengths?")

4. Reflect on what you learn from this experiment; write this down.
5. How can you use what you learned to improve your future learning prospects, whether self-directed or in consultation with another therapist?

Another reflective exercise therapists can do is to conceptualize a personal issue and identify their own strengths and integrate these within the conceptualization. Paulina is an intermediate-level CBT therapist who has had a chronic tendency to let sessions go over time. This is a problem because she has other clinical tasks that need to be done between appointments. When sessions run late her entire schedule starts to run late, and she does not have time to make telephone calls and write her case notes between sessions. She ends up working an extra hour or more each evening as a result of her chronic lateness. Paulina observes herself in her sessions for a week and notices several common triggers for running late: intense client emotion, her own dissatisfaction with a session's progress, and starting a therapy session late. In these circumstances, she identifies the following underlying assumptions as ones maintaining her chronic lateness:

"If a client is in distress, then I should continue the session until she feels better; otherwise therapy is counterproductive."
"If I have not accomplished as much as is ideal, then I should meet a bit longer with the client until they get their money's worth."
"If my clients think I operate according to the clock, they will think I don't care for them."
"If I start a session late and then end it on time, then the client will get the impression that he is less important to me than my previous client."

Next Paulina identifies her strengths. She characterizes herself as someone who:

- Genuinely cares for clients.
- Has excellent interpersonal skills, especially empathy and communication.

- Collaborates well with clients.
- Uses empirical methods such as behavioral experiments in session.

Paulina decides to see how her strengths might help her deal more effectively with session timeliness. She knows that underlying assumptions are usually evaluated using behavioral experiments. Construction of behavioral experiments is one of her strengths. Therefore Paulina decides to construct behavioral experiments to test her underlying assumptions. After some consideration she decides her third underlying assumption, that clients will interpret ending on time as not caring for them, is central to her difficulties. Pauline reviews her strengths one more time to see how these might guide her experiments. Looking simultaneously at her problems, assumptions, and strengths, it occurs to Paulina that this problem can be addressed collaboratively with her clients by employing good communication and empathy to set up behavioral experiments and get feedback.

The next week Paulina selects five clients with whom she has a good therapy alliance. She plans to do an experiment in their sessions which begins with saying the following to them at the beginning of the session:

"You may have noticed that I have had a history of running late in my sessions. Sometimes we start late, other times we end late. This is not really good for me, and I imagine it may not be good for you. Do you have any thoughts or feelings about this? (*At this point, Paulina will listen to the client's feedback and process any reactions he or she has to her observation. If it is relevant to the client's concerns, Paulina will give more details about why running late is not good for her and how the minutes between appointments are spent writing notes, reviewing notes for the next session, etc.*) Starting this week, I have a goal to keep my appointments on schedule. This means I will be looking at my watch or the clock on the wall more than usual. I also may remind you when we have just 15 minutes left so you and I can make sure we target the most important information in the final minutes before our session is over. How do you think this will be for you? (*Paulina will discuss any client reactions and enlist their collaboration with her.*) At the end of the session, I'll check and see how this worked out for you."

It is obvious how Paulina is drawing on her strengths. She decides to communicate openly with her clients about her experiment, with an empathic recognition that her change may have an impact on them. She maintains a therapeutic focus by seeking client reactions, collaboratively exploring any meanings this change may hold for the clients, and promising to get feedback from them at the end of their sessions. She may even call this a behavioral experiment when speaking with clients who are familiar with this terminology. It may encourage her clients to know she uses the same methods to work on her own issues as she uses with them.

A final area of learning regarding incorporation of client strengths pertains to client and therapist values. Most therapists experience empathy for many different types of client distress. However, a therapist's values can sometimes impede appreciation of the client's strengths. Consider the following consultation interchange.

Edward: A Case Example in Values

Edward is a very religious man who suffers with OCD in which he experiences intrusive thoughts that conflict with his faith. This leads him to avoid church attendance. Instead, Edward prays many hours each day, yet he still feels distant from God. His main concern is that he is not the person he thinks he should be. Edward's therapist discusses this issue with her supervisor.

SUPERVISOR: Update me on the work you are doing with Edward.

THERAPIST: I am getting a bit stuck, actually. He is feeling better, less bothered by the unwanted thoughts. He is actually praying less, which is good because he was praying primarily to show he was a good person, and he has gone back to attending church. Last session we reviewed his goals and he said his goal is to be closer to God. This is really difficult for me because I do not believe in God, so I think I am not the right person to help him with this goal.

SUPERVISOR: That sounds important to address today. Would you like to talk about this?

THERAPIST: I would like that, if you think it would help. I am really stuck.

SUPERVISOR: Can you put it into words what you mean by "stuck"?

THERAPIST: Well, because I don't believe, I feel uneasy about helping someone work toward being closer to God. It does not seem like it is my business, really.

SUPERVISOR: How do you think Edward would feel if he was closer to God?

THERAPIST: I think he would feel better and his life would be more fulfilling. He really values his faith and his church community.

SUPERVISOR: So if he felt better, his life was more fulfilling, and he felt closer to God, how would you feel about Edward's future?

THERAPIST: Better, I suppose.

SUPERVISOR: Have you helped people work toward goals where they are trying to improve their social networks or feel better about themselves before?

THERAPIST: Well ... I often help people get to the gym, or try and meet people socially.

SUPERVISOR: OK, so if he wanted to go to the gym or make close friends how would that be different from what Edward wants—to get closer to God?

THERAPIST: I don't know, really. It does feel different to me. Yet I don't go to a gym, and that doesn't stop me from encouraging clients who want to. I guess my own feelings about religion are getting in the way. (*Looks thoughtful.*) When I think about it, it doesn't matter what I think about God. If it is something Edward feels is important, I should be working toward helping him achieve it. I could recommend he use his church resources to figure out how to get closer to God, just like I would recommend someone talk to people about gyms in their area.

SUPERVISOR: So how stuck do you feel now in terms of your work with Edward?

THERAPIST: Much less. I think if I separate my values from his I'll have a much easier time supporting his goal.

Therapists are encouraged to reflect on how their own values can enhance or impede therapy progress, especially when these values diverge from client values.

Step 4: Evaluate Learning Progress to Determine Further Learning Needs

The same methods can be used to evaluate learning progress whether goals have been set in the area of collaborative empiricism, levels of conceptualization, incorporation of client strengths, or some combination of these principles. Just as Clarissa did earlier in this chapter, therapists can rate progress on goals for learning via self-appraisal as well as feedback from clients, colleagues, a supervisor, or a consultant. Recall that Clarissa rated her performance conceptualizing auditory hallucinations in a recorded interview a 3 on a 5-point scale, and this rating matched that given her by her role-play colleague. Subsequent client feedback indicated that a collaborative conceptualization of "voices" rated a 75% fit with the client's experience. In Clarissa's view, as well as that of a knowledgeable therapist with whom she consulted, she successfully met her initial learning goals in the area of conceptualizing "voices."

Therapists are encouraged to rate their learning progress on a regular basis, at least every few weeks. Progress and success can be self-determined. For example, even an awkward attempt to use functional analysis that leads to an ABC model might be rated "success" by a novice therapist. An intermediate therapist might only rate such an intervention as successful if it was collaboratively derived and yielded a model that the client endorsed as a "good fit" to the presenting issue. Comparison of ratings over time allows therapists to see their progress in acquiring conceptualization skills. If learning is not progressing as expected then additional learning modalities can be considered. For example, a therapist might initially plan to learn more about cross-sectional conceptualization through self-study involving reading and review of session recordings. If self-study does not lead to the desired progress, this therapist may decide to seek consultation to get help in developing this skill.

It can help to set "target dates" to provide motivation for integrating new skills into clinical practice. In addition, periodic review dates remind the therapist to revisit learning priorities and reset learning goals as necessary. Therapists who set periodic learning goals and use the learning methods outlined in the previous sections will begin to master component skills of case conceptualization. In the end, however, facility with component skills is not sufficient.

Therapists will want to seamlessly integrate collaboration, empiricism, and incorporation of client strengths within each level of conceptualization and move fluidly among these levels as therapy requires. Fortunately, it is not necessary to reach an advanced level of skill in each area before such integration can occur. Even novice therapists integrate skills that they acquire, often without even being aware of it. For example, a therapist who wants to collaboratively co-construct a conceptual model needs to know at least one descriptive conceptualization model in order to begin practicing this task.

Optimal learning requires both a focus on the development of specific skills and reflection on how best to implement these skills within a given therapy context with a particular client. For this reason we recommend that therapists continue over their career to read, attend workshops, and practice component skills outside therapy sessions. Component practice can occur in role plays and by analyzing session recordings with peers or a supervisor. Once moderately fluent with several individual skills, therapists can practice role plays that mimic actual therapy situations, combining skills such as collaborative empiricism within one of the levels of conceptualization. Additional knowledge and competencies can be targeted for improvement over time. We recommend that therapists work on areas initially in isolation using the four-step model described in this chapter and then integrate new learning with other skills in one's clinical practice.

EVALUATING OVERALL CONCEPTUALIZATION COMPETENCY

In order to evaluate one's overall CBT competencies in case conceptualization, therapists may want to use a standardized measure of competence instead of or in addition to self-defined ratings. There are a number of options. The most widely used general measure of CBT therapist competence is the Cognitive Therapy Rating Scale (Barber, Liese, & Abrams, 2003), which assesses several domains of competence relevant to CBT case conceptualization, most notably the principles of collaboration and empiricism and many relevant micro skills such as structuring therapy. It also explicitly assesses therapists' theoretical understanding. Therapists and supervisors can use the scale as they listen to therapy session recordings and consider therapist strengths and targets for learning. A number of formal measures of the quality of case conceptualizations have been developed (Eells et al., 2005; Kuyken, Fothergill, et al., 2005). Although these were primarily developed for research purposes they offer a starting point for evaluating what makes a high-quality case conceptualization.

Along with research criteria, therapists can use self-assessment checklists to set goals for self-study, consultation, and supervision. For example, Butler (1998) offers 10 tests of a formulation that could be rated. Therapists, supervisors, and instructors can also consider the general criteria in Box 8.5 to evaluate particular conceptualizations. These criteria tap higher-order concepts for evaluating case conceptualizations such as comprehensiveness and coherence. They suggest that high-quality conceptualizations balance a number of inherent tensions. For example, conceptualizations strive to combine theory and client experience in a way that is coherent and meaningful to the client. Ideally, a conceptualization is as simple as possible without losing important meaning. Conceptualizations should also fit with all the available data. Inferences are best if developed collaboratively with clients and if they make sense to therapist, client, and consulting therapists.

PROMOTING LEARNING THROUGH SUPERVISION
AND CONSULTATION

Supervision and consultation are valuable opportunities to reflect on strengths and identify the boundaries of therapist skill and knowledge

---

Box 8.5. Criteria for Judging the Quality of Case Conceptualizations

To consider the quality of a case conceptualization, ask whether it is:

- **Comprehensive:** Does it cover the key issues? Is important relevant information included and irrelevant information excluded?
- **Parsimonious:** Is it as simple as possible without loss of important information, meaning, or treatment utility?
- **Coherent:** Are the elements linked together well? Do they make overall sense of the individual's presenting issues?
- **Precisely worded:** Is the language exact, specific, and sufficiently thorough with regard to what is meaningful to the client and to relevant theory?
- **Meaningful to the client:** Does the case conceptualization resonate fully with the client?

(Falender & Shafranske, 2004). Novice and intermediate therapists are often in supervision while they are learning CBT. All licensed therapists, including advanced-level CBT therapists, can benefit from consultation on particular cases. Most readers of this book participate in consultation or supervision either as a learning therapist or as a consultant/supervisor. Therefore we briefly address how the learning principles discussed in this chapter apply to these relationships. Consider the following supervision excerpt, in which a novice therapist and his supervisor assess knowledge and skill regarding conceptualization of a new case:

THERAPIST: I'm not sure what is going on with this client.

SUPERVISOR: What ideas do you have so far?

THERAPIST: This client is certainly very anxious. I think she might have social anxiety because her anxiety started after she had an embarrassing episode when she had to give a report at work. But she also has panic attacks, so maybe she has panic disorder. I'm not sure.

SUPERVISOR: Have you studied social anxiety and the other anxiety disorders very much?

THERAPIST: Not really. I attended a workshop that taught us basic principles and I've looked in my books to review diagnostic criteria, but most of my CBT clinical experience so far has been with depression. Actually, if it is social anxiety I'm not really sure what to do to help her.

SUPERVISOR: Based on what you said so far, social anxiety is a possible diagnosis. People with social anxiety can have panic attacks. Panic attacks do not necessarily mean panic disorder. However, it is also possible she has social anxiety and panic disorder. Let me take some of our time today to give you a primer on anxiety assessment and treatment. I'm also going to recommend some readings for you to do this week. Is that OK with you?

THERAPIST: (*Appears relieved.*) Sure.

SUPERVISOR: Let's start with a review of diagnostic differences among anxiety disorders, because your conceptualization and treatment will vary depending on the type of anxiety she is experiencing. Then we can explore what information you need to gather in the next session to help decide her diagnosis. We'll also review conceptualizations for several likely anxiety disorders so you have some idea where you may be headed with this client.

THERAPIST: Thanks. I do feel really lost with what to do next.

In this particular supervision session, the supervisor discovers that the therapist lacks basic empirical knowledge regarding anxiety disorder diagnosis and treatment. Without this knowledge, case conceptualization is difficult, if not impossible. Thus the focus of supervision begins with helping the therapist accumulate this knowledge via didactic instruction and reading. Later in this same session, the supervisor shifts to developing basic procedural skills in the use of this knowledge. The supervisor and therapist set up a role play to rehearse new skills, and the supervisor agrees to role-play the client:

THERAPIST: Tell me, Margaret, what goes through your mind when you are having a panic attack?

SUPERVISOR: Let's stop for a minute. Remember, part of a establishing a good therapy alliance and enlisting collaboration is to give the client a rationale for why you are asking certain questions.

THERAPIST: Oh, right!

SUPERVISOR: Think what rationale you might give Margaret and let's begin again.

THERAPIST: (*Thoughtful pause while checking notes.*) Margaret, when we met last time you told me about the anxiety and panic you have been experiencing. Before I can know the best way to help you, I need to ask you some more questions so you and I know in a bit more detail what this anxiety is about. Would that be OK with you?

SUPERVISOR: Before I answer as Margaret and we continue this role play, what do you think about that rationale? How did you feel giving it?

THERAPIST: Actually, that felt much better. The rationale would probably help her and it also will probably help me feel a bit more comfortable asking the questions.

More advanced therapists who are in consultation often take a lead in structuring the consultation session. They identify learning goals, ask specific consultation questions, and discuss issues with greater knowledge and expertise. The following excerpt illustrates a consultation session with an advanced therapist:

THERAPIST: So my consultation question is "How can I get to a conceptualization with Elizabeth that is as simple as possible?" She has a lot going on, and I have a tendency to overcomplicate things. I really want to develop a skill of forming simpler conceptualizations.

CONSULTANT: That's a great question. First, what's your sense of why you want to keep things simple?

THERAPIST: (*Thinks about this for a while.*) I guess it will help us focus. Simple models are easier to understand, remember, test, and apply in everyday situations. Also, Elizabeth has borderline personality disorder and tends to get highly emotional. A simple conceptualization will be easier for her to remember when she is emotionally aroused.

CONSULTANT: Yes, I agree. Are there any risks in trying to develop a simple conceptualization?

THERAPIST: She's very bright, and I don't want her to think I am patronizing her. I also don't want to miss any crucial information that is important to helping us reach her goals. But she and I work well together, so I think if we check the fit of the conceptualization it will be all right.

CONSULTANT: Good, so collaboration and checking on your conceptualization's fit are strengths you have.

THERAPIST: (*lightheartedly*) Yes, I guess so. You know me—I have the opposite of a self-serving bias and focus more on what I need to develop than what I am already good at. (*Consultant nods and laughs.*) But yes, that's right. These are strengths of mine.

CONSULTANT: So, thinking about your consultation question, can you think about cases you've worked with before where quite simple conceptualizations have managed to capture the richness of clients' presenting issues?

THERAPIST: Yes, loads.

CONSULTANT: What did these conceptualizations have in common?

THERAPIST: (*Thinks for a moment and then laughs.*) Bad pictures. No, seriously, where we developed a picture or image not only of the problem but also of what the clients wanted, their biggest dreams.

This advanced-level therapist is aware of her strengths (working collaboratively, checking a conceptualization's fit) and her weaknesses (overcomplicating conceptualizations). When she reflects on previous therapy experiences that have gone well she is able to extrapolate useful principles to keep her on track with pursuing a simpler conceptualization with Elizabeth. Notice that the consultant trusts this therapist's knowledge and strengths and uses guided discovery more than didactic teaching.

RECOMMENDATIONS FOR SUPERVISORS AND INSTRUCTORS

Readers who are CBT supervisors and instructors can use guidelines in this chapter as well as the learning exercises in Appendices 8.1, 8.2, and 8.3 to tailor programs for all therapist skill levels. Classes or supervision for graduate students will generally follow the guidelines offered for novice therapists. Postgraduate teaching and supervision can implement exercises described for either novice, intermediate, or advanced therapists depending on the individual or group skill level. Keep in mind that highly experienced therapists who are relatively new to CBT may need to start at the novice level of learning case conceptualization despite years of clinical practice. Therapists benefit from novice-level training until they accumulate empirical knowledge regarding CBT theory and research, develop skills of collaborative empiricism, and learn specific CBT methods for each level of conceptualization.

Sometimes postgraduate instructors teach workshops or seminars to groups that include therapists who range from novice to advanced skill and knowledge. Construction of learning exercises in mixed-skill-level groups is more challenging than teaching groups with more homogeneous levels of competency. In this instance, learning exercises such as role plays need to be constructed to offer learning benefit to all skill levels. Exercises can be designed with enough structure that novice therapists can complete the task and yet include enough complexity to challenge the more advanced therapists in attendance.

An example of such an exercise would be to create a very specific client case description that outlines the presenting issues list along with specific guidelines for the person role-playing the client. Beginning therapist teams could be assigned to complete an ABC functional analysis

with this client for a particular issue. At the same time, advanced therapists could be asked to complete a functional analysis for two separate
situations and look for common themes. Therapists attending the course
can be encouraged to work with therapists of similar skill level so that
reflective learning discussions after the role plays are at a level that will
benefit all members of the role-play team.

Therapists and supervisors may want to use this text as part of a
learning curriculum. If so, we recommend that chapter reading assignments be linked to active learning tasks as described in this chapter.
For example, Chapter 3 can be paired with practice of skills related to
collaboration (e.g., setting agendas, giving rationales for interventions,
asking clients to identify and rate the impact of presenting issues) or
empiricism (e.g., use of Socratic dialogue, setting up behavioral experiments), and Chapter 4 to incorporation of client strengths (e.g., practice
of questions that help clients identify strengths). Skills practice can be
self-reflective (e.g., searching for strengths within oneself), procedural
(e.g., role-play practice), and declarative (e.g., class observation of a
DVD recording of an expert therapist with discussion to identify good
practice principles). The didactic learning that comes from reading a
book is greatly enhanced when paired with active learning practice.

When this text is used in supervision, supervisees can be assigned to
read the entire book (paired with practice assignments in supervision and
therapy sessions) or particular sections that pertain to assessed learning
needs. For example, a supervisor might assign Chapter 5 to a supervisee
who would benefit from examples of how to collaboratively develop a list
of presenting issues and guide a client to make impact and priority ratings. References throughout this text alert supervisors to supplementary
readings that can enhance supervisor and supervisee knowledge.

Beliefs and Biases in Teaching and Supervision

Therapists who are learning case conceptualization, as well as supervisors and instructors who are teaching it, are subject to the same heuristic thinking errors and biases that were described in Chapter 2. These
beliefs and biases can create roadblocks to learning and teaching CBT
case conceptualization. In addition, professionals sometimes hold specific underlying assumptions that can interfere with the practice, teaching, or learning of case conceptualization as we describe it in this text.
Consider the following beliefs:

> "If my client is relatively low functioning then he or she won't be
> able to participate in case conceptualization. It is best if I do it
> for my client."

"If a therapist whom I am supervising/teaching does not have a good understanding of fundamental therapy processes, then he or she can't even begin to learn case conceptualization."

"CBT has successful treatment protocols, but when it comes to case conceptualization, psychodynamic theories get more to the root of problems."

"As long as *I* understand what is going on, I can begin to treat my client; it is not necessary for him or her to participate in case conceptualization."

"If my supervisees do not understand case conceptualization, then it is better to simply teach them to diagnose and then give them an empirically supported conceptual model for each diagnosis."

"It is impossible to teach case conceptualization. With experience, each therapist will naturally learn to do it."

Reflective practice helps us identify beliefs such as these and actively examine them. It is best not to lightly dismiss such beliefs. Instead, these beliefs can be empirically examined just as we test client beliefs. Therapists, instructors, and supervisors are encouraged to identify such beliefs and devise behavioral experiments to test them. For example, a therapist who believes client participation in case conceptualization is unimportant or impossible can conduct an experiment in which a conceptualization is constructed with client collaboration. Prior to this experiment, the therapist should make predictions (based on his or her beliefs) of what the outcomes will be. Once the experiment is done, client and consultant feedback can be obtained and therapist predictions compared with actual outcomes. Feedback from clients and a consultant reduce the likelihood of a biased interpretation of outcomes. Similarly, instructors, supervisors, and consultants can strive to be aware of their own biases and test these out with behavioral experiments by obtaining feedback from students, supervisees, and peers.

CONCLUSION

We opened this chapter with comments by therapists at three different skill levels reacting to the case of Mark in previous chapters. Each therapist expressed a different learning need. Regardless of skill level, development as a CBT therapist requires having a sense of what knowledge and competencies we already possess and what knowledge and skills we want to acquire. Self-reflection is crucial in the assessment of competency. This chapter is designed to help therapists identify learning needs, organize learning goals, and track progress in acquiring the knowledge and skills required by our three case conceptualization principles. Therapists are encouraged to conduct an ongoing appraisal of strengths and their current limitations in knowledge and skills.

Improving competency in case conceptualization can be a career-long process. And yet even in its early stages this learning incorporates rich rewards in terms of the quality of therapy one can offer. As knowledge and skills are added and strengthened, therapists can enjoy the many benefits of interactions among competencies. Therapists who adopt a learning focus in their own practice also gain a deeper understanding of CBT theory, empirical processes, and the processes of personal curiosity and discovery that lie at CBT's core. Whether you are novice, intermediate, or advanced in conceptualization competencies, this chapter can guide your learning and development to the next level of expertise.

Chapter 8 Summary

- Bennett-Levy (2006) describes three related learning processes (declarative, procedural, and reflective) that guide therapists in learning CBT.
- We incorporate Bennett-Levy's model into a four-stage learning cycle for learning and teaching case conceptualization:
  —Assess learning needs.
  —Set personal learning goals.
  —Participate in declarative, procedural, and reflective learning processes.
  —Evaluate learning progress to determine additional learning needs.
- To assess learning needs, therapists are encouraged to rate their knowledge and competencies in areas linked to the three principles of collaborative case conceptualization: collaborative empiricism, levels of conceptualization, and incorporation of client strengths.
- Personal learning goals should be specific, observable, and measurable, as well as prioritized to tackle one or two at a time so learning is not overwhelming.
- It is helpful to set moderate learning goals that can be achieved in a few months' time.
- Exercises that rely on various learning modalities (e.g., reading, role play, feedback on session recordings) are described for therapists at each skill level, from novice to advanced.
- Self-ratings; client, supervisor, and consultant feedback; as well as standardized measures are used to evaluate learning progress.
- Therapists are encouraged to incorporate reflective practice, including case conceptualization with oneself, to boost ongoing awareness of strengths and learning needs.

Learning Exercises to Develop Competence in Collaborative Empiricism

NOVICE LEVEL

- Read books and journal articles, and attend workshops to learn specific CBT conceptualizations for common disorders in one's clinical practice.
- Observe written and recorded session examples to identify questions that elicit the relevant client information necessary for CBT conceptualizations.
- Observe and discuss clinical demonstrations of case conceptualization (e.g., Padesky, 1997a).
- Practice both micro skills (e.g., explain rationales for aspects of conceptualization or use objective language to make summary statements or describe a client behavior) and macro skills (e.g., use five-part model for descriptive conceptualization, help client devise a behavioral experiment).
- Practice four stages of Socratic dialogue (Padesky, 1993).
- Rehearse methods for introducing the idea of empiricism to clients.
- Work collaboratively with clients and get feedback from a supervisor or consultant on how to do this more effectively.
- Write down client observations and draw relevant links among them.

INTERMEDIATE LEVEL

- Focus on development of conceptualization skills that are relatively weaker; consider using the above novice exercises to do this.
- Note client examples that fit or contradict "standard" case conceptualizations.
- Attend to similarities and differences among models for related disorders.
- Watch recordings of expert therapists conducting case conceptualizations;

identify strategies that seem to facilitate collaboration and consider what client information they elicit as well as why this information might be important.

- Collect written examples of case conceptualization from books, journal articles, and one's own practice.
- Role-play practice of relevant skills with feedback from "client" and supervisory observer.
- Strive to maximize client participation in the conceptualization process.
- Introduce clients to empirically supported models by using client data to personalize standard models.
- Practice a variety of metaphors for explaining key CBT ideas.
- Express curiosity and elicit client curiosity regarding observations made in and outside of session that are relevant to conceptual models.
- Design behavioral experiments to gather relevant information for conceptualization.
- Participate in live or electronic case conference discussions of client presentations that deviate from standard models.

ADVANCED LEVEL

- Consider any exercise in the novice or intermediate sections above that might strengthen relatively weaker skills.
- Read books and journal articles, talk to colleagues, and attend workshops to refine one's understanding of new findings regarding empirically supported models.
- Read, consult with colleagues, or attend workshops to learn how to collaborate with clients who pose challenges to standard methods of collaboration.
- Discuss with other advanced therapists how to reconcile differences between empirically derived models and divergent client experiences.
- Study how empirical methods are used differentially with various client problems (e.g., Bennett-Levy et al., 2004).
- Practice clear communication during therapy impasses; negotiate collaborative solutions to barriers encountered during case conceptualization.
- Note client observations that contradict empirical models; highlight these observations in session for collaborative examination.
- Listen to session recordings for relevant client comments neglected by the case conceptualization.
- Obtain feedback from all clients on the utility of case conceptualizations.
- Make conceptualization-based predictions of potential problems that might occur in therapy.
- Show case conceptualization diagrams to peer therapists for feedback and discussion.
- Teach methods of collaborative empiricism to less-experienced therapists.

Learning Exercises to Develop Competence in Levels of Conceptualization

NOVICE LEVEL

- Observe clinical demonstrations, preferably by CBT instructors or experts, that show how to implement conceptualization tasks such as forming a presenting issues list, goal setting, and linking client experience to CBT theory using the five-part model or functional analysis.
- Practice these same skills via role play as both "therapist" and "client" with feedback from a knowledgeable therapist.
- Self-practice; construct descriptive or explanatory CBT conceptualizations for a personal issue such as performance anxiety or procrastination.
- Focus on descriptive conceptualizations until adept at describing a wide variety of client issues using functional analysis or the five-part model.
- Once skilled in descriptive conceptualizations, practice identifying triggers and maintenance factors.
- Practice both micro skills (e.g., identifying underlying assumptions) and macro skills (e.g., constructing conceptual models for client concerns in CBT terms).
- Bring conceptualization dilemmas to supervision or consultation for discussion and role play.

INTERMEDIATE LEVEL

- Focus on development of conceptualization skills that are relatively weaker; consider using the above novice exercises to do this.
- Role-play levels of conceptualization with multiproblem clients.
- Emphasize use of client language in conceptualization, especially incorporation of metaphors, imagery, and other symbolism.

- Practice incorporating relevant cultural factors into case conceptualizations.
- Practice testing the "fit" of conceptualizations both in and out of session through behavioral experiments and careful analysis of client experiences.

ADVANCED LEVEL

- Role-play practice with clients who tightly cling to unhelpful case conceptualizations (e.g., everyone in my family is anxious; my anxious DNA means change is not possible); practice searching for information within the client's experience that will broaden an otherwise narrow perspective.
- Actively search for themes that link client presenting issues.
- Help clients construct simple conceptualizations that account for a broad range of client experiences.
- Evaluate the "fit" of conceptualizations through active searches for contradictory evidence in the client's experience; these data can lead to meaningful personalization of existing conceptual models.
- Link descriptive, explanatory, and longitudinal conceptualizations for a client's issues in a flowchart similar to those in Figures 7.6 and 7.7 in order to discern common themes.
- Show case conceptualization diagrams to peer therapists for feedback and discussion.
- Teach case conceptualization skills to less-experienced therapists.

Learning Exercises to Develop Competence in Incorporation of Client Strengths

NOVICE LEVEL

Therapists just beginning to develop skill in incorporating client strengths into case conceptualizations are encouraged to:

- Observe clinical demonstrations and identify unspoken client strengths.
- Role-play asking questions to elicit strengths; ask for feedback.
- Practice writing strengths within or parallel to descriptive case conceptualizations (see Figure 4.1 for an example).
- Conceptualize one's own strengths using CBT models.
- Identify client strengths while observing demonstrations or listening to session recordings.

INTERMEDIATE LEVEL

As a strengths focus becomes second nature, therapists reach an intermediate level of competency in which they are encouraged to:

- Incorporate a search for client strengths within written and verbal assessment procedures.
- Observe strengths in clients and bring these strengths to the client's attention.
- Actively ask about strengths in most therapy sessions.
- Integrate identified client strengths into conceptual models.
- Help clients identify ways they can use strengths to bolster treatment interventions.

ADVANCED LEVEL

Therapists who possess advanced competence in incorporating client strengths into case conceptualization are encouraged to:

- Identify strengths for several clients and consider whether these have been optimally integrated into conceptualizations.
- Present one or two of the case analyses above to peers or a consultant to get feedback about the integration of strengths within the conceptualization.
- Actively infer strengths for new clients and use guided discovery to see if the client identifies similar or additional strengths.
- Integrate client strengths into each level of conceptualization when constructive to do so.
- Integrate identified strengths into treatment plans.

Chapter 9

Appraising the Model

Learning never ends; instead it progresses to ever deeper levels of understanding. This final chapter revisits themes introduced earlier in this book to see what new perspectives are gained through our conceptualization approach. In addition, we suggest directions for future research that can help us appraise and understand this model more deeply. Specifically, the following sections (1) review distinctive aspects of our conceptualization model, (2) discuss how the model can fulfill the functions of case conceptualization, and (3) offer suggestions for how to evaluate the model conceptually and empirically. The key tests of our model are how useful it is to therapists and clients and also how well it stands up to carefully conducted research.

KEY CHARACTERISTICS OF THE MODEL

What are the distinctive characteristics of our model and how are they helpful to CBT therapists and clients?

The Model Is a Response to Clinical and Empirical Challenges

Therapists often find case conceptualization one of the most challenging aspects of CBT (Chapter 8). The evidence base for case conceptualization provides only weak support for the assumption that conceptualization-driven therapy has advantages. At best, research suggests that we need to refine our approach to case conceptualization (Chapter 1; Bieling &

Kuyken, 2003). Our conceptualization model is a response to these clinical and empirical challenges. The model's three principles answer these challenges by explicitly addressing how case conceptualization can integrate theory and the particularities of client experience. Collaborative empiricism builds on the best available evidence and maximizes the likelihood that conceptualizations will make sense to clients. We propose that the combination of a collaborative, stepped, and strengths-focused approach makes it more likely that clients will experience conceptualization as constructive. The principles taught in this text can guide therapists' conceptualization practice to help maximize their effectiveness as therapists, consultants, supervisors, and trainers.

The Model Is Embedded in the Broader Science and Practice of CBT

Cognitive-behavioral therapy encompasses many empirically supported theories and protocols (Beck, 2005; Box 1.3). Therapists face multiple choice points with each client. Our model builds on CBT's strong foundations by providing an approach therapists can use to integrate empirically supported theory with clients' experience and strengths to inform these therapy choice points. Thus our case conceptualization approach sits firmly within the broader science and practice of CBT; it can serve as the linchpin between science and practice (Butler, 1998).

The Therapist and Client Co-Create the Conceptualization

Most contemporary CBT approaches advocate conceptualization as an activity that occurs inside the therapist's head or as an activity directed by the therapist. Our approach advocates that therapist and client co-create conceptualizations that evolve throughout therapy at a pace and in a manner determined by both client and therapist. In this way therapist and client are likely to agree on their description of the client's issues and goals. Moreover, they will have a shared understanding of what causes and maintains the presenting issues. This shared understanding provides clients with a rationale for change.

In the early phases of therapy, the therapist is heavily engaged in building and facilitating this collaborative process; as therapy progresses the client takes more and more responsibility for the cycle of conceptualization and change. In our sample case, Mark initially described his presenting issues in detail, and his therapist captured these within a descriptive CBT framework (Chapter 5). By the end of therapy Mark took the initiative in developing rich metaphors to conceptualize both his vulnerability and his growing resilience (Chapter 7). Collaborative co-creation of a conceptualization incorporates both the clients' surface and deeper presenting issues. This requires the therapist to build a high degree of trust and be sensitive to clients' subtler agendas, worries, memories, and concerns. For example, issues that arouse shame or involve discussions of sexuality may be difficult for some clients to voice.

Client Strengths Are Emphasized

From the initial assessment therapists look for client strengths that can be incorporated into conceptualizations so treatment plans can build on these strengths. In later phases of therapy strengths are heavily emphasized to help clients cope resiliently and to prevent relapse. Clients build their resilience through experiences of coping effectively with challenges and also through commitment to meaningful activities that broaden strengths. Initial attempts to draw out Mark's strengths were hampered by Mark's depression. However, by the end of therapy Mark independently articulated beliefs and strategies for coping with adversity that were summarized by his resilient image of a grizzly bear (Figure 7.5). He also resumed his dedication to music and other positive activities that enriched his life.

Therapists use the clients' own language to ensure that evolving conceptualizations are a good fit with clients' experience and sense of their own strengths. The therapist uses client words, metaphors, and images to create a sense of hope and point to pathways for change (Chapter 3). Over the course of therapy clients begin to use language in the same way. Mark described the grizzly bear in this way:

"He represents all the ways my grandfather taught me to be. He is active and figures things out and uses a lot of creativity with a 'can-do' attitude."

Conceptualization Is an Evolving Process

We do not think of conceptualization as a fixed entity that is derived and settled in the early or middle stages of therapy. Instead, we see conceptualization as a process that evolves throughout therapy. Conceptualizations are not only provisional subject to new data but they also evolve into forms that serve different functions. Initially, their functions are to describe, set the scene, and provide education and normalization. The function of cross-sectional conceptualizations is to explain presenting issues in terms of triggers and maintenance factors. These can be targeted for intervention, and clients learn alternative ways to think and behave. Longitudinal conceptualizations evolve from a developmental understanding of maintenance cycles. These conceptualizations help explain the more enduring beliefs and behaviors that leave a client vulnerable to future difficulties. In turn, longitudinal conceptualizations can guide relapse management and development of client resilience.

The Model Incorporates Clients' Cultural Contexts and Personal Values

Clients' beliefs and behaviors are inevitably shaped by their cultural contexts. CBT therapists incorporate clients' cultural contexts and personal values into conceptualizations because these are an integral part of clients' beliefs and behavioral repertoires. Rose's case conceptualization (Chapter 3) made sense of her presenting issues as a conflict between her professional work context in the United States and her Mexican American cultural values regarding gender roles and emotional expression. Rose's conceptualizations provided her with an empowering choice—she could choose when to operate from her family's cultural values and when to adopt the prevailing values of her workplace. Similarly, Zainab's therapist (Chapter 4) used his relative lack of knowledge about the Muslim faith to unpack the implicit beliefs that underpinned a conflict between Zainab and her husband, Muhammad. In a couples session, Muhammad reframed Zainab's worry that she was not teaching their children the Muslim faith:

> "Zainab is an example of one of the pillars of Islam. There is the pillar of Zakah, which you might understand as generosity to others. Always she has done this, not just with money but with her time and heart as well. This is why we call her a pillar."

Zainab and Muhammad used this conceptualization to agree about their mutual strengths as parents.

In Mark's case, he recognized that some of his values were learned from his grandfather, who grew up in a generation when men had to be responsible and provide uncomplainingly for their families (Chapters 6 and 7). Mark's father's struggle with bipolar illness made it difficult for him to provide for his own family. This multigenerational history provided a helpful context for understanding Mark's beliefs about responsibility. Thus our model readily accommodates cultural beliefs and personal values as part of the emerging case conceptualization. Moreover, we encourage therapists to use language in conceptualizations that honors the client's values and culture.

The Model Is a Heuristic Framework

Our model is best used as a heuristic framework. Because case conceptualization is a higher order, complex skill therapists are helped by having "rules of thumb." Our approach builds on an extensive body of decision-making evidence that shows heuristic approaches work best when someone is faced with complex or incomplete data (Garb, 1998; Kahneman, 2003). However, research also suggests heuristic decision making is prone to a range of biases. Therefore our model incorporates (1) methods to minimize these biases (Box 2.2) and (2) guidelines for learning case conceptualization skills (Chapter 8).

THE USEFULNESS AND APPLICABILITY OF THE MODEL

If the case conceptualization crucible is a useful model, it should help therapists achieve conceptualization's primary functions and prove applicable in a variety of settings. The following sections address these issues.

Does the Model Fulfill the Functions of Case Conceptualization?

Does our approach accomplish the functions commonly attributed to case conceptualization (Butler, 1998; Denman, 1995; Eells, 2007; Box 1.1)? Does it meet therapists' needs (Flitcroft et al., 2007)? We revisit these key functions in Box 9.1, which also shows how these functions are illustrated in Mark's therapy. The conceptualizations Mark co-created throughout therapy were integral to describing his presenting issues in CBT terms, improving his understanding of these presenting issues, and informing therapy interventions.

Other case examples throughout the book also illustrate the functions of case conceptualization specifically in relation to collaborative empiricism and incorporation of client strengths. Katherine's case (Chapter 3) offers a puzzling interplay of psychological (panic attacks) and physical (fainting) factors. Her therapist works empirically and collaboratively with Katherine to resolve this puzzle. Initially they develop a cognitive conceptualization and use a standard protocol for panic disorder. However, the outcomes of cognitive interventions do not entirely "fit" this conceptualization. The mismatch between the existing conceptualization and Katherine's experiences alerts her therapist to the need for a new conceptualization, one that reconsiders possible physical causes for Katherine's problems. In the first contact with her therapist, Zainab (Chapter 4) identifies herself as "not broken." Zainab's therapist follows this lead and focuses early conceptualizations on her strengths using a metaphor that she and her husband offer of a "pillar."

These are just a few of the cases that illustrate how our model can fulfill the functions of case conceptualization. The next section illustrates additional contexts in which our model can be applied.

Box 9.1. Revisiting the Functions of Conceptualization

Function of formulation	Case illustrations
1. Synthesizes client experience, CBT theory, and research	Mark's depression, OCD, and health concerns were understood and treated by drawing on evidence-based models and interventions (see Chapter 6 for examples).
2. Normalizes and validates presenting issues	Mark's therapist was able to understand and normalize Mark's health concerns when the fear of acquiring HIV was identified. This led to interventions normalizing intrusive thoughts (see Chapter 6).
3. Promotes client engagement	Mark's curiosity and involvement were harnessed by gathering examples of changes in mood over the week to help establish whether the evolving conceptualizations were a good fit (Chapters 5 and 6). By the end of therapy Mark's high level of engagement meant he was refining the conceptualization independently (Chapter 7).
4. Makes numerous complex problems more manageable	Mark's presentation was complex and at times the conceptualization reflected this complexity (Figures 7.6 and 7.7). Throughout therapy, efforts were made to distill this complexity into simpler forms that were more manageable for Mark and the therapist to use in the long term.
5. Guides the selection, focus, and sequence of interventions	Mark's therapy illustrates the progression from an initial descriptive conceptualization that shapes presenting issues and goals (Chapter 5), to a cross-sectional conceptualization that guides choices of behavioral and cognitive interventions (Chapter 6), to cognitive-behavioral work focused on pervasive and enduring beliefs and behavior patterns (Chapter 7).
6. Identifies client strengths and suggests ways to build client resilience	Mark's strengths were part of the presenting issues list (Chapter 5), thereafter integrated into interventions (Chapter 6), and a conceptualization of resilience that promoted Mark's long-term growth (Chapter 7).
7. Enables the simplest and most cost-efficient interventions	Although progress using disorder-specific models was encouraging (Chapter 6), Mark and his therapist recognized they needed to address more pervasive and underlying issues (transdiagnostic processes of responsibility and high standards) to reduce residual symptoms, lessen Mark's vulnerability, and build his resilience (Chapter 7).

(cont.)

Box 9.1 (cont.)

8. Anticipates and responds to therapeutic difficulties	Like many clients with mood disorders, Mark experiences all-or-nothing thinking about his problems and expresses hopelessness. The therapist looks for variation in Mark's experiences to identify exceptions to his low mood and to identify potential areas of strength and resilience that can help increase hope.
9. Helps understand nonresponse in therapy and suggests alternative routes for change	After making significant gains Mark has a "blowout" at home, which he regards as evidence that he is a "waste of space at work *and at home*." The therapist uses the conceptualization work up to that point to help Mark reframe the setback as "I have a lot to offer; I am capable and take responsibility" (Chapter 7).
10. Enables high-quality supervision	See illustrative examples of supervision and consultation linked to conceptualization in Chapter 8.

Broader Applications of the Model

Couples and Families

Nearly all case examples in this book describe individual adult clients. However, the model can be used equally well with couples (Beck, 1989) and families. For example, the case of Zainab and her husband Muhammad illustrates how individual and shared beliefs can be made explicit and reframed to move toward a couple's shared goal of effective coparenting (Chapter 4).

With each additional person, conceptualizations can become more multilayered and complex. Family case conceptualizations often incorporate two parental perspectives and several child perspectives on the same events (see, e.g., Burbach & Stanbridge, 2006). The same model and principles apply, but therapists need to be flexible and skilled to capture and work with several different perspectives simultaneously. Therapists also need to find ways to distill this complexity into simpler formats. For example, during conceptualization of an ongoing family conflict, an adolescent daughter learned that her father's rage about her study habits was fueled by his anxious image of her as an unemployed and poverty-stricken adult. When she learned that fear rather than judgment fueled her father's rage, they were able to talk together more constructively. In later stages of therapy the father described how he had dropped out of high school at age 14 and felt "lost and isolated" for several years. This longitudinal conceptualization helped the family understand the emotional intensity of his reactions.

Working Indirectly through Staff, Family, and Caretakers

Conceptualizations are usually actively developed with the individuals, couples, and families concerned who provide the primary sources of information about personal experiences. However, sometimes clients are unable to participate in this way. As an example, people with serious cognitive impairment may be unable to collaboratively construct a conceptualization (James, 1999). In these cases, caretakers and support staff can collaborate on the person's behalf. James, Kendell, and Reichelt (1999) describe working with staff groups to create conceptualizations to understand the sometimes confusing behavior of people with dementia.

Consider the case of George, a man with dementia who each evening wanders around the residential unit where he lives, checking all the doors, walking into people's rooms, and setting off the exit alarms. Staff and residents find George's behavior disruptive. Using functional analysis, the staff identify antecedents to George's behavioral patterns, yet due to his dementia, staff members are unable to interview George to understand the meaning of his behavior. In this instance the staff works collaboratively with George's family to conceptualize what might be going on. His family links George's behavior to a lifetime pattern of locking up his house each night. Hence George's behavior is understood in context of his desire to keep his home and family safe. This conceptualization leads staff and the residents to reinterpret George's behavior as a sign of his caring about others' well-being rather than an intention to create disruption. This conceptualization normalizes George's behavior, changes attitudes toward him, and suggests treatment plans such as accompanying him in the evening to assure him that everyone is safe (James, 1999).

This work by James and his colleagues demonstrates that cognitive conceptualizations can be extended to working with caregivers and staff groups in order to create a more empathic view of a person's behavior. Of course, adapting the model in this way means that therapists need to make a greater effort to incorporate checks and balances against possible heuristic biases. The person concerned cannot always comment on evidence of "fit." As always, conceptualizations must be considered as hypotheses to be tested carefully against the outcomes of an intervention.

SUGGESTIONS FOR EVALUATING THE MODEL

Just as a case conceptualization needs to be tested, our model needs to be objectively evaluated and empirically tested. What criteria can we use to judge our model? How can we evaluate whether this model leads to better CBT outcomes? There are two related sets of criteria that can help and we discuss them in the next sections. The first is conceptual—Eells's (2007) description of the dialectical challenges faced by therapists. The second, from Bieling and Kuyken (2003), is empirical and leads to a suggested research agenda. We begin with a discussion of dialectics in case conceptualization.

Conceptual Criteria: Dialectics in Case Conceptualization

Dialectic is defined as "an argument that juxtaposes opposed or contradictory ideas and seeks to resolve their conflict" (Allen, 2000). In the seminal *Handbook of Psychotherapy Case Formulation* (Eells, 2007), Tracy Eells elegantly sets out some of the key dialectics therapists face when constructing case conceptualizations. Here we consider our model of collaborative case conceptualization in relation to these dialectics.

Dialectic 1: Nomothetic versus Idiographic

The first dialectic is between nomothetic and idiographic considerations. That is, to what extent does what we know in general about a disorder match or conflict with what we know about our client's individual experience? Clinical decisions often balance between the two poles of this dimension. At one extreme, some clinicians are overly wedded to CBT theory and become Procrustean: unnaturally fitting the person to a theory. Other clinicians immerse themselves in clients' accounts of difficulties and disregard relevant theory and research. Both of these polarized positions shortchange the client by losing important descriptive and explanatory information.

Sometimes this dialectic is argued between adherents of two approaches: those who advocate closely following evidence-based treatment protocols and those who promote treatment guided by pragmatic individualized case conceptualizations. The first practice group suggests that therapists should use evidence-based CBT conceptualizations linked to protocols that have been extensively shown to be effective (e.g., Chambless & Ollendick, 2001). Others posit that this ideal is impractical; the reality is that most CBT therapists use a pragmatic individualized approach to treatment (Persons, 2005). Models that rely on primary diagnoses and sequenced interventions have been proposed to resolve this dilemma by individualizing therapy without moving too far away from evidence-based practice (e.g., Fava et al., 2003; Kendall & Clarkin, 1992).

We argue that the protocol-driven versus conceptualization-driven dichotomy is largely illusory. In the Schulte et al. (1992) study comparing manualized and individualized therapy, post hoc analyses of the audiotapes of the manualized condition suggested that therapists could not help but individualize the manual. No client fits a protocol exactly, and protocols tend to be written as guiding frameworks. One of the rationales for a case conceptualization approach is that many client presentations include significant comorbidity and do not easily fit an established evidence-based approach, even one based on sequential use of protocols. Comorbidity appears to be the norm rather than the exception to the rule (Zimmerman, McGlinchey, Chelminski, & Young, 2008). It is likely that most CBT therapists use an individualized case conceptualization approach with such cases.

We propose that when client presentations are relatively straightforward, evidence-based CBT theories and protocols should be used as the primary source for conceptualization and treatment planning. This is for the very simple reason that these approaches work in the context of randomized controlled trials *and, in contrast to clinical lore, also work in clinically representative settings* (Shadish, Matt, Navarro, & Phillips, 2000). Manualized approaches bring value by helping define the territory most relevant for clinical attention. Furthermore, they encourage sustained application of techniques and close monitoring of the results.

However, even within evidence-based manualized approaches there are multiple decision points that require an individualized understanding of clients' presenting issues. As presentations become more idiosyncratic or complex, therapists can increasingly rely on individualized case conceptualization to add to the best available theory and protocols. Viewed in this way, therapists are expected to use at least a small degree of individualized conceptualization in all cases and rely on this process more as cases become increasingly complex or when clients do not respond to standardized protocols.

As such, our model proposes that case conceptualization serves as a linchpin between clinical practice decisions and the best available theory and protocols. Its role becomes more significant when greater individualized decision making is required. Choice points requiring an individualized case conceptualization are limited for relatively straightforward cases for which a theory and treatment manual are excellent fits. With complex cases or when no single theory or manual fits, an individualized conceptualization is essential to draw together disparate theoretical perspectives and integrate these with case particularities. Our model requires that therapists' decisions about when to deviate from therapy manuals be made (1) empirically and (2) collaboratively. For example, when clients do not show progress toward their goals and expected improvement on standardized outcome measures, it is reasonable to conceptualize this and respond appropriately. Indeed, doing so is crucial to improving outcomes (Lambert et al., 2003).

How did this approach help Mark's therapy? Mark's therapist used empirically supported behavioral and cognitive-behavioral models (Beck et al., 1979; Dobson, 1989; Martell et al., 2001) to help describe, understand, and intervene with Mark's depression. Similarly, empirically tested models of OCD (van Oppen & Arntz, 1994) and health anxiety (Williams, 1997) were used to understand his checking behavior. At the same time, throughout therapy Mark and his therapist carefully examined the match between Mark's unique experience and CBT theory. Disorder-specific models contributed to cross-sectional conceptualizations and a treatment plan that yielded significant progress toward Mark's goals. However, there were still significant residual symptoms of both anxiety and depression (Chapter 6). Subsequent therapy drew on a more generic CBT model to understand the factors that predisposed and protected Mark so that further interventions could target these pivotal cognitive and behavioral processes and reduce residual symptoms of anxiety and depression. These pivotal processes were vital to understanding the comorbidity in Mark's presentation (Chapter 7). Finally, an individualized conceptualization of strengths and resilience helped Mark manage relapse and maintain his gains in the face of life stressors.

Dialectic 2: Complex versus Simple

A case conceptualization approach to CBT is particularly useful when clients' presenting issues are multidiagnostic or too complex to represent within a single theoretical framework. Therapists are sometimes prone to develop overly elaborate and complex case conceptualizations under these circumstances. In consideration of the dialectic of complexity versus simplicity, our model suggests that case conceptualizations should be as simple as pragmatically possible without losing essential meaning. An overly complex conceptualization is likely to lack focus and overwhelm both the therapist and client. On the other hand, an overly simplistic case conceptualization misses important aspects of the person's presentation, and this omission may lead to avoidable difficulties. Thus the goal is a conceptualization that includes all the necessary components but not extraneous ones.

The proposal that the simpler of two functional conceptualizations is likely to be best is not meant to deny the complexity of the experiences of each person seeking help. However, the task of case conceptualization is not to understand everything about a person but rather to work together toward his or her therapy goals. When more than one case conceptualization applies, the simplest conceptualization is preferred because simple models are easier to comprehend, remember, test, and apply in everyday situations. Thus while brain functioning might help explain certain memory aspects of posttraumatic stress disorder, these would not be included in a case conceptualization unless these more complicated ideas were necessary to understand client experiences.

Achieving simplicity in the face of genuine complexity requires a high level of skill; it must capture the essence of the client's presenting issues without "cutting off" important information in a Procrustean way. As therapists progress from novice to intermediate levels of competence it can be helpful to distill complex conceptualizations into much simpler ones with input from supervisors and consultants (Chapter 8). Both highly complex (Figure 7.5) and much simpler conceptualizations (Figures 7.6 and 7.7) were presented to understand Mark's presenting issues. Metaphors, images, and diagrams co-created with clients are particularly effective ways to achieve this distillation.

Early in therapy, Mark used an evocative term: "waste of space." This self-image was a key part of his cross-sectional and longitudinal conceptualizations. Furthermore, in the process of understanding and developing his resilience Mark produced simple conceptual images of a caged and a wild grizzly bear to represent his vulnerability and resilience (Figure 7.5). Mark's progression from more complex to simpler conceptualizations is a common process in therapy. Complexity of understanding is gradually distilled with clients into ever simpler conceptualizations that clients can use to prevent relapse and build resilience.

Dialectic 3: Subjective versus Objective

Our experience working with CBT therapists in workshops and supervision or consultation suggests that many therapists consider case conceptualization more art than science. After a workshop, one therapist said, "Thank you for today. I've never really given much thought to how I conceptualize. I tend to get good client outcomes and it's something I've always done intuitively. I have a better sense now of what I have been doing intuitively all these years."

In the same way that expert piano tuners employ both art and science in their trade, case conceptualization is a high-level skill that is both art and science. Piano tuners have to ensure that all the keys are in tune and that the whole is in harmony. To do this they use a systematic approach to ensure each key is in tune and, at the same time, intuitively draw on musical skill and technical expertise to ensure the piano as a whole is in harmony. There are steps in this process, but the steps are used flexibly. This echoes Kahneman's (2003) theoretical distinction between intuitive and rational decision making (Figure

2.9), as well as contemporary views on advanced conceptualization skills (Eells et al., 2005). Similarly, our model views case conceptualization as a dynamic process that evolves over time (levels of conceptualization) and demands a high degree of knowledge, rational decision making, and rigor (science), as well as humanity and intuition (art).

The dialectical challenges therapists face are resolved in our model by the integration of theory, research, and client experience in the case conceptualization crucible. Over time and across levels, conceptualizations are gradually distilled into the simplest model that enables progress toward client goals. For therapists this requires high levels of skill as they use collaborative empiricism to balance intuitive and rational decision making.

Empirical Tests: A Research Agenda

In Chapter 1 we critically reviewed the existing evidence base for case conceptualization by using a set of criteria suggested by Bieling and Kuyken (2003). We argued there that, just like Nasruddin looks for his keys under a street light, research to date has examined conceptualization primarily in ways that are easier to study. These have perhaps missed aspects of conceptualization which may be most important. In the discussion that follows, we again use the Bieling and Kuyken (2003) criteria to suggest an agenda for future research.

Top-Down Research Criterion: Is the Conceptualization's Theory Evidence Based?

This first research criterion concerns the evidence base for the CBT theories and protocols that are a key ingredient in our case conceptualization crucible. CBT's commitment to research and evidence-based practice makes it inevitable that the next few decades will bring theoretical and therapeutic refinements that increase the specificity of models and the effectiveness of treatment protocols (for a review of 40 years of such development see Beck, 2005). Furthermore, there is an increasing focus on CBT comorbidity (Clarkin & Kendall, 1992), with evidence that more competent therapists achieve better outcomes with clients who present with comorbid diagnoses (Kuyken & Tsivrikos, 2008). Future research can examine whether therapist success treating comorbidity is partially mediated by the ability to use case conceptualization effectively with these clients to understand central cognitive and behavioral processes.

The "top-down" research agenda provides an opportunity to examine intriguing research questions linking CBT theory with case conceptualization. How often are the mechanisms described in theories of disorders implicated in individual case conceptualizations of people presenting with these disorders? What are the nuances in these mechanisms at the level of the individual case conceptualization? When mechanisms are apparently not present, how can we understand these individual differences? This information can be used to refine theory and design experimental clinical work to explain individual differences. In clients with comorbid presentations do the mechanisms implicated in cross-sectional and longitudinal conceptualizations match our understanding of transdiagnostic processes (Harvey, Watkins, Mansell, & Shatran, 2004)? How does this improve our understanding of comorbidity and transdiagnostic cognitive and behavioral processes? How does this improved understanding inform therapy choices?

Bottom-Up Criteria

These criteria include questions about conceptualization's reliability, validity, whether it improves outcomes, and whether it is acceptable and useful to both client and therapist. To date, research addressing these "bottom-up" criteria is more limited (Chapter 1; Bieling & Kuyken, 2003). The relative sparseness of data in these areas offers great scope for innovation and was one of the drivers for our new approach. Consistent with our commitment to evidence-based practice, it is vital that our new approach be submitted to empirical testing. However, before such testing can yield useful answers, a range of preliminary questions need to be addressed.

Defining and Operationalizing Case Conceptualization

An obvious and initial question is, "How do cognitive therapists conduct case conceptualization in real-world practice?" Clinical lore (e.g., Butler, 1998; Eells, 2007) and recent research (Flitcroft et al., 2007) suggest that the key functions of case conceptualization set out in Chapter 1 (Box 1.1) are generally endorsed by therapists. But which of these functions do therapists regard as most important, and in what contexts? To what extent do CBT therapists already use the principles outlined in our model, and in what contexts? Do they already progress through levels of conceptualization, work collaboratively, underpin their practice with empiricism, and incorporate client strengths? How much do clients collaborate in creating case conceptualizations? Is client collaboration implicit or explicit? How are the principles we set out in this book already demonstrated in therapy sessions? These initial questions are primarily descriptive and exploratory. They can be answered using methods such as interviews, surveys, and questionnaires, as well as observation and coding of therapy sessions.

Measuring the Quality of Case Conceptualizations

A psychometrically robust measure of the quality of case conceptualizations is needed to meet the needs of clinical researchers as well as instructors. There have been two recent attempts to create such measures (Eells et al., 2005; Kuyken, Fothergill, et al., 2005). The impressive work of Tracy Eells and his colleagues relies on painstaking coding of client data and therapy transcripts (Eells et al., 2005; Eells & Lombart, 2003). They stress eight criteria: comprehensiveness, elaboration, precision of language, complexity, coherence, goodness-of-fit, treatment plan elaboration, and the extent to which the therapist appears to follow a systematic formulation process across all cases. Fothergill and Kuyken (2002) developed a measure of the quality of CBT case conceptualization that emphasizes parsimony, coherence, and the conceptualization's explanatory power. Their rating system has good evidence of interrater reliability and convergent validity.

Nevertheless, simpler, easy-to-use, psychometrically robust measures are required to evaluate our conceptualization model. Our model suggests the following dimensions should be included in such a measure: inclusion of theory and research, appropriate use of levels of conceptualization, evidence of collaborative empiricism, and an appropriate focus on strengths and resilience. In addition to providing a necessary research tool, the utility of such a measure in training and practice is clear. It would help therapists and trainers assess knowledge and skills, set learning goals, and evaluate learning progress.

What Therapist, Client, and Contextual Factors Are Associated with Good-Quality Case Conceptualization?

Do therapist competence, training, experience, professional accreditation status, intelligence, openness, curiosity, or as-yet unspecified factors affect case conceptualization? How do decision-making processes affect the quality of case conceptualization? How does the decision making involved in case conceptualization differ across novice, intermediate, and advanced therapists? A potential research program could ask, "What factors affect clinical decision making in case conceptualization?" There is an opportunity to take the extensive expert decision-making literature and extrapolate it to clinical decision making generally (Garb, 1998) and case conceptualization specifically (Eells & Lombart, 2003).

How widespread is decision-making bias among novice, intermediate, and advanced therapists? In relation to our model, we have argued that our three principles, especially collaborative empiricism, should provide a check and balance on common problematic heuristic biases. Do they? If a therapist interviews a client in a collaborative and empirical manner, does this increase corrective feedback and reduce heuristic biases? Are there other ways to minimize problematic heuristic biases?

What client and contextual factors improve the quality of conceptualizations (Eells, 2007)? Client factors to consider include: complexity of presentation, motivation for therapy, degree of distress, psychological-mindedness, and openness to experimentation and new experience. Contextual factors include length of therapy, time and availability of supervision and consultation, and therapist–client similarities and differences. Regarding our specific model, does hope increase when a client's strengths are highlighted? If conceptualization is at the appropriate level, does it increase clients' understanding and minimize the chances of the client and therapist feeling overwhelmed?

Do Training, Supervision, and Consultation Improve Case Conceptualization Skills?

Once we better understand the therapist, client, and contextual factors that improve case conceptualization we can use these findings to develop training programs. Does training in our approach lead to demonstrated improvements in the use of the principles set out in the model? Kendjelic & Eells (2007) demonstrated that training aimed at improving therapists' use of a systematic approach to conceptualization led to improvements in overall quality of conceptualization. Drawing on such methods, we could establish whether training in our model reduces therapists' tendency to use problematic heuristics or improves the likelihood of higher-quality conceptualizations. Similarly, research can examine whether particular supervision and consultation models improve the quality of conceptualization processes.

Once some of these preliminary questions are addressed, we can examine whether our approach improves the reliability and validity of conceptualizations.

Reliability and Validity of Conceptualization

Our model proposes a rather different relationship between reliability and validity than that proposed by Bieling and Kuyken (2003). First it suggests that a primary goal of collaborative empiricism is to ensure that the conceptualization is *a good fit for clients*. Given that there are a number of different valid conceptualizations that could emerge from available theory and client experience, the key test of reliability and validity is whether the client and the therapist *agree with each other* in generating a conceptualization that fits with the best available theory and client experience. Second the model suggests that conceptualizations evolve over time, and therefore different conceptualizations are expected at different phases of therapy. The research designs looking at reliability to date have not considered either collaborative empiricism or levels of conceptualization (Kuyken, Fothergill, et al., 2005; Persons, Mooney, & Padesky, 1995).

Within our model, the most appropriate test of reliability is whether a therapist and client agree on the content of the conceptualization and whether the level of agreement is maintained over the course of therapy. A first consideration is whether therapists and clients can independently agree on a list of presenting issues and therapy goals after several therapy sessions. In early phases of therapy, reliability could be a measure of how well the therapist and client can independently identify or produce similar descriptive conceptualizations. As appropriate, this would be replicated later in therapy for cross-sectional and longitudinal conceptualizations. These tests would assess whether therapists and clients who use our conceptualization model agree with each other and continue to agree as the conceptualization evolves over the course of therapy.

Rather like an archer who repeatedly misses the target even while shooting arrows into the same vicinity, it is quite possible for the therapist and client to show high levels of agreement on an erroneous conceptualization. An important initial question relating to validity is whether collaboratively derived case conceptualizations relate meaningfully to presenting issues and the factors underlying them. In essence, do the conceptualizations derived using our model demonstrate convergent validity with other sources of data such as, standardized measures of client history, beliefs and behaviors, or the reliable accounts of knowledgeable informants?

Conceptualization's Relationship to Treatment Processes and Outcomes

How does conceptualization affect therapy processes and outcomes? A powerful design used in the 1980s to evaluate the impact of case conceptualization (especially functional analysis) was the randomized controlled trial (Jacobson et al., 1989; Schulte et al., 1992). In this design, clients are randomized to therapists matched on every key variable except whether they use an enhanced model of case conceptualization (the experimental group) or a standardized approach (the control group). Therapy processes and outcomes are the dependent variables.

Key research questions include: Do clients in an enhanced conceptualization condition based on our model report (1) a more normalized understanding of their issues, (2) more feelings of validation, (3) more engagement and motivation, (4) greater ability to identify and use their strengths, (5) earlier therapy gains, and (6) more substantial gains maintained over longer time periods?

A further example of how to study the value of conceptualization is informed by research examining therapist and client factors that predict outcomes (Hamilton & Dobson, 2002). Can the content and quality of conceptualizations derived in the first, middle, and later phases of therapy predict overall treatment response? If so, this finding would surely indicate the utility and value of conceptualization in helping alleviate distress and build resilience.

In an impressive research program Michael Lambert has shown that outcomes are improved when they are measured and reported back to therapists (Lambert et al., 2003; Okiishi et al., 2006). An extension of this research is to measure outcomes as Lambert does and then, when outcomes are not as good as expected, to support therapists in their work with clients to refine the conceptualizations. The impact of this refinement on outcomes can then be examined. Within our model of conceptualization, we would hypothesize that therapists who receive additional support to collaboratively refine the conceptualization would achieve improved outcomes over therapists not provided with this additional support.

Randomized controlled trials with embedded process outcome questions typically require large numbers of participants (Kraemer, Wilson, Fairburn, & Agras, 2002). Before designing larger-scale studies, it is arguably more appropriate to refine research questions using alternative smaller-scale designs. Single-case designs provide alternative approaches to answering some of the questions above (Barlow, Hayes, & Nelson, 1984; Hayes, 1981). There have already been some single-case design studies in the area of case conceptualization (e.g., Chadwick et al., 2003; Moras, Telfer, & Barlow, 1993; Nelson-Gray et al., 1989). To evaluate our model, therapists could be asked to switch on and off different elements of conceptualization. Clients as well as blind independent raters could assess the effects of these switches on key processes and outcomes over time. For example, in an additive design the therapist adds (switches on) a new element (e.g., focusing on client strengths), and the client and independent raters assess the impact (e.g., on client's sense of hope and engagement). In a dismantling design key components are removed (e.g., collaborative empiricism), and blind independent raters as well as the client assess the impact (e.g., evidence of heuristic errors). These switches could be made during parts of therapy sessions, whole therapy sessions, or phases of therapy.

Analogue studies can also be used to answer many of the questions set out above. Therapists working with role-play clients can use the single-case designs described above in workshop and training settings. Components of our model can be studied via vignettes or session recordings that manipulate variables of interest and then examine the effects of these manipulations. For example, what is the effect on therapist hope and treatment planning when client vignettes either omit or include client strengths?

Naturalistic studies use data collected from clients in regular therapy settings (e.g., Persons, Roberts, Zalecki, & Brechwald, 2006). Many outpatient settings routinely collect outcome data. These data can be used as a resource for answering questions such as: "Does training in case conceptualization affect client outcomes?" Client outcomes before and after therapists receive training in case conceptualization can be compared. Such studies would ideally match clients in the two cohorts on initial demographic and psychiatric variables and strive to minimize attrition of therapists across the two study phases.

A Note on Methodology

One of the reasons case conceptualization research to date is so underdeveloped is because these types of questions require careful consideration of methodology. Process–outcome research regarding our model of case conceptualization needs to account for a number of complex factors:

- Case conceptualization occurs in the context of a number of other factors that constitute CBT. For example, the therapeutic alliance and competent delivery of CBT interventions are prerequisites for change. Any research into case conceptualization must take these contextual factors into account.
- Our conceptualization model contains several different elements: Are they all relevant to the research question being asked? What is the impact of (1) moving progressively through levels of conceptualization, (2) employing collaborative empiricism, and (3) focusing on client strengths? Each of these aspects of the model might be expected to have slightly different effects on therapy processes and outcomes. For example, one might predict a focus on client strengths would increase clients' and therapists' hope, reduce stigma, improve the working alliance, and reduce relapse. Focusing progressively on levels of conceptualization could enhance clients' and therapists' sense of mastery and reduce the possibility of client distress compared with making overly inferential hypotheses early in therapy. In summary, research needs to

address these principles separately and together in terms of their impact on understanding and change.

- Are the measures of case conceptualization, therapy process, and therapy outcome appropriate and psychometrically robust? For example, to test our model, researchers need to incorporate measures of achieving personally defined goals and resilience in addition to changes on standardized instruments that measure alleviation of distress.
- Chadwick et al. (2003) show that therapists and clients can report discrepancies in the impact of conceptualization. It follows that the assessment of both therapist and client versions of therapy processes and outcomes could be necessary. In addition, both positive and negative effects of conceptualization should be measured. That being said, we hypothesize that the discrepancies between client and therapist reports on the impact of conceptualization will be reduced if the client and therapist co-create conceptualizations over time, especially if these conceptualizations explicitly incorporate strengths and are attuned to client resilience.

Therapy process and outcome research methodology has become more sophisticated in recent years. A number of recently published seminal papers could inform the research agenda we set out above (Garratt, Ingram, Rand, & Sawalani, 2007; Hayes, Laurenceau, Feldman, Strauss, & Cardaciotto, 2007; Holmbeck, 2003; Kraemer et al., 2002; Laurenceau, Hayes, & Feldman, 2007; Pachankis & Goldfried, 2007; Perepletchikova & Kazdin, 2005).

CONCLUSION

We have outlined an approach to CBT case conceptualization that bridges theory and practice, informs therapy, and has the potential to stand up to empirical scrutiny. This model takes a step toward resolving the challenges faced by therapists using conceptualization in their everyday practice as well as some of the challenges presented by research examining CBT case conceptualization. We hope therapists, as a result of reading this text, now have a deeper understanding of case conceptualization. Furthermore, we hope therapists who follow the practice guidelines provided in earlier chapters experience noticeable improvements in their conceptualization skills.

Case conceptualization is a collaborative, dynamic, and constructive process. We have presented our case that the primary function of case conceptualization is *to guide therapy in order to relieve client distress and build client resilience*. We believe the conceptualization processes we describe enhance CBT in ways that will accomplish these goals more effectively than current conceptualization practices. Our model encourages therapists and clients to work together to integrate the best scientific understandings with the most personal client observations regarding difficulties and strengths. As we have shown, this process occurs iteratively over the course of therapy. We offer our model as a map to guide this shared adventure of discovery.

Appendix

Aid to History Taking Form

AID TO HISTORY TAKING

The purpose of this questionnaire is to obtain some information about your background, which may help us to understand your situation. We will have the opportunity to discuss your difficulties with you in detail, but we may not have the time to discuss all aspects of your history and situation. This form gives you the chance to provide us with a fuller picture and to do this at your pace. Some questions are quite factual, whereas others are of a more subjective nature. If you find any parts of the form difficult, please leave these blank and we can discuss these at your appointment. In the meantime, if you have any trouble completing any of the sections please do not hesitate to contact us. **All of the information you provide on this form is confidential.**

YOUR PERSONAL DETAILS

Name		Marital status	
Date of birth		Religion	
Sex		Date	
Occupation		Telephone	

YOUR DIFFICULTIES AND GOALS

Please briefly list the three main issues that have led you to seek help.

1.
2.
3.

Please state what you want to achieve by attending our center.

1.

YOU AND YOUR FAMILY

1. Where was your place of birth? _____

2. Could you please give some detail about your **FATHER** (if known)
   - What is his age now? _____
   - If he is no longer alive, at what age did he die? _____
   - How old were you when he died? _____
   - What is, or was, his occupation? _____

Please tell something about your father, his character or personality, and your relationship with him.

3. Could you please give some details about your **MOTHER** (if known)
   - What is her age now? _____
   - If she is no longer alive, at what age did she die? _____
   - How old were you when she died? _____
   - What is, or was, her occupation? _____

Please tell something about your mother, her character or personality, and your relationship with her.

4. If there were/are any problems in your relationship with your parents, please describe the most important one(s).

How much does this bother you now? (please circle)

Not at all   A little   Moderately   Very much   Couldn't be worse

Your brothers and sisters (if known)

5. How many children, including yourself, are there in your family? _____

Please give us their names and other details listed below. Include yourself and please start with the **eldest**. Please also include any step- or half-siblings or any other children adopted by your parents and indicate who they are.

Name	Occupation	Age	Sex	Comments
			M/F	
			M/F	
			M/F	
			M/F	
			M/F	
			M/F	

6. Please describe any important relationships with your siblings, whether helpful or problematic for you.

7. What was the general atmosphere like at home?

8. Were there any important changes, for example, moves or any other significant events, during your childhood or adolescence? Include any separations from the family. Please give approximate ages and details.

9. Was there someone else who was important to you during your childhood (e.g., grandparents, aunts/uncles, family friend, etc.)? If so, could you tell us something about them?

10. Has anyone in your family ever received psychiatric treatment?   Yes   No   Not sure

11. Does anyone in your family have a history of mental illness, alcohol, or drug abuse?   Yes   No   Not sure

If yes, please complete:

	Family member	List specific psychiatric, alcohol, or drug problem
1		
2		
3		
4		

12. Has any member of your family ever made a suicide attempt?   Y/N

If yes, how is this person related to you?   _____

13. Has any member of your family died from suicide?   Y/N

If yes, how is this person related to you?   _____

YOUR EDUCATION

1. (a) Please tell us something about your schooling and education.

   (b) How did you enjoy school? Were there any particular achievements or difficulties? Which were the most important ones?

How much does this bother you now? (please circle)

Not at all	A little	Moderately	Very much	Couldn't be worse

YOUR WORK HISTORY

1. What job or main role do you currently do?

2. Please tell us something about your past working life, including the jobs and trainings you have done.

3. Have there been any particular difficulties? Which were the most important ones?

EXPERIENCES OF UPSETTING EVENTS

1. Sometimes things happen to people that are extremely upsetting—things like being in a life-threatening situation like a major disaster, very serious accident, or fire; being physically assaulted or raped; or seeing another person killed, badly hurt, or hearing about something horrible that has happened to someone you are close to. At any time during your life, have any of these kinds of things happened to you?

   (a) If "no," please check here. ____

   (b) If "yes," please list the traumatic events.

Brief description	Date (month/year)	Age
1.		
2.		
3.		
4.		
5.		
6.		

If *any* events listed: Sometimes these things keep coming back in night-mares, flashbacks, or thoughts that you can't get rid of. Has this ever happened to you?   Yes   No

If "no": What about being very upset when you were in a situation that reminded you of one of these terrible things?   Yes   No

2. Did you ever experience physical abuse as a child?   Yes   No   Not sure

3. Have you ever experienced physical abuse as an adult?   Yes   No   Not sure

4. Did you ever experience sexual abuse as a child?   Yes   No   Not sure

5. Have you ever experienced rape, including date or marital rape?   Yes   No   Not sure

6. Did you ever experience emotional or verbal abuse as a child?   Yes   No   Not sure

7. Have you ever experienced emotional or verbal abuse as an adult?   Yes   No   Not sure

YOUR PARTNER AND YOUR PRESENT FAMILY

1. About your **partner(s)** (if applicable)

   (a) Please briefly describe any previous important relationship(s), in chronological order. Please include how long they lasted and why you think the relationship(s) ended.

   (b) Do you have a partner now? If yes,

   How old is s/he? _____

   What is her/his occupation? _____

   How long have you been together? _____

   (c) Please tell us something about your partner, her/his character or personality, and your relationship with her/him. What do you like about the relationship?

   (d) If there are any problems in your relationship with your partner, please describe the most important one(s).

   How much does this bother you now? (please circle)

   Not at all   A little   Moderately   Very
   much   Couldn't
   be worse

2. How is your sex life? Do you have any difficulties in your sexual life? If so, please try to describe these.

How much does this bother you now? (please circle)

Not at all   A little   Moderately   Very much   Couldn't be worse

3. About your **children** (if known)

(a) If you have children, please list them in order of age. Please indicate any children from previous marriage(s) and adopted children; indicate who they are.

Name	Occupation	Age	Sex	Comments
			M/F	
			M/F	
			M/F	
			M/F	
			M/F	

(b) Please describe your relationship with your children. If there are any difficulties with your children, please describe the most important one(s).

How much does this bother you now? (please circle)

Not at all   A little   Moderately   Very much   Couldn't be worse

YOUR PSYCHIATRIC HISTORY

1. Have you ever been hospitalized for any emotional or psychiatric reason?   Y/N

If yes, how many times have you been hospitalized?   _____

Date	Name of hospital	Reason for hospitalization	Was it helpful?

2. Have you ever received outpatient psychiatric or psychological treatment?   Y/N

If yes, please complete the following:

Date	Name of professional	Reason for treatment	Was it helpful?
			Y/N
			Y/N
			Y/N
			Y/N

3. Are you taking any medication for psychiatric reasons?   Y/N

If yes, please complete the following:

Medication	Dosage	Frequency	Name of prescribing doctor

4. Have you ever made a suicide attempt?   Y/N

If yes, how many times have you attempted suicide? __

Approx. date	What exactly did you do to hurt yourself?	Were you hospitalized?
		Y/N
		Y/N
		Y/N
		Y/N

YOUR MEDICAL HISTORY

1. Who is your general practitioner?

Name	
Practice address	

2. When was the last time you had a physical checkup?   _____

3. Have you been treated by your GP or been hospitalized in the past year?   Y/N

If yes, please specify.   _____

4. Has there been any change in your general health in the past year?   Y/N

If yes, please specify.   _____

5. Are you taking any nonpsychiatric medications or over-the-counter drugs at the moment?   Y/N

	Medications	Dosage	Frequency	Reason
1.				
2.				
3.				
4..				

6. Have you ever had or have a history of (check all that apply)

☐ Stroke   ☐ Rheumatic fever   ☐ Heart surgery

☐ Asthma   ☐ Heart murmur   ☐ Heart attack

☐ Tuberculosis   ☐ Anemia   ☐ Angina

☐ Ulcers   ☐ High or low blood pressure ☐ Thyroid problems

☐ Diabetes

7. Are you pregnant or do you think you may be pregnant?   Yes   No

8. Have you ever had fits, seizures, convulsions, or epilepsy?   Yes   No

9. Do you have prosthetic heart valve?   Yes   No

10. Do you have any current medical conditions?   Yes   No

If yes, please specify:

_____

11. Do you have any medication or food allergies?   Yes   No

If yes, please specify:

_____

ALCOHOL AND DRUG USE HISTORY

1. Has your alcohol use ever caused any problems for you?   Y/N

2. Has anyone ever told you that alcohol has caused a problem for you or complained about your drinking?   Y/N

3. Has your drug use ever caused any problems for you?   Y/N

4. Has anyone ever told you that drugs have caused a problem for you or complained about your drug use?   Y/N

5. Have you ever been "hooked" on a prescribed medication or taken a lot more of it than you were supposed to?   Y/N   *If yes, please list those medications:*

_____

6. Have you ever been hospitalized, entered a detox program, or been in a rehabilitation

program because of a drug or alcohol problem?   Y/N   *If yes, when and where were you hospitalized?*

YOUR FUTURE

1. Please mention any particular satisfaction that you draw from your family life, your work life, or any other areas that are important to you.

2. Could you tell us something about your plans, hopes, and expectations for the future?

3. Please could you let us know how you felt completing this questionnaire?

Thank you.

References

Abramowitz, J. S. (1997). Effectiveness of psychological and pharmacological treatments for obsessive–compulsive disorder: A quantitative review. *Journal of Consulting and Clinical Psychology, 65*, 44–52.

Addis, M. E., & Martell, C. R. (2004). *Overcoming depression one step at a time: The new behavioral activation approach to getting your life back.* Oakland, CA: New Harbinger.

Allen, R. (2000). (Ed.). *The new Penguin English dictionary* (Penguin Reference Books). New York: Penguin Books.

American Psychiatric Association. (2000). *Diagnostic and statistical manual of mental disorders* (4th ed.). Arlington, VA: Author.

American Psychological Association. (2000). Guidelines for psychotherapy with lesbian, gay, and bisexual clients. *American Psychologist, 55*, 1440–1451.

American Psychological Association. (2003). Guidelines on multicultural education, training, research, practice, and organizational change for psychologists. *American Psychologist, 58*, 377–402.

Aspinwall, L. G., & Staudinger, U. M. (Eds.). (2002). *A psychology of human strengths: Fundamental questions and future directions for a positive psychology.* Washington, DC: American Psychological Association.

Barber, J. P., Liese, B. S., & Abrams, M. J. (2003). Development of the cognitive therapy adherence and competence scale. *Psychotherapy Research, 13*, 205–221.

Barber, J. P., Luborsky, L., Crits-Christoph, P., & Diguer, L. (1998). Stability of the CCRT from before psychotherapy starts to the early sessions. In L. Luborsky & P. Crits-Christoph (Eds.), *Understanding transference: The Core Conflictual Relationship Theme method* (2nd ed., pp. 253–260). New York: Basic Books.

Barlow, D. H. (Ed.). (2001). *Clinical handbook of psychological disorders* (3rd ed.). New York: Guilford Press.

Barlow, D. H., Hayes, S. C., & Nelson, R. O. (1984). *The scientist–practitioner: Research and accountability in clinical and educational settings.* Oxford, UK: Pergamon Press.

Barnard, P. J., & Teasdale, J. D. (1991). Interacting cognitive subsystems: A systemic approach to cognitive-affective interaction and change. *Cognition and Emotion, 5,* 1–39.

Baucom, D. H., Shoham, V., Mueser, K. T., Daiuto, A. D., & Stickle, T. R. (1998). Empirically supported couple and family interventions for marital distress and adult mental health problems. *Journal of Consulting and Clinical Psychology, 66,* 53–88.

Beck, A. T. (1967). *Depression: Causes and treatment.* Philadelphia: University of Pennsylvania Press.

Beck, A. T. (1976). *Cognitive therapy and the emotional disorders.* New York: Meridian.

Beck, A. T. (1989). *Love is never enough: How couples can overcome misunderstandings, resolve conflicts, and solve relationship problems through cognitive therapy.* New York: HarperCollins.

Beck, A. T. (1996). Beyond belief: A theory of modes, personality, and psychopathology. In P. M. Salkovskis (Ed.), *Frontiers of cognitive therapy* (pp. 1–25). New York: Guilford Press.

Beck, A. T. (2002). Prisoners of hate. *Behaviour Research and Therapy, 40,* 209–216.

Beck, A. T. (2005). The current state of cognitive therapy: A 40-year retrospective. *Archives of General Psychiatry, 62,* 953–959.

Beck, A. T., & Beck, J. S. (1991). *The Personality Belief Questionnaire.* Philadelphia: Beck Institute. [Unpublished manuscript]

Beck, A. T., Brown, G., Epstein, N., & Steer, R. A. (1988). An inventory for measuring clinical anxiety—psychometric properties. *Journal of Consulting and Clinical Psychology, 56,* 893–897.

Beck, A. T., Brown, G., Steer, R. A., & Weissman, A. N. (1991). Factor analysis of the Dysfunctional Attitude Scale. *Psychological Assessment, 3,* 478–483.

Beck, A. T., Emery, G., & Greenberg, R. L. (1985). *Anxiety disorders and phobias: A cognitive perspective.* New York: Basic Books.

Beck, A. T., Freeman, A., Davis, D. D., Pretzer, J., Fleming, B., Arntz, A., Butler, A., Fusco, G., Simon, K. M., Beck, J. S., Morrison, A., Padesky, C. A., & Renton, J. (2004). *Cognitive therapy of personality disorders* (2nd ed.). New York: Guilford Press.

Beck, A. T., & Rector, N. A. (2003). A cognitive model of hallucinations. *Cognitive Therapy, 27,* 19–52.

Beck, A. T., Rush, A. J., Shaw, B. F., & Emery, G. (1979). *Cognitive therapy of depression.* New York: Guilford Press.

Beck, A. T., Steer, R. A., & Brown, G. K. (1996). *The Beck Depression Inventory— Second Edition.* San Antonio, TX: The Psychological Corporation.

Beck, A. T., Wright, F. D., Newman, C. F., & Liese, B. S. (1993). *Cognitive therapy of substance abuse.* New York: Guilford Press.

Beck, J. S. (1995). *Cognitive therapy: Basics and beyond.* New York: Guilford Press.

Beck, J. S. (2005). *Cognitive therapy for challenging problems.* New York: Guilford Press.

Beck, R., & Fernandez, E. (1998). Cognitive-behavioral therapy in the treatment of anger: A meta-analysis. *Cognitive Therapy and Research, 22,* 63–74.

Bennett-Levy, J. (2006). Therapist skills: A cognitive model of their acquisition and refinement. *Behavioural and Cognitive Psychotherapy, 34,* 57–78.

Bennett-Levy, J., Butler, G., Fennell, M., Hackmann, A., Mueller, M., & Westbrook, D. (2004). *The Oxford guide to behavioural experiments in cognitive therapy.* Oxford, UK: Oxford University Press.

Bennett-Levy, J., Turner, F., Beaty, T., Smith, M., Paterson, B., & Farmer, S. (2001). The value of self-practice of cognitive therapy techniques and self-reflection in the training of cognitive therapists. *Behavioural and Cognitive Psychotherapy, 29,* 203–220.

Beynon, S., Soares-Weiser, K., Woolacott, N., Duffy, S., & Geddes, J. R. (2008). Psychosocial interventions for the prevention of relapse in bipolar disorder: Systematic review of controlled trials. *British Journal of Psychiatry, 192,* 5–11.

Bieling, P. J., Beck, A. T., & Brown, G. K. (2000). The sociotropy–autonomy scale: Structure and implications. *Cognitive Therapy and Research, 24,* 763–780.

Bieling, P. J., & Kuyken, W. (2003). Is cognitive case formulation science or science fiction? *Clinical Psychology: Science and Practice, 10,* 52–69.

Blenkiron, P. (2005). Stories and analogies in cognitive-behaviour therapy: A clinical review. *Behavioural and Cognitive Psychotherapy, 33,* 45–59.

Borkovec, T. D. (2002). Life in the future versus life in the present. *Clinical Psychology: Science and Practice, 9,* 76–80.

Boyce, W. T., & Ellis, B. J. (2005). Biological sensitivity to context: I. An evolutionary-developmental theory of the origins and functions of stress reactivity. *Development and Psychopathology, 17,* 271–301.

Brewin, C. R., Dalgleish, T., & Joseph, S. (1996). A dual representation theory of posttraumatic stress disorder. *Psychological Review, 103,* 670–686.

Burbach, F., & Stanbridge, R. (2006). Somerset's family interventions in psychosis service: An update. *Journal of Family Therapy, 28,* 39–57.

Burns, D. D. (1989). *The feeling good handbook: Using the new mood therapy in everyday life.* New York: HarperCollins.

Burns, L. R., Dittmann, K., Nguyen, N. L., & Mitchelson, J. K. (2001). Academic procrastination, perfectionism, and control: Associations with vigilant and avoidant coping. *Journal of Social Behavior and Personality, 15,* 35–46.

Butler, A. C., Chapman, J. E., Forman, E. M., & Beck, A. T. (2006). The empirical status of cognitive-behavioral therapy: A review of meta-analyses. *Clinical Psychology Review, 26,* 17–31.

Butler, G. (1998). Clinical formulation. In A. S. Bellack & M. Hersen (Eds.), *Comprehensive clinical psychology* (pp. 1–24). New York: Pergamon Press.

Chadwick, P., Williams, C., & Mackenzie, J. (2003). Impact of case formulation in cognitive-behaviour therapy for psychosis. *Behaviour Research and Therapy, 41,* 671–680.

Chambless, D. L., & Gillis, M. M. (1993). Cognitive therapy of anxiety disorders. *Journal of Consulting and Clinical Psychology, 61,* 248–260.

Chambless, D. L., & Ollendick, T. H. (2001). Empirically supported psychological interventions: Controversies and evidence. *Annual Review of Psychology, 52,* 685–716.

Clark, D. A., Beck, A. T., & Alford, B. A. (1999). *Scientific foundations of cognitive theory and therapy of depression.* New York: Wiley.

Clark, D. M. (1986). A cognitive approach to panic. *Behaviour Research and Therapy, 24,* 461–470.

Clark, D. M. (1997). Panic disorder and social phobia. In D. M. Clark & C. G. Fairburn (Eds.), *Science and practice of cognitive behaviour therapy* (pp. 121–153). New York: Oxford University Press.

Clark, D. M., & Wells, A. (1995). A cognitive model of social phobia. In R. G. Heimberg, M. Liebowitz, D. Hope, & F. Scheier (Eds.), *Social phobia: Diagnosis, assessment and treatment* (pp. 69–93). New York: Guilford Press.

Clarkin, J. F., & Kendall, P. C. (1992). Comorbidity and treatment planning: Summary and future directions. *Journal of Consulting and Clinical Psychology, 60,* 904–908.

Craske, M. G., & Barlow, D. H. (2001). Panic disorder and agoraphobia. In D. H. Barlow (Ed.), *Clinical handbook of psychological disorders: A step-by-step treatment manual* (3rd ed., pp. 1–59). New York: Wiley.

Crits-Christoph, P. (1998). Changes in the CCRT pervasiveness during psychotherapy. In L. Luborsky & P. Crits-Christoph (Eds.), *Understanding transference: The Core Conflictual Relationship Theme method* (2nd ed., pp. 151–164). New York: Basic Books.

Crits-Christoph, P., Cooper, A., & Luborsky, L. (1988). The accuracy of therapists' interpretations and the outcome of dynamic psychotherapy. *Journal of Consulting and Clinical Psychology, 56,* 490–495.

Davis, D., & Padesky, C. (1989). Enhancing cognitive therapy for women. In A. Freeman, K. M. Simon, H. Arkowitz, & L. Beutler (Eds.), *Comprehensive handbook of cognitive therapy* (pp. 535–557). New York: Plenum Press.

Davis, N. (1999). *Resilience: Status of the research and research-based programs* [working draft]. Rockville, MD: U.S. Department of Health and Human Services, Substance Abuse, and Mental Health Services Administration, Center for Mental Health Services. As of October 2008, available from *www.mentalhealth.samhsa.gov/schoolviolence/5-28resilience.asp*

Denman, C. (1995). What is the point of a case formulation? In C. Mace (Ed.), *The art and science of assessment in psychotherapy* (pp. 167–181). London: Routledge.

DeRubeis, R. J., Brotman, M. A., & Gibbons, C. J. (2005). A conceptual and methodological analysis of the nonspecifics argument. *Clinical Psychology: Science and Practice, 12,* 174–183.

Dimidjian, S., Hollon, S.D., Dobson, K.S., Schmaling, K.B., Kohlenberg, R., Addis, M., Gallop, R., McGlinchey, J., Markley, D., Gollan, J.K., Atkins, D.C., Dunner, D.L., & Jacobson, N.S. (2006). Randomized trial of behavioral activation, cognitive therapy, and antidepressant medication in the acute treatment of adults with major depression. *Journal of Consulting and Clinical Psychology, 74*(4), 658–670.

Dobson, K. S. (1989). A meta-analysis of the efficacy of cognitive therapy for depression. *Journal of Consulting and Clinical Psychology, 57,* 414–419.

Eells, T. D. (Ed.). (2007). *Handbook of psychotherapy case formulation* (2nd ed.). New York: Guilford Press.

Eells, T. D., & Lombart, K. G. (2003). Case formulation and treatment concepts among novice, experienced, and expert cognitive-behavioral and psychodynamic therapists. *Psychotherapy Research, 13,* 187–204.

Eells, T. D., Lombart, K. G., Kendjelic, E. M., Turner, L. C., & Lucas, C. P. (2005). The quality of psychotherapy case formulations: A comparison of expert, experienced, and novice cognitive-behavioral and psychodynamic therapists. *Journal of Consulting and Clinical Psychology, 73,* 579–589.

Ehlers, A., & Clark, D. M. (2000). A cognitive model of posttraumatic stress disorder. *Behaviour Research and Therapy, 38,* 319–345.

Ehlers, A., Clark, D. M., Hackmann, A., McManus, F., & Fennell, M. (2005). Cognitive therapy for posttraumatic stress disorder: Development and evaluation. *Behaviour Research and Therapy, 43,* 413–431.

Ehlers, A., Hackmann, A., & Michael, T. (2004). Intrusive reexperiencing in posttraumatic disorder: Phenomenology, theory, and therapy. *Memory, 12,* 403–415.

Eifert, G. H., Schulte, D., Zvolensky, M. J., Lejucz, C. W., & Lau, A. W. (1997). Manualized behavior therapy: Merits and challenges. *Behavior Therapy, 28,* 499–509.

Emmelkamp, P. M. G., Visser, S., & Hoekstra, R. J. (1988). Cognitive therapy and exposure in vivo in the treatment of obsessive–compulsives. *Cognitive Therapy and Research, 12,* 103–114.

Epstein, N., & Baucom, D. H. (1989). Cognitive-behavioral marital therapy. In A. Freeman & K. M. Simon (Eds.), *Comprehensive handbook of cognitive therapy* (pp. 491–513). New York: Plenum Press.

Evans, J., & Parry, G. (1996). The impact of reformulation in cognitive-analytic therapy with difficult-to-help clients. *Clinical Psychology and Psychotherapy, 3,* 109–117.

Fairburn, C. G., Cooper, Z., & Shafran, R. (2003). Cognitive-behaviour therapy for eating disorders: A "trans-diagnostic" theory and treatment. *Behaviour Research and Therapy, 41,* 509–528.

Falender, C. A., & Shafranske, E. P. (2004). *Clinical supervision: A competency-based approach.* Washington, DC: American Psychological Association.

Fava, G. A., Ruini, C., & Belaise, C. (2007). The concept of recovery in major depression. *Psychological Medicine, 37,* 307–317.

Fava, M., Rush, A. J., Trivedi, M. H., Nierenberg, A. A., Thase, M. E., Sackeim, H. A., et al. (2003). Background and rationale for the Sequenced Treatment Alternatives to Relieve Depression (STAR*D) study. *Psychiatric Clinics of North America, 26,* 457–494.

Felsman, J. K., & Vaillant, G. E. (1987). Resilient children as adults: A 40-year study. In E. J. Anthony & B. J. Cohler (Eds.), *The invulnerable child* (pp. 289–314). New York: Guilford Press.

Ferster, C. B. (1973). A functional analysis of depression. *American Psychologist, 28,* 857–870.

Flitcroft, A., James, I. A., Freeston, M., & Wood-Mitchell, A. (2007). Determining what is important in a good formulation. *Behavioural and Cognitive Psychotherapy, 35,* 325–333.

Fothergill, C. D., & Kuyken, W. (2002). *The quality of cognitive case formulation rating scale*. Exeter, UK: Mood Disorders Centre. [Unpublished manuscript]

Fowler, D., Garety, P., & Kuipers, E. (1995). *Cognitive behavior therapy for psychosis: Theory and practice*. New York: Wiley.

Fredrickson, B. L. (2001). The role of positive emotions in positive psychology: The broaden-and-build theory of positive emotions. *American Psychologist, 56*, 218–226.

Frost, R., Steketee, G., Amir, N., Bouvard, M., Carmin, C., Clark, D. A., et al. (1997). Cognitive assessment of obsessive–compulsive disorder. *Behaviour Research and Therapy, 35*, 667–681.

Garb, H. N. (1998). *Studying the clinician: Judgment research and psychological assessment*. Washington, DC: American Psychological Association.

Garratt, G., Ingram, R. E., Rand, K. L., & Sawalani, G. (2007). Cognitive processes in cognitive therapy: Evaluation of the mechanisms of change in the treatment of depression. *Clinical Psychology: Science and Practice, 14*, 224–239.

Ghaderi, A. (2006). Does individualization matter? A randomized trial of standardized (focused) versus individualized (broad) cognitive-behavior therapy for bulimia nervosa. *Behaviour Research and Therapy, 44*, 273–288.

Gladis, M. M., Gosch, E. A., Dishuk, N. M., & Crits-Christoph, P. (1999). Quality of life: Expanding the scope of clinical significance. *Journal of Consulting and Clinical Psychology, 67*, 320–331.

Greenberger, D., & Padesky, C. A. (1995). *Mind over mood: Change how you feel by changing the way you think*. New York: Guilford Press.

Hackmann, A., Bennett-Levy, J., & Holmes, E. A. (in press). *The Oxford guide to imagery in cognitive therapy*. Oxford, UK: Oxford University Press.

Hamilton, K. E., & Dobson, K. S. (2002). Cognitive therapy of depression: Pretreatment patient predictors of outcome. *Clinical Psychology Review, 22*, 875–893.

Harper, A., & Power, M. (1998). Development of the World Health Organization WHOQOL-BREF quality of life assessment. *Psychological Medicine, 28*, 551–558.

Harvey, A. G., Bryant, R. A., & Tarrier, N. (2003). Cognitive-behaviour therapy for posttraumatic stress disorder. *Clinical Psychology Review, 23*, 501–522.

Harvey, A. G., Watkins, E., Mansell, W., & Shafran, R. (2004). *Cognitive-behavioural processes across psychological disorders: A transdiagnostic approach to research and treatment*. Oxford, UK: Oxford University Press.

Hayes, A. M., Laurenceau, J. P., Feldman, G., Strauss, J. L., & Cardaciotto, L. (2007). Change is not always linear: The study of nonlinear and discontinuous patterns of change in psychotherapy. *Clinical Psychology Review, 27*, 715–723.

Hayes, S. C. (1981). Single-case experimental design and empirical clinical practice. *Journal of Consulting and Clinical Psychology, 49*, 193–211.

Hayes, S. C., & Follette, W. C. (1992). Can functional analysis provide a substitute for syndromal classification? *Behavioral Assessment, 14*, 345–365.

Hays, P. A. (1995). Multicultural applications of cognitive-behavioral therapy. *Professional Psychology: Research and Practice, 25*, 309–315.

Hays, P. A., & Iwamasa, G. Y. (2006). *Culturally responsive cognitive-behavior therapy: Assessment, practice, and supervision*. Washington, DC: American Psychological Association.

Hollon, S. D., DeRubeis, R. J., Shelton, R. C., Amsterdam, J. D., Salomon, R. M., O'Reardon, J. P., et al. (2005). Prevention of relapse following cognitive therapy vs. medications in moderate to severe depression. *Archives of General Psychiatry, 62*, 417–422.

Holmbeck, G. N. (2003). Toward terminological, conceptual, and statistical clarity in the study of mediator and moderators: Examples from the child clinical and pediatric literatures. In A. E. Kazdin (Ed.), *Methodological issues and strategies in clinical research* (3rd ed., pp. 77–105). Washington, DC: American Psychological Association.

Horvath, A. O. (1994). Research on the alliance. In A. O. Horvath & L. S. Greenberg (Eds.), *The working alliance: Theory, research and practice* (pp. 259–287). New York: Wiley.

Horvath, A. O., & Greenberg, L. S. (Eds.). (1994). *The working alliance: Theory, research, and practice*. New York: Wiley.

Jacobson, N. S., Dobson, K. S., Truax, P. A., Addis, M. E., Koerner, K., Gollan, J. K., et al. (1996). A component analysis of cognitive-behavioral treatment for depression. *Journal of Consulting and Clinical Psychology, 64*, 295–304.

Jacobson, N. S., Martell, C. R., & Dimidjian, S. (2001). Behavioral activation treatment for depression: Returning to contextual roots. *Clinical Psychology: Science and Practice, 8*, 255–270.

Jacobson, N. S., Schmaling, K. B., Holtzworthmunroe, A., Katt, J. L., Wood, L. F., & Follette, V. M. (1989). Research-structured vs. clinically flexible versions of social learning-based marital therapy. *Behaviour Research and Therapy, 27*, 173–180.

James, I. (1999). Using a cognitive rationale to conceptualize anxiety in people with dementia. *Behavioural and Cognitive Psychotherapy, 27*, 345–351.

James, I. (2001). Psychological therapies and approaches in dementia. In C. G. Ballard, J. O'Brien, I. James, & A. Swann (Eds.), *Dementia: Management of behavioural and psychological symptoms*. New York: Oxford University Press.

James, I., Kendell, K., & Reichelt, F. K. (1999). Using a cognitive rationale to conceptualise anxiety in people with dementia. *Behavioural and Cognitive Psychotherapy, 27*, 345–351.

Judd, L. L., Paulus, M. P., Zeller, P., Fava, G. A., Rafanelli, C., Grandi, S., et al. (1999). The role of residual subthreshold depressive symptoms in early episode relapse in unipolar major depressive disorder. *Archives of General Psychiatry, 56*, 764–765.

Kabat-Zinn, J. (2004). *Wherever you go, there you are*. New York: Piatkus Books.

Kahneman, D. (2003). A perspective on judgment and choice: Mapping bounded rationality. *American Psychologist, 58*, 697–720.

Kendall, P. C., & Clarkin, J. F. (1992). Comorbidity and treatment implications: Introduction. *Journal of Consulting and Clinical Psychology, 60*, 833–834.

Kendjelic, E. M., & Eells, T. D. (2007). Generic psychotherapy case formulation training improves formulation quality. *Psychotherapy, 44*, 66–77.

Kernis, M. H., Brockner, J., & Frankel, B. S. (1989). Self-esteem and reactions to failure: The mediating role of overgeneralization. *Journal of Personality and Social Psychology, 57*, 707–714.

Kingdon, D. G., & Turkington, D. (2002). *A case study guide to cognitive therapy of psychosis.* Chichester, UK: Wiley.

Kohlenberg, R. J., & Tsai, M. (1991). *Functional analytic psychotherapy: Creating intense and curative therapeutic relationships.* New York: Springer.

Kraemer, H. C., Wilson, G. T., Fairburn, C. G., & Agras, W. S. (2002). Mediators and moderators of treatment effects in randomized clinical trials. *Archives of General Psychiatry, 59*, 877–883.

Kuyken, W. (2004). Cognitive therapy outcome: The effects of hopelessness in a naturalistic outcome study. *Behaviour Research and Therapy, 42*, 631–646.

Kuyken, W. (2006). Evidence-based case formulation: Is the emperor clothed? In N. Tarrier (Ed.), *Case formulation in cognitive behaviour therapy* (pp. 12–35). Hove, UK: Brunner-Routlege.

Kuyken, W., Fothergill, C. D., Musa, M., & Chadwick, P. (2005). The reliability and quality of cognitive case formulation. *Behaviour Research and Therapy, 43*, 1187–1201.

Kuyken, W., Kurzer, N., DeRubeis, R. J., Beck, A. T., & Brown, G. K. (2001). Response to cognitive therapy in depression: The role of maladaptive beliefs and personality disorders. *Journal of Consulting and Clinical Psychology, 69*, 560–566.

Kuyken, W., & Tsivrikos, D. (in press). Therapist competence, comorbidity and cognitive-behavioral therapy for depression. *Psychotherapy and Psychosomatics.*

Kuyken, W., Watkins, E., & Beck, A. T. (2005). Cognitive-behavior therapy for mood disorders. In G. Gabbard, J. S. Beck, & J. Holmes (Eds.), *Psychotherapy in psychiatric disorders* (pp. 113–128). Oxford, UK: Oxford University Press.

Lambert, M. J. (Ed.). (2004). *Bergin and Garfield's handbook of psychotherapy and behavior change* (5th ed.). New York: Wiley.

Lambert, M. J., Whipple, J. L., Hawkins, E. J., Vermeersch, D. A., Nielsen, S. L., & Smart, D. W. (2003). Is it time for clinicians to routinely track patient outcome? A meta-analysis. *Clinical Psychology: Science and Practice, 10*, 288–301.

Lau, M. A., Segal, Z. V., & Williams, J. M. (2004). Teasdale's differential activation hypothesis: Implications for mechanisms of depressive relapse and suicidal behaviour. *Behaviour Research and Therapy, 42*, 1001–1017.

Laurenceau, J. P., Hayes, A. M., & Feldman, G. C. (2007). Some methodological and statistical issues in the study of change processes in psychotherapy. *Clinical Psychology Review, 27*, 682–695.

Lewis, G. (2002). *Sunbathing in the rain: A cheerful book about depression.* London: Flamingo, HarperCollins.

Lewis, S. Y. (1994). Cognitive-behavioral therapy. In L. Comas-Díaz & B. Greene (Eds.), *Women of color: Integrating ethnic and gender identities in psychotherapy* (pp. 223–238). New York: Guilford Press.

Linehan, M. M. (1993). *Cognitive-behavioral treatment of borderline personality disorder.* New York: Guilford Press.

Lopez, S. J., & Synder, C. R. (2003). *Positive psychological assessment: A handbook of models and measures.* Washington, DC: American Psychological Association.

Luborsky, L., & Crits-Christoph, P. (1998). *Understanding transference: The Core Conflictual Relationship Theme method* (2nd ed.). New York: Basic Books.

Luborsky, L., Crits-Christoph, P., & Alexander, K. (1990). Repressive style and relationship patterns: Three samples inspected. In J. A. Singer (Ed.), *Repression and disassociation: Implications for personality theory, psychopathology, and health.* Chicago: University of Chicago Press.

Luborsky, L., & Diguer, L. (1998). The reliability of the CCRT measure: Results from eight samples. In L. Luborsky & P. Crits-Christoph (Eds.), *Understanding transference: The Core Conflictual Relationship Theme method* (2nd ed., pp. 97–108). New York: Basic Books.

Luthar, S. S., Cicchetti, D., & Becker, B. (2000). The construct of resilience: A critical evaluation and guidelines for future work. *Child Development, 71,* 543–562.

Lyubomirsky, S. (2001). Why are some people happier than others? The role of cognitive and motivational processes in well-being. *American Psychologist, 56,* 239–249.

Lyubomirsky, S., Sheldon, K. M., & Schkade, D. (2005). Pursuing happiness: The architecture of sustainable change. *Review of General Psychology, 9,* 111–131.

Martell, C. R., Addis, M. E., & Jacobson, N. S. (2001). *Depression in context: Strategies for guided action.* New York: Norton.

Martell, C. R., Safran, S. A., & Prince, S. E. (2004). *Cognitive-behavioral therapies with lesbian, gay, and bisexual clients.* New York: Guilford Press.

Masten, A. S. (2001). Ordinary magic: Resilience processes in development. *American Psychologist, 56,* 227–238.

Masten, A. S. (2007). Resilience in developing systems: Progress and promise as the fourth wave rises. *Development and Psychopathology, 19,* 921–930.

McCullough, J. P. (2000). *Treatment for chronic depression: Cognitive behavioural analysis system of psychotherapy (CBASP).* New York: Guilford Press.

Monroe, S. M., & Harkness, K. L. (2005). Life stress, the "kindling" hypothesis, and the recurrence of depression: Considerations from a life stress perspective. *Psychological Review, 112,* 417–445.

Mooney, K. A., & Padesky, C. A. (2002, July). *Cognitive therapy to build resilience.* Workshop presented at the annual meetings of British Association of Cognitive and Behavioural Psychotherapies, Warwick, UK.

Moras, K., Telfer, L. A., & Barlow, D. H. (1993). Efficacy and specific effects data on new treatments: A case study strategy with mixed anxiety-depression. *Journal of Consulting and Clinical Psychology, 61,* 412–420.

Morrison, A. (2002). *A casebook of therapy for psychosis.* New York: Brunner-Routledge.

Mumma, G. H., & Mooney, S. R. (2007). Comparing the validity of alternative cognitive case formulations: A latent variable, multivariate time series approach. *Cognitive Therapy and Research, 31,* 451–481.

Mumma, G. H., & Smith, J. L. (2001). Cognitive–behavioral–interpersonal scenarios: Interformulator reliability and convergent validity. *Journal of Psychopathology and Behavioral Assessment, 23,* 203–221.

Needleman, L. D. (1999). *Cognitive case conceptualization: A guidebook for practitioners.* Mahwah, NJ: Erlbaum.

Nelson-Gray, R. O., Herbert, J. D., Herbert, D. L., Sigmon, S. T., & Brannon, S. E. (1989). Effectiveness of matched, mismatched, and package treatments of depression. *Journal of Behavior Therapy and Experimental Psychiatry, 20,* 281–294.

Newman, C. F., Leahy, R. L., Beck, A. T., Reilly-Harrington, N. A., & Gyulai, L. (2002). *Bipolar disorder: A cognitive therapy approach.* Washington, DC: American Psychological Association.

Nolen-Hoeksema, S. (1991). Responses to depression and their effects on the duration of depressive episodes. *Journal of Abnormal Psychology, 100,* 569–582.

Nolen-Hoeksema, S. (2000). The role of rumination in depressive disorders and mixed anxiety/depressive symptoms. *Journal of Abnormal Psychology, 109,* 504–511.

Okiishi, J. C., Lambert, M. J., Nielsen, S. L., & Ogles, B. M. (2003). Waiting for supershrink: An empirical analysis of therapist effects. *Clinical Psychology and Psychotherapy, 10,* 352–360.

Okiishi, J. C., Lambert, M. J., Eggett, D., Nielsen, L., Dayton, D. D., & Vermeersch, D. A. (2006). An analysis of therapist treatment effects: Toward providing feedback to individual therapists on their clients' psychotherapy outcome. *Journal of Clinical Psychology, 62,* 1157–1172.

Ost, L. G., & Breitholtz, E. (2000). Applied relaxation vs. cognitive therapy in the treatment of generalized anxiety disorder. *Behaviour Research and Therapy, 38,* 777–790.

Pachankis, J. E., & Goldfried, M. R. (2007). On the next generation of process research. *Clinical Psychology Review, 27,* 760–768.

Padesky, C. A. (1990). Schema as self-prejudice. *International Cognitive Therapy Newsletter, 6,* 6–7. Retrieved October 13, 2008, from *www.padesky.com/clinicalcorner/pubs.htm*

Padesky, C. A. (1993, September). *Socratic questioning: Changing minds or guiding discovery?* Invited keynote address presented at the 1993 European Congress of Behaviour and Cognitive Therapies, London. Retrieved October 13, 2008, from *www.padesky.com/clinicalcorner/pubs.htm*

Padesky, C. A. (1994a). Schema change processes in cognitive therapy. *Clinical Psychology and Psychotherapy, 1,* 267–278. Retrieved October 13, 2008, from *www.padesky.com/clinicalcorner/pubs.htm*

Padesky, C. A. (1994b). For Milton H. Erickson Foundation and Center for Cognitive Therapy (co-producers). *Cognitive therapy for panic disorder: A client session* [DVD]. Huntington Beach, CA: Center for Cognitive Therapy. Available from *www.padesky.com.*

Padesky, C. A. (1996). Developing cognitive therapist competency: Teaching and supervision models. In P. M. Salkovskis (Ed.), *Frontiers of cognitive therapy* (pp. 266–292). New York: Guilford Press.

Padesky, C. A. (1997a). Center for Cognitive Therapy (Producer). *Collaborative case conceptualization: A client session* [DVD]. Huntington Beach, CA: Center for Cognitive Therapy. Available from *www.padesky.com*.

Padesky, C. A. (1997b). *Behavioral experiments: Testing the rules that bind* (Audio CD No. BEHX). Huntington Beach, CA: Center for Cognitive Therapy. Available from *www.padesky.com*.

Padesky, C. A. (2000). *Therapists' beliefs: Protocols, personalities, and guided exercises* (Audio CD No. TB1). Huntington Beach, CA: Center for Cognitive Therapy. Available from *www.padesky.com*.

Padesky, C. A. (2004). Center for Cognitive Therapy (Producer). *Constructing NEW underlying assumptions and behavioral experiments* [DVD]. Huntington Beach, CA: Center for Cognitive Therapy. Available from *www.padesky.com*.

Padesky, C. A. (2005, June). *The next phase: Building positive qualities with cognitive therapy.* Invited address at the International Congress of Cognitive Psychotherapy, Göteborg, Sweden.

Padesky, C. A. (2008). Center for Cognitive Therapy (Producer). *CBT for social anxiety* [DVD]. Huntington Beach, CA: Center for Cognitive Therapy. Available from *www.padesky.com*.

Padesky, C. A., & Greenberger, D. (1995). *Clinician's guide to Mind over Mood.* New York: Guilford Press.

Padesky, C. A., & Mooney, K. A. (1990). Clinical tip: Presenting the cognitive model to clients. *International Cognitive Therapy Newsletter, 6,* 13–14. Retrieved October 13, 2008, from *www.padesky.com/clinicalcorner/pubs.htm*

Padesky, C. A., & Mooney, K. A. (2006). *Uncover strengths and build resilience using cognitive therapy: A four-step model.* Workshop presented for the New Zealand College of Clinical Psychologists in Auckland, New Zealand.

Perepletchikova, F., & Kazdin, A. E. (2005). Treatment integrity and therapeutic change: Issues and research recommendations. *Clinical Psychology: Science and Practice, 12,* 365–383.

Persons, J. B. (1989). *Cognitive therapy in practice: A case formulation approach.* New York: Norton.

Persons, J. B. (2005). Empiricism, mechanism, and the practice of cognitive-behavior therapy. *Behavior Therapy, 36,* 107–118.

Persons, J. B., & Bertagnolli, A. (1999). Interrater reliability of cognitive-behavioral case formulations of depression: A replication. *Cognitive Therapy and Research, 23,* 271–283.

Persons, J. B., Mooney, K. A., & Padesky, C. A. (1995). Interrater reliability of cognitive-behavioral case formulations. *Cognitive Therapy and Research, 19,* 21–34.

Persons, J. B., Roberts, N. A., Zalecki, C. A., & Brechwald, W. A. G. (2006). Naturalistic outcome of case formulation-driven cognitive-behavior therapy for anxious depressed outpatients. *Behaviour Research and Therapy, 44,* 1041–1051.

Power, M. J., & Dalgleish, T. (1997). *Cognition and emotion: From order to disorder.* Hove, UK: Psychology Press.

Raue, P. J., & Goldfried, M. R. (1994). The therapeutic alliance in cognitive-behavioral therapy. In A. O. Horvath & L. S. Greenberg (Eds.), *The working alliance: Theory, research and practice* (pp. 131–152). New York: Wiley.

Riskind, J. H., Williams, N. L., Gessner, T. L., Chrosniak, L. D., & Cortina, J. M. (2000). The looming maladaptive style: Anxiety, danger, and schematic processing. *Journal of Personality and Social Psychology, 79*, 837–852.

Roth, A., & Fonagy, P. (2005). *What works for whom?: A critical review of psychotherapy research* (2nd ed.). New York: Guilford Press.

Roth, A., & Pilling, S. (2007). *The CBT competences framework for depression and anxiety disorders.* London: Centre for Outcome Research and Evaluation.

Rutter, M. (1987). Psychosocial resilience and protective mechanisms. *American Journal of Orthopsychiatry, 57*, 316–331.

Rutter, M. (1999). Resilience concepts and findings: Implications for family therapy. *Journal of Family Therapy, 21*, 119–144.

Ryff, C. D., & Singer, B. (1996). Psychological well-being: Meaning, measurement, and implications for psychotherapy research. *Psychotherapy and Psychosomatics, 65*, 14–23.

Ryff, C. D., & Singer, B. (1998). The contours of positive human health. *Psychological Inquiry, 9*, 1–28.

Safran, J. D., Segal, Z. V., Vallis, T. M., Shaw, B. F., & Samstag, L. W. (1993). Assessing patient suitability for short-term cognitive therapy with an interpersonal focus. *Cognitive Therapy and Research, 17*, 23–38.

Salkovskis, P. M. (1999). Understanding and treating obsessive–compulsive disorder. *Behaviour Research and Therapy, 37*, S29–S52.

Salkovskis, P. M., & Warwick, H. M. C. (2001). Making sense of hypochondriasis: A cognitive model of health anxiety. In G. J. G. Admundson, S. Taylor, & B. J. Cox (Eds.), *Health anxiety: Clinical and research perspectives on hypochondriasis and related conditions* (pp. 46–63). New York: Wiley.

Sanavio, E. (1980). Obsessions and compulsions: The Padua Inventory. *Behaviour Research and Therapy, 26*, 169–177.

Schneider, B. H., & Byrne, B. M. (1987). Individualizing social skills training for behaviour-disordered children. *Journal of Consulting and Clinical Psychology, 55*, 444–445.

Schulte, D., & Eifert, G. H. (2002). What to do when manuals fail? The dual model of psychotherapy. *Clinical Psychology: Science and Practice, 9*, 312–328.

Schulte, D., Kunzel, R., Pepping, G., & Shulte-Bahrenberg, T. (1992). Tailor-made versus standardized therapy of phobic patients. *Advances in Behaviour Research and Therapy, 14*, 67–92.

Seligman, M. E. P. (2002). *Authentic happiness: Using the new positive psychology to realize your potential for lasting fulfillment.* New York: Free Press.

Seligman, M. E. P., & Csikszentmihalyi, M. (2000). Positive psychology: An introduction. *American Psychologist, 55*, 5–14.

Shadish, W. R., Matt, G. E., Navarro, A. M., & Phillips, G. (2000). The effects of psychological therapies under clinically representative conditions: A meta-analysis. *Psychological Bulletin, 126*, 512–529.

Shaw, B. F., Elkin, I., Yamaguchi, J., Olmsted, M., Vallis, T. M., Dobson, K. S., et al. (1999). Therapist competence ratings in relation to clinical outcome in cognitive therapy for depression. *Journal of Consulting and Clinical Psychology, 67*, 837–846.

Sloman, L., Gilbert, P., & Hasey, G. (2003). Evolved mechanisms in depression: The role and interaction of attachment and social rank in depression. *Journal of Affective Disorders, 74*, 107–121.

Snyder, C. R., & Lopez, S. J. (2005). *Handbook of positive psychology*. New York: Oxford University Press.

Strauman, T. J., Vieth, A. Z., Merrill, K. A., Kolden, G. G., Woods, T. E., Klein, M. H., et al. (2006). Self-system therapy as an intervention for self-regulatory dysfunction in depression: A randomized comparison with cognitive therapy. *Journal of Consulting and Clinical Psychology, 74*, 367–376.

Tang, T. Z., & DeRubeis, R. J. (1999). Sudden gains and critical sessions in cognitive-behavioral therapy for depression. *Journal of Consulting and Clinical Psychology, 67*, 894–904.

Tarrier, N. (2006). *Case formulation in cognitive behaviour therapy: The treatment of challenging and complex cases*. Hove, UK: Routledge.

Tarrier, N., & Wykes, T. (2004). Is there evidence that cognitive behaviour therapy is an effective treatment for schizophrenia? A cautious or cautionary tale? *Behaviour Research and Therapy, 42*, 1377–1401.

Teasdale, J. D. (1993). Emotion and two kinds of meaning: Cognitive therapy and applied cognitive science. *Behavior Research and Therapy, 31*, 339–354.

Thich Nhat Hahn. (1975). *The miracle of mindfulness*. Boston: Beacon Press.

Truax, C. B. (1966). Reinforcement and nonreinforcement in Rogerian psychotherapy. *Journal of Abnormal Psychology, 71*, 1–9.

van Oppen, P., & Arntz, A. (1994). Cognitive therapy for obsessive–compulsive disorder. *Behaviour Research and Therapy, 32*, 79–87.

van Oppen, P., de Haan, E., van Balkom, A. J. L., Spinhoven, P., Hoogduin, K., & van Dyck, R. (1995). Cognitive therapy and exposure in vivo in the treatment of obsessive–compulsive disorder. *Behavior Research and Therapy, 33*, 379–390.

Warwick, H. M., Clark, D. M., Cobb, A. M., & Salkovskis, P. M. (1996). A controlled trial of cognitive-behavioural treatment of hypochondriasis. *British Journal of Psychiatry, 169*, 189–195.

Watkins, E., & Moulds, M. (2005). Distinct modes of ruminative self-focus: Impact of abstract versus concrete rumination on problem solving in depression. *Emotion, 5*, 319–328.

Watkins, E., Scott, J., Wingrove, J., Rimes, K., Bathurst, N., Steiner, H., et al. (2007). Rumination-focused cognitive behaviour therapy for residual depression: A case series. *Behaviour Research and Therapy, 45*, 2144–2154.

Weissman, A. N., & Beck, A. T. (1978). *Development and validation of the Dysfunctional Attitudes Scale: A preliminary investigation*. Paper presented at the American Educational Research Association, Toronto, Canada.

Wells, A. (2004). A cognitive model of GAD. In R. G. Heimberg, C. L. Turk, & D. S. Mennin (Eds.), *Generalized anxiety disorder: Advances in research and practice* (pp. 164–186). New York: Guilford Press.

Wells-Federman, C. L., Stuart-Shor, E., & Webster, A. (2001). Cognitive therapy: Applications for health promotion, disease prevention, and disease management. *Nursing Clinics of North America, 36*, 93–113.

Westbrook, D., Kennerley, H., & Kirk, J. (2007). *An introduction to cognitive behaviour therapy: Skills and applications*. London: Sage.

Wheatley, J., Brewin, C. R., Patel, T., Hackmann, A., Wells, A., Fisher, P., et al. (2007). "I'll believe it when I can see it": Imagery rescripting of intrusive sensory memories in depression. *Journal of Behavior Therapy and Experimental Psychiatry, 38*, 371–385.

Williams, C. (1997). A cognitive model of dysfunctional illness behaviour. *British Journal of Health Psychology, 2*, 153–165.

Wright, J. H., Kingdon, D. G., Turkington, D., & Basco, M. R. (2008). *CBT for severe mental illness*. Arlington, VA: American Psychiatric Publishing.

Young, J. E. (1999). *Cognitive therapy for personality disorders: A schema-focused approach* (3rd ed.). Sarasota, FL: Professional Resource Press.

Zigler, E., & Phillips, L. (1961). Psychiatric diagnosis: A critique. *Journal of Abnormal and Social Psychology, 63*, 607–618.

Zimmerman, M., McGlinchey, J. B., Chelminski, I., & Young, D. (2008). Diagnostic comorbidity in 2,300 psychiatric outpatients presenting for treatment evaluated with a semistructured diagnostic interview. *Psychological Medicine, 38*, 199–210.

Zimmerman, M., McGlinchey, J. B., Posternak, M. A., Friedman, M., Attiullah, N., & Boerescu, D. (2006). How should remission from depression be defined?: The depressed patient's perspective. *American Journal of Psychiatry, 163*, 148–150.

Index

ABC Model. *See also* Functional analysis
  levels of conceptualization and, 43*f*
  low mood and, 174–176, 176*f*,
    180–181, 180*f*
  overview, 139–144, 142*f*, 173
  resilience and, 188–189, 188*f*
  supervision and consultation and,
    296–297
Aid to History Taking Form, 135–137,
  160–170, 224–225, 327–339
Alliance, therapy. *See* Therapy alliance
Antecedents, 139–140, 177*f*, 188*f*. *See also*
  ABC Model; Triggers
Anxiety
  assessment and, 137
  automatic thoughts related to, 77
  case examples of, 31–35, 75–82
  cognitive models of, 5, 16, 18
  collaboration and, 269
  collaborative empiricism and, 71–72
  competencies and, 261–262, 273, 280,
    293–294
  health anxiety, 43–44, 209–213, 212*f*,
    221, 234
  modes and, 13
  obsessive–compulsive disorder (OCD)
    and, 205–206, 206*f*
  physical factors and, 85
  social anxiety, 77, 293–294
Anxiety disorders, 13, 17–18
Assessment
  biopsychosocial assessment, 133–135
  case conceptualization and, 9
  collaboration during, 133–137

descriptive conceptualization and, 27,
    83
  diagnosis and, 151–152
  levels of conceptualization and, 27
  measures of, 65, 135–137, 137–138,
    160–170. *See also specific measures*
  presenting issues and, 133–138
  strengths and, 56, 126, 304, 308–309
Assumptions, underlying. *See also* Beliefs
  developmental view of, 229*f*
  identifying, 87–88
  levels of conceptualization and, 42*f*, 43*f*
  longitudinal conceptualization and,
    232*f*, 234–236, 245*f*, 246*f*
  overview, 14–15, 87–88
  resilience and, 108
Automatic thoughts. *See also* Beliefs;
    Intrusive thoughts; Thought Record
  case example of, 36–39, 37*f*, 38*f*
  core beliefs and, 88
  empiricism and, 75
  identifying, 86–87
  longitudinal conceptualization and, 221
  overview, 12, 14, 16–18, 85, 86–87
  positive automatic thoughts, 198–199
  underlying assumptions and, 15
Avoidance
  ABC Model and, 140–144, 147
  automatic thoughts and, 251
  core beliefs and, 89
  curiosity and, 69
  generalized anxiety disorder and, 18
  identifying, 124–125
  low mood and, 154, 182–192

Avoidance (*cont.*)
    maintenance factors and, 39, 158, 183,
        184–189, 185*f*, 187*f*, 188*f*, 190, 194,
        198, 205–206
    nonresponse to therapy and, 9
    OCD and, 211

B

Beck Anxiety Inventory (BAI), 137–138
Beck Depression Inventory—II (BDI-II),
    137–138
Beck scales, 115, 137–138
Behavior. *See also* ABC Model;
    Maintenance factors; Safety
    behaviors
    assessment and, 137, 139
    automatic thoughts and, 16
    biopsychosocial assessment and, 134
    case conceptualization and, 7–8, 19,
        308–309, 313, 322
    collaborative empiricism and, 44, 279
    cross-sectional conceptualization and,
        35–39, 172
    cultural context and, 309
    descriptive conceptualization and,
        31–35, 33*f*, 149–151, 150*f*, 158
    developmental history and, 12, 225,
        233
    diagnosis and, 152
    empiricism and, 68
    fit and, 184
    in the five-part model, 146–147
    five-part model and, 83–84, 144,
        146–147, 148
    goal setting and, 154
    interventions and, 235, 311
    learning to conceptualize and, 256, 275,
        276, 277, 277*f*, 287
    levels of conceptualization and, 27, 31,
        42–44, 43*f*
    longitudinal conceptualization and, 242
    low mood and, 177*f*, 181, 188*f*, 198,
        205–206, 206*f*
    metaphors, stories and images and, 109,
        113*f*
    modes and, 13
    nonresponse to therapy and, 9
    OCD and, 207, 209–211, 212–213, 214
    overview, 85–91, 91*f*, 140
    presenting issues and, 223
    resilience and, 180, 180*f*, 240
    strategies and, 15–16
    strengths and, 97, 99, 103, 105–107,
        106*f*, 120, 284
    therapy structure and, 65–66
    top-down criteria and, 318, 319
    triggers and, 176–177, 177*f*
    underlying assumptions and, 15
    values and, 240
Behavioral activation, 9, 114, 132, 190
Behavioral experiments
    behavioral activation, 190–191
    case conceptualization and, 92
    case example of, 70–71, 80–82, 81*f*, 82*f*
    client observation and, 83
    collaborative empiricism and, 278
    competencies and, 261, 262, 265
    empiricism and, 75–82, 80*f*, 81*f*, 82*f*
    interventions based on
        conceptualizations and, 234
    learning to conceptualize and, 276,
        288–289, 297, 298
    low mood and, 198–199
    OCD and, 221, 222
    outside of sessions, 83
    overview, 192
    strengths and, 101
    underlying assumptions and, 192–193
Behavioral theory, 139
Beliefs. *See also* Automatic thoughts; Biases;
        Core beliefs; Underlying assumptions
    alternative, 234–236, 239
    automatic thoughts, 16–18, 86–87
    case example of, 80–82, 81*f*, 82*f*
    core beliefs, 13–14, 88–89, 229*f*, 232*f*,
        245*f*, 246*f*
    levels of conceptualization and, 42*f*, 43*f*
    longitudinal conceptualization and,
        224–225, 234–236
    low mood and, 195, 196–200, 196*f*, 197*f*
    resilience and, 107–108, 118–119
    strategies and, 15–16
    strengths and, 97
    in teaching and supervision, 297–298
    top-down criteria and, 12–13
    underlying assumptions, 14–15, 87–88
Bennett-Levy model of learning, 253,
    254*f*, 299
Biases
    case conceptualization crucible and,
        320–321
    decision-making errors, 45–49, 48*f*,
        69–70, 317–318, 320–321

heuristic bias, 45–46, 71, 158, 313, 321
in teaching and supervision, 297–298
Biopsychosocial assessment, 133–138
Bottom-up criteria, 12, 18–23, 319–325

C

Case Conceptualization Diagram, 19
Case conceptualization in general. *See also* Collaborative empiricism; Crucible model; Descriptive conceptualizations; Empiricism; Explanatory conceptualizations; Levels of conceptualization; Longitudinal conceptualizations
applicability of, 310–313
characteristics of, 306–310
cross-sectional, 35–39, 37*f*, 38*f*
defined, 3–5, 3*f*, 319–320
descriptive, 31–35, 33*f*, 121–122
evaluating, 313–325
fit, 184–189, 185*f*, 187*f*, 188*f*, 209, 241–244, 245*f*–246*f*
functions, 5–10, 149
goal setting and, 152–157
longitudinal, 39–41, 40*f*
measuring, 320
models of, 42–43, 43*f*
operationalizing, 319–320
overview, 306–310, 325–326
principles, 26–29
resilience and, 105–114, 106*f*, 112*f*, 113*f*, 114–117
strengths and, 101–103, 102*f*
Cognitive Therapy Rating Scale, 292
Cognitive-behavioral therapy research
case conceptualization crucible and, 3–5, 3*f*, 307, 311
descriptive conceptualization and, 138–152, 142*f*, 145*f*, 150*f*
empiricism and, 49–50
functions of case conceptualization and, 5
improvements in therapy and outcomes and, 20–22
nonresponse to therapy and, 9
resilience and, 105
Cognitive-behavioral therapy theory
case conceptualization crucible and, 3–5, 3*f*, 307, 311
descriptive conceptualization and, 138–152, 142*f*, 145*f*, 150*f*

empiricism and, 49–50
functions of case conceptualization and, 5, 56
longitudinal conceptualization and, 224–234, 229*f*, 232*f*
resilience and, 105
top-down criteria and, 12–18
Collaboration. *See also* Collaborative empiricism
during assessment, 133–137
competencies and, 250
goal setting and, 152–157
learning to conceptualize and, 260, 263–264, 278–282, 300–301
longitudinal conceptualization and, 243
overview, 28, 52–54, 61–68, 92, 307–308
Collaborative empiricism. *See also* Collaboration; Empiricism
case conceptualization crucible and, 3*f*, 4–5, 307–308
case example of, 70–71, 75–82, 279–281
descriptive conceptualization and, 158
five-part model and, 83–92, 91*f*
learning to conceptualize and, 260, 263–264, 278–282, 300–301
overview, 28, 44–54, 48*f*, 92
Comorbidity, 1, 2, 7, 23, 45, 315, 318–319
Competencies
anxiety and, 261–262, 273, 280, 293–294
assessment, 298–299
behavioral experiments and, 261, 262, 265
case conceptualization crucible and, 320–321
case example of, 269, 276–278
collaboration and, 250
conceptualization as a high-level skill and, 249–253, 249*f*
diagnosis and, 265
evidence base and, 262, 265, 266
five-part model and, 261, 264, 265, 300, 302
functional analysis and, 261, 265
imagery and, 266, 303
individualized treatment and, 262, 314
maintenance factors and, 302
metaphors and, 266, 301, 303

Competencies (*cont.*)
  obsessive–compulsive disorder (OCD)
    and, 265, 267
  outcomes and, 250, 266
  panic disorder and, 265
  personality disorder and, 267
  presenting issues and, 250–251, 261,
    262, 263, 265, 266, 267, 270–271,
    272, 302–303
  relapse and, 250, 262, 264, 265, 266
  safety behaviors and, 265
  Socratic dialogue and, 261, 262, 300
  strategies and, 258–292, 277*f*, 301, 308
  supervision and, 292–294
  therapist, 249–253, 249*f*, 258–292,
    277*f*, 320–321
  training and, 249–250
  triggers and, 253, 256, 302
Conceptualization. *See* Case
  conceptualization in general
Consultation
  case conceptualization crucible and,
    312, 321
  case example of, 46–48
  decision-making errors and, 51
  functions of case conceptualization and,
    9–10
  learning to conceptualize and, 273–275,
    292–298
  longitudinal conceptualization and,
    244, 245*f*–246*f*
  reflective learning and, 256
Coping methods, 182–184, 198–199, 229,
  236–239, 237*f*
Core beliefs. *See also* Beliefs
  developmental view of, 229*f*
  longitudinal conceptualization and,
    232*f*, 245*f*, 246*f*
  overview, 13–14, 88–89
Core Conflictual Relationship Theme
  (CCRT), 10–11, 19–20, 23
Cross-sectional conceptualizations. *See also*
  Explanatory conceptualizations
  development of, 172–173, 173*f*
  flexibility and, 43
  interventions based on, 189–192
  learning to conceptualize and, 264–267
  linking of presenting issues and,
    213–214, 213*f*
  longitudinal conceptualization and, 222
  low mood and, 174–200, 176*f*, 177*f*,
    180*f*, 185*f*, 187*f*, 188*f*, 196*f*, 197*f*
  outcomes of, 214–215

overview, 35–39, 37*f*, 38*f*, 171–172,
  215–216
resilience and, 105, 120
Crucible model. *See also* Case
  conceptualization in general
  applicability of, 310–313
  case conceptualization and, 3–5, 3*f*, 23
  CBT and, 18
  characteristics of, 306–310
  clients and, 83–92, 91*f*
  collaborative empiricism and, 158
  descriptive conceptualization and,
    122–138
  empiricism and, 68, 75
  evaluating, 313–325
  explanatory conceptualization and, 172,
    184, 206, 214–215
  outcomes of, 214–215
  overview, 25–58, 60–61, 159, 325–326
  principles of case conceptualization and,
    26–29
  theory and research and, 138–152
  usefulness and applicability of, 310–313
Culture
  case conceptualization crucible and, 309
  case example of, 75–82, 80*f*, 81*f*, 82*f*
  overview, 84–85
  as a source of strength, 100–101
Curiosity, 69–71, 128–129

D

Decision-making errors, 45–49, 48*f*, 51,
  69–70, 317–318. *See also* Biases
Declarative learning, 254–255, 254*f*,
  259–260, 271–272
Depression
  case example of, 31–35
  CBT and, 17
  cognitive models of, 16
  explanatory conceptualization and,
    174–200, 176*f*, 177*f*, 180*f*, 185*f*,
    187*f*, 188*f*, 196*f*, 197*f*
  longitudinal conceptualization and,
    233–234, 242–243
  nonresponse to therapy and, 9
  onset, 181–182, 233–234
  prioritization of presenting issues and,
    131–132
Descriptive conceptualizations, 121–170.
  See also Case conceptualization in
  general
  Aid to History Taking Form, 160–170

cognitive-behavioral therapy theory
and, 138–152, 142*f*, 145*f*, 150*f*
goal setting and, 152–157
learning to conceptualize and, 264–267
overview, 31–35, 33*f*, 121–122,
157–159
presenting issues and, 122–138
resilience and, 105, 120
Developmental history, 39–41, 40*f*,
224–234, 229*f*, 232*f*, 245*f*, 246*f*
Diagnosis. *See also specific diagnoses*
biopsychosocial assessment and, 134
case conceptualization and, 2, 25–26,
30, 77, 210, 314
clinical summary and, 151–152
collaborative empiricism and, 269
comorbidity and, 2, 318–319
competencies and, 265
declarative learning, 254
evidence-based theories and, 203
explanatory conceptualization and,
203–204
multiple, 75, 318
strengths and, 285
supervision and consultation and, 294,
298
Dysfunctional Attitude Scale, 50

E

Emotional factors, 77, 85–91, 91*f*,
144–146, 145*f*
Empiricism. *See also* Collaborative
empiricism
case conceptualization crucible and, 3*f*,
4, 318–325
learning to conceptualize and, 260,
263–264, 278–281, 300–301
overview, 28, 44–54, 48*f*, 68–83, 80*f*,
81*f*, 82*f*, 92
Engagement, 6–7, 115–116, 311
Environmental factors, 144–146, 145*f*
Evidence base. *See also* Research
bottom-up criteria and, 18–23, 319
case conceptualization and, 11–12,
26, 45, 50, 77–78, 138–139, 311,
314–316
client experience and, 172–173
competencies and, 262, 265, 266
curiosity and, 71
descriptive conceptualization and, 31
empiricism and, 68–69, 71–75
fit and, 184–189, 185*f*, 187*f*, 188*f*

learning to conceptualize and, 279,
282
levels of conceptualization and, 41–42
overview, 5, 11–23
prioritization of presenting issues and,
131–132
top-down criteria and, 12–18, 318–319
treatment manuals, 25
treatment plans, 145
triggers and, 216
Expertise, therapist, 258–292, 277*f*,
320–321. *See also* Competencies
Explanatory conceptualizations, 171–216.
See also Case conceptualization
in general; Cross-sectional
conceptualizations
case example of, 37–39
interventions based on, 189–192
learning to conceptualize and, 264–267
levels of conceptualization and, 43
linking of presenting issues and,
213–214, 213*f*
longitudinal conceptualization and, 222
low mood and, 174–200, 176*f*, 177*f*,
180*f*, 185*f*, 187*f*, 188*f*, 196*f*, 197*f*
obsessional worries and, 200–213, 203*f*,
206*f*, 212*f*
outcomes of, 214–215
overview, 16–18, 171–172, 215–216
resilience and, 105, 120

F

Families and couples, 312–313
Family history, 134, 328–331. *See also*
Developmental history; Personal
history
Five-part model
case example of, 47–48
competencies and, 261, 264, 265, 300,
302
descriptive conceptualization and, 138,
157
goal setting and, 152, 154–155
heuristics and, 47
learning needs and, 264
levels of conceptualization and, 43*f*
low mood and, 176–177
overview, 31–35, 33*f*, 83–92, 91*f*, 139,
144–151, 145*f*, 150*f*, 173
presenting issues and, 159, 255
reflective learning and, 277, 278
strengths and, 105, 106, 106*f*

Functional analysis
    ABC Model, 139–144, 142*f*
    case conceptualization and, 322–323
    competencies and, 261, 265
    cross-sectional conceptualization and,
        36, 174, 176*f*
    descriptive conceptualization and, 138,
        157, 159
    goal setting and, 152, 154
    learning needs and, 291
    learning to conceptualize and, 302
    levels of conceptualization and, 43*f*, 264
    low mood and, 150, 174–176, 176*f*
    maintenance factors and, 180*f*, 228–229
    overview, 139–140, 141–142, 142*f*,
        144, 313
    procedural learning, 255
    resilience and, 105
    supervision and consultation and,
        296–297

G

Goal setting, 152–157, 269–271
Goals of therapy
    Aid to History Taking Form, 160–161,
        328
    assessment of progress towards, 44
    biopsychosocial assessment and, 134
    case conceptualization and, 8, 24,
        27–28, 250, 258, 307, 311, 315,
        316–317, 318, 320, 322, 325, 326
    collaboration and, 53, 61, 64, 65
    collaborative empiricism and, 290–291
    descriptive conceptualization and, 122,
        137, 143, 158
    engagement and, 6
    explanatory conceptualization and,
        214–215
    goal setting and, 152–157
    learning to conceptualize and, 258, 264,
        269–272, 278, 279, 283, 290–291,
        298–299
    levels of conceptualization and, 42
    longitudinal conceptualization and, 41,
        222, 247
    metaphors, stories and images and, 112
    outcomes and, 21
    overview, 5, 114–117, 159
    presenting issues and, 224, 240, 241
    strengths and, 55–56, 95–97, 101,
        114–119, 120

    therapy alliance and, 106
    values and, 240
Guided discovery, 179, 284

H

Health anxiety
    case conceptualization and, 316
    onset, 234
    overview, 43–44, 209–213, 212*f*, 221, 225
Heuristics. *See also* Biases; Decision-
        making errors
    case conceptualization and, 214,
        309–310, 313
    collaborative empiricism and, 158, 321
    empiricism and, 45–46, 48, 49, 51, 71
    learning to conceptualize and, 321
    outcomes and, 323
    reflective learning and, 275
    teaching and supervision and, 297
History. *See* Developmental history; Family
        history; Personal history
Homework assignments
    ABC Model, 176
    collaboration and, 54, 63
    completion of, 251, 253, 256, 257
    OCD and, 207–208
    strengths and, 103
    therapy structure and, 65
    Thought Record and, 196*f*
Hypothesis testing, 30–31, 50, 72–74,
        76–80, 80*f*

I

Idiographic dialectic, 314–316
Imagery
    anxiety and, 70, 147, 252, 253–254,
        258
    competencies and, 266, 303
    longitudinal conceptualization and, 236
    overview, 89–91, 91*f*
    resilience and, 109–114, 112*f*, 113*f*, 237
Interrater agreement. *See* Reliability
Interventions. *See also* Therapy
    based on explanatory
        conceptualizations, 189–192,
        206–208
    case conceptualization crucible and, 311
    longitudinal conceptualization and,
        223–244, 224*f*, 229*f*, 232*f*, 234–244,
        237*f*, 245*f*–246*f*

low mood and, 189–200, 196f, 197f
obsessional worries and, 206–208
strengths and, 103
Intrusive thoughts, 202–203, 203f,
205–208, 206f. *See also* Automatic
thoughts

L

Learning to conceptualize. *See also*
Teaching
assess learning needs, 259–269
case example of, 269, 276–278,
279–281, 289–290
collaborative empiricism and, 300–301
conceptualization as a high-level skill,
249–253, 249f
declarative learning, 254–255, 254f
evaluating competency/learning
progress, 290–293
levels of conceptualization and,
302–303
overview, 248–249, 253–258, 254f,
258f, 298–299
procedural learning, 254f, 255–256
professional development and, 257–258
reflective learning, 254f, 256–257
strategies for developing expertise,
258–292, 277f
strengths and, 304–305
supervision and consultation and,
292–298
Levels of conceptualization
cross-sectional, 35–39, 37f, 38f
descriptive, 31–35, 33f
flexibility in, 41–44, 42f, 43f
learning to conceptualize and, 264–267,
281–282, 302–303
longitudinal, 39–41, 40f
overview, 4–5, 27–44, 30f, 33f, 37f, 38f,
40f, 42f, 43f
strengths and resilience and, 119, 120
Longitudinal conceptualizations, 217–247.
See also Case conceptualization in
general
construction of, 223–244, 224f, 229f,
232f, 237f, 245f–246f
fit and, 241–244, 245f–246f
flexibility and, 43
interventions based on, 234–244, 237f
overview, 39–41, 40f, 217–221, 220f,
244, 247

reasons to use, 222–223
resilience and, 105, 120
strengths and, 308–309

M

Maintenance factors
case conceptualization and, 52, 56, 60,
158, 273–274
competencies and, 302
cross-sectional conceptualization and,
176–189, 177f, 185f, 187f, 188f,
191, 192–193, 197f, 199, 204, 211,
215–216
developmental view of, 228–229, 229f
explanatory conceptualization and,
42–43, 172, 173
fit and, 184–189, 185f, 187f, 188f
identifying, 204–206
learning to conceptualize and, 264–
267
longitudinal conceptualization and,
222–223, 245f, 246f
low mood and, 182–184, 191–192
OCD and, 207, 213
overview, 35–39, 37f, 38f, 172, 194
presenting issues and, 213–214, 213f,
308
procedural learning, 255–256
resilience and, 105, 119–120
strengths and, 101
Manualized treatment, 21, 22, 314–316
Metacompetencies, 249f, 250. *See also*
Competencies, therapist
Metaphors
case conceptualization and, 284
clients and, 83
collaboration and, 308–309, 317
competencies and, 266, 301, 303
cross-sectional conceptualization and,
212
learning to conceptualize and, 270, 280,
281
overview, 89–91, 91f, 92
resilience and, 109–114, 112f, 113f
Mind Over Mood (Greenberger & Padesky,
1995), 83
Modes
declarative learning, 254
learning modes, 271
overview, 12, 13, 14–15
values and, 240

Moods
    explanatory conceptualization and,
        174–200, 176f, 177f, 180f, 185f,
        187f, 188f, 196f, 197f
    in the five-part model, 145f
    longitudinal conceptualization and,
        242–243

N

Nonresponse to therapy, 9, 64, 312
Normalization of client's experiences, 5–6,
    149, 208–209, 311, 323
Notebook, therapy, 103, 127

O

Obsessional worries, 200–213, 203f, 206f,
    212f, 242–243
Obsessive–compulsive disorder (OCD)
    case conceptualization and, 311
    case example of, 289–290
    competencies and, 265, 267
    diagnosis and, 152
    empiricism and, 316
    explanatory conceptualization and,
        203–213, 203f, 206f, 212f, 214–215
    health anxiety and, 149
    longitudinal conceptualization and,
        221, 233, 242–243
    onset, 234
    resilience and, 236–237
    values and, 289
Outcomes
    assessment and, 44, 137–138, 315–316
    bottom-up criteria and, 18–19, 319
    case conceptualization and, 12, 20–22,
        51–52, 55–56, 310, 313–314, 317
    case conceptualization crucible and,
        214–215, 322–325
    CCRT and, 11
    collaboration and, 66–67, 71
    competencies and, 250, 266
    explanatory conceptualization and, 172,
        188–189, 192
    flexibility and, 250
    goal setting and, 154, 156
    improvements in, 20–22
    interventions and, 223
    longitudinal conceptualization and,
        222, 223
    nonresponse to therapy and, 9
    research and, 159

resilience and, 114, 114–117, 115,
    188–189
strengths and, 4, 8, 283
supervision and consultation and, 10
therapy alliance and, 65
therapy structure and, 67
top-down criteria and, 318
underlying assumptions, 88

P

Panic disorder
    case conceptualization and, 310
    case example of, 70–71
    cognitive models of, 17, 72
    competencies and, 265
    learning to conceptualize and, 293–294
    overlapping nature of, 210
    panic attacks and, 293–294
Personal history, 5, 134–135, 278. See
    also Developmental history; Family
    history
Personal values, 99–100, 114, 240–241,
    309
Personality Belief Questionnaire (PBQ),
    243
Personality disorder
    CBT and, 17
    cognitive models of, 16
    competencies and, 267
    declarative learning and, 254
    longitudinal conceptualization and,
        222, 243–244, 247, 295
    overview, 13–14
    Personality Belief Questionnaire (PBQ)
        and, 243
    top-down criteria and, 18
Physiological factors, in the five-part
    model, 85, 145f, 146
Posttraumatic stress disorder (PTSD)
    case conceptualization and, 317
    case example of, 2, 5, 8
    CBT and, 17
    declarative learning, 255
    levels of conceptualization and, 43–44
Predisposing factors. See also Vulnerability
    biopsychosocial assessment and, 135
    cross-sectional conceptualization and,
        209
    learning to conceptualize and, 264–267
    levels of conceptualization and, 29–30
    longitudinal conceptualization and,
        40–42, 40f, 231–233, 232f

Presenting issues
  case conceptualization and, 2, 30–31, 293, 315, 316–317, 319
  case conceptualization crucible and, 3, 3f, 310, 311
  collaboration and, 307, 322
  competencies and, 250–251, 261, 262, 263, 265, 266, 267, 270–271, 272, 302–303
  in context, 133–138
  cross-sectional conceptualization and, 211–212, 216, 308–309
  descriptive conceptualization and, 122–138, 131, 136–137, 138–140, 158, 159
  empiricism and, 75–76
  evidence-based theories and, 45, 49–50, 57, 69, 71
  explanatory conceptualization and, 173, 189–190, 200
  five-part model and, 35–39, 83, 85–90, 144, 149–151, 278
  functions of case conceptualization and, 5–10, 21, 24
  goal setting and, 152–157
  identifying, 122–128
  impact of, 128–133
  learning to conceptualize and, 264, 279, 281, 284, 291
  levels of conceptualization and, 27, 281
  linking of, 213–214, 213f, 224–234
  list, 127–128, 138, 322
  longitudinal conceptualization and, 221, 223, 233–234, 240, 241–242, 245f, 246f, 247
  maintenance factors and, 172
  onset, 181, 181–182, 233–234
  origins of, 41–43, 42f
  overview, 121–125
  principle driven approach and, 29
  prioritization of, 131–133
  procedural learning, 255
  strengths and, 56, 96, 101, 114, 116, 117, 119, 284
  supervision and consultation and, 244, 295–297
  therapy structure and, 65–66
  top-down criteria and, 18
Problem list. *See* Presenting issues
Procedural learning, 254f, 255–256, 271, 272–275, 282
Procrustean dilemma, 1, 4–5, 46–48, 70, 314

Professional development, 257–258. *See also* Learning to conceptualize
Protective factors
  case conceptualization and, 4, 60
  evidence-based theories and, 18
  learning to conceptualize and, 264–267
  levels of conceptualization and, 27, 29–30
  longitudinal conceptualization and, 39–41, 40f, 44, 199, 231, 232f, 233, 244, 245f, 246f
  presenting issues and, 214
Psychosis
  case example of, 279–281
  CBT and, 17
  cognitive models of, 16
  evidence-based theories and, 21, 60
  learning to conceptualize and, 269, 280–281
  strengths and, 96, 100, 104, 113

R

Rational systems, 48–49, 48f, 317–318
Reassurance seeking, 209–213, 212f
Reflective learning
  case example of, 276–278
  overview, 254f, 256–257, 271, 275–278, 277f, 298–299
  strengths and, 286–287
  teaching and supervision and, 297–298
Relapse
  case conceptualization and, 324
  competencies and, 250, 262, 264, 265, 266
  explanatory conceptualization and, 215
  longitudinal conceptualization and, 222, 223, 236–239, 237f, 244
  nonresponse to therapy and, 9
  prevention of, 9, 236–239, 237f
  strengths and, 308–309, 316–317
  therapy structure and, 66
Reliability
  bottom-up criteria and, 319–322
  case conceptualization and, 282
  collaboration and, 52
  Core Conflictual Relationship Theme (CCRT), 11
  heuristics and, 51
  overview, 19, 321–322

Research. *See also* Evidence base
  case conceptualization crucible and,
    3–5, 3*f*, 307, 311
  descriptive conceptualization and,
    138–152, 142*f*, 145*f*, 150*f*
  empiricism and, 49–50
  functions of case conceptualization
    and, 5
  improvements in therapy and outcomes
    and, 20–22
  nonresponse to therapy and, 9
  resilience and, 105
Resilience. *See also* Strengths
  automatic thoughts and, 198–199
  beliefs and, 198–199
  building as a function of therapy, 5,
    114–117
  case conceptualization crucible and, 311
  CBT and, 17
  explanatory conceptualization and, 215
  functions of case conceptualization
    and, 8
  levels of conceptualization and, 119,
    120
  longitudinal conceptualization and,
    40–41, 40*f*, 236–239, 237*f*, 240–241,
    246*f*
  overview, 104–114, 106*f*, 112*f*, 113*f*, 120
  strengths and, 28, 54–55, 97
Risk factors
  biopsychosocial assessment and, 135
  learning to conceptualize and, 264–267
  levels of conceptualization and, 29–30
  longitudinal conceptualization and,
    40–41, 40*f*, 231, 232*f*, 233, 245*f*
Rumination, 187–189, 187*f*, 188*f*,
    228–229

S

Safety behaviors, 13–14, 70–71, 135, 207,
    265. *See also* Maintenance factors
Schema. *See* Beliefs
Self-reflection
  overview, 254*f*, 256–257, 271, 275–
    278, 277*f*, 298–299
  strengths and, 286–287
  teaching and supervision and, 297–298
Social anxiety, 77, 293–294
Socratic dialogue
  case example of, 72–74, 174–176
  client observation and, 83

competencies and, 261, 262, 300
empiricism and, 69, 72–75, 75–82, 80*f*,
    81*f*, 82*f*, 83, 92
hypothesis testing and, 50
learning to conceptualize and, 297, 300
overview, 173
Standardized assessment tools, 137–138.
  See also Assessment
Stories, resilience and, 109–114, 112*f*,
    113*f*
Strategies
  automatic thoughts and, 87
  case conceptualization and, 19, 39, 101
  collaborative empiricism and, 75
  competencies and, 258–292, 301, 308
  core beliefs and, 89
  cross-sectional conceptualization and,
    173, 181, 189, 211
  developmental history and, 224–225,
    228–233
  levels of conceptualization and, 42*f*,
    43*f*
  longitudinal conceptualization and,
    43, 221, 223, 232*f*, 234–237, 239,
    241–243, 245*f*, 246*f*
  metaphors, stories and images and, 90,
    109, 112–114
  modes and, 12
  overview, 14, 15–16
  reflective learning and, 256
  resilience and, 107–108, 117, 240
  strengths and, 118–119, 308
Strengths. *See also* Resilience
  case conceptualization crucible and, 5,
    308–309, 311
  cultural, 100–101
  distress and, 117–119
  functions of case conceptualization
    and, 8
  identifying, 95–101, 125–127
  incorporating into conceptualizations,
    54–56, 101–103, 102*f*, 125–127
  learning to conceptualize and, 268–269,
    282–290, 304–305
  levels of conceptualization and, 119
  longitudinal conceptualization and,
    40–41, 40*f*, 230–231
  overview, 28, 84, 120
  personal values, 99–100
  resilience and, 104, 114
Structure of therapy, 63, 65–66, 66–68,
    69–82, 80*f*, 81*f*, 82*f*

Supervision
bottom-up criteria and, 321
case conceptualization and, 6, 9–10, 312, 317
case conceptualization crucible and, 312, 321
case example of, 46–48
competencies and, 292–294
decision-making errors and, 51
functions of case conceptualization and, 9–10
learning to conceptualize and, 23, 26, 248–249, 259–260, 271, 273–275, 292–298
longitudinal conceptualization and, 244, 245f–246f, 302
procedural learning and, 282
reflective learning and, 256

T

Teaching. *See also* Learning to conceptualize
case example of, 269, 276–278, 279–281, 289–290
conceptualization as a high-level skill, 249–253, 249f
overview, 23, 248–249, 257–258, 298–299
procedural learning, 271
recommendations regarding, 296–298
strengths and, 111–112
therapy structure and, 65–66
Theory, cognitive-behavioral therapy
case conceptualization crucible and, 3–5, 3f, 307, 311
descriptive conceptualization and, 138–152, 142f, 145f, 150f
empiricism and, 49–50
functions of case conceptualization and, 5, 56
longitudinal conceptualization and, 224–234, 229f, 232f
resilience and, 105
top-down criteria and, 12–18
Therapist. *See also* Competencies; Learning to conceptualize
case conceptualization crucible and, 320–321
conceptualization as a high-level skill and, 249–253, 249f
empiricism and, 68–83, 80f, 81f, 82f
metacompetencies, 249f

reflection and, 275–278, 277f
strategies for developing expertise, 258–292, 277f
Therapy. *See also* Interventions; Treatment planning
alliance, 64–65, 66–68
case conceptualization crucible and, 322–324
evidence-based, 11–23, 12–18, 18–23, 68–69, 71–75, 131–132, 184–189, 185f, 187f, 188f, 314–316
resilience and, 114–117
set-backs, 9, 312
structure, 65–66, 66–68, 69–82, 80f, 81f, 82f
treatment plans, 7–9, 64, 65–66, 114–117, 199
Therapy alliance, 64–65, 66–68
Therapy notebook, 103, 127
Thought Record
case example of, 36–39, 37f, 38f
Dysfunctional Thought Record, 50
longitudinal conceptualization and, 219, 220f, 221
low mood and, 194, 196f, 198–199
maintenance factors and, 228–229
overview, 87
Thoughts. *See also* Automatic thoughts
cognitive specificity theory and, 77
explanatory conceptualization and, 202–203, 203f
in the five-part model, 145f
interventions and, 206–208
OCD and, 205–206, 206f
Top-down criteria, 11, 12–18, 318–319
Training. *See also* Learning to conceptualize
case conceptualization and, 19–20, 22, 23, 51, 279, 296
case example of, 285–289
competencies and, 249–250
decision-making errors and, 48–49
declarative learning, 254
overview, 2, 320–321, 324
reflective learning and, 256
supervision and consultation and, 244
Treatment planning. *See also* Therapy
collaboration and, 64
explanatory conceptualization and, 199
functions of case conceptualization and, 7–9
resilience and, 114–117
therapy structure and, 65–66

Triggers
    ABC Model and, 139–140
    case conceptualization and, 9–10, 18,
        27–28, 29–30, 56
    cognitive factors and, 86–87
    competencies and, 253, 256, 302
    cross-sectional conceptualization and,
        174–175, 191–193, 199–202, 211,
        212–214, 215–216, 308
    cultural factors and, 84–85
    explanatory conceptualization and, 60,
        172–173
    fit and, 184–189, 185f, 187f, 188f
    identifying, 204–206
    learning to conceptualize and, 264–267,
        273, 277
    longitudinal conceptualization and,
        42–44, 222–223, 224, 228, 236–237,
        240, 244, 245f, 246f
    low mood and, 176–182, 177f, 180f,
        191–192, 195, 197f
    modes and, 13
    overview, 35–39, 37f, 38f
    resilience and, 105, 120
    strengths and, 101, 119, 120

U

Underlying assumptions. *See also* Beliefs
    developmental view of, 229f
    identifying, 87–88
    levels of conceptualization and, 42f,
        43f
    longitudinal conceptualization and,
        232f, 234–236, 245f, 246f
    overview, 14–15, 87–88
    resilience and, 108

V

Validity
    bottom-up criteria and, 18, 319
    case conceptualization and, 19–20, 51,
        52–53, 58
    cognitive-behavioral theories and, 16
    cross-sectional conceptualization and,
        208–209
    empiricism and, 49, 51
    overview, 11, 320, 321–322
Values, personal, 8, 41, 82, 99–101,
        109–110, 114, 116, 240–241,
        289–290, 309
    case examples of, 75–80, 104–107,
        110–114, 240–241
Vulnerability. *See also* Predisposing factors
    case conceptualization and, 311, 317
    collaboration and, 307–308
    cross-sectional conceptualization and,
        178
    descriptive conceptualization and, 158
    learning to conceptualize and, 264
    levels of conceptualization and, 27
    longitudinal conceptualization and,
        221, 236, 237f, 239
    overview, 39–41, 40f, 245f
    resilience and, 240

W

Working Alliance Inventory, 65
World Health Organization Quality of Life
        Brief scale (WHOQOL), 138
Worries, obsessional, 200–213, 203f,
        206f, 212f, 242–243. *See also* Health
        anxiety
    case example of, 32–35